Advances in Neurosurgery 22

B. L. Bauer, M. Brock, M. Klinger (Eds.)

Cerebellar Infarct

Midline Tumors

Minimally Invasive Endoscopic Neurosurgery (MIEN)

With 116 Figures

Springer-Verlag
Berlin Heidelberg New York London Paris
Tokyo Hong Kong Barcelona Budapest

Proceedings of the 44th Annual Meeting
of the Deutsche Gesellschaft für Neurochirurgie
Marburg, May, 2-5, 1993

Prof. Dr. Bernhard L. Bauer
Klinikum der Philipps-Universität Marburg
Zentrum für Operative Medizin I
Klinik für Neurochirurgie
Baldingerstr., 35033 Marburg, Germany

Prof. Dr. Dr. h.c. Mario Brock
Neurochirurgische Klinik und Poliklinik
Universitätsklinikum Steglitz, Freie Universität Berlin
Hindenburgdamm 30, 12200 Berlin, Germany

Prof. Dr. Margareta Klinger
Neurochirurgische Klinik der Universität Erlangen-Nürnberg
Schwabachanlage 6, (Kopfklinikum), 91054 Erlangen, Germany

ISBN 3-540-57668-1 Springer-Verlag Berlin Heidelberg NewYork
ISBN 0-387-57668-1 Springer-Verlag NewYork Berlin Heidelberg

CIP data applied for

Typesetting: M. Masson-Scheurer, Homburg/Saar

SPIN: 10423739 25/3130-5 4 3 2 1 0 – Printed on acid-free paper

Contents

Minimally Invasive Endoscopic Neurosurgery (MIEN)

Experimental Neurosurgery

Neurosurgery of the Spine

Winning Poster Presentations

List of Contributors

You will find the addresses at the beginning of the respective contribution

Introduction

B. L. Bauer[1]

It is an honor for me and my staff to have had been entrusted with the organization of the 44th Annual Meeting of the German Neurosurgical Society of here in Marburg on the occasion of the 15th anniversary of the Neurosurgery Division at the University Hospital. The Neurosurgery Division at the Philipps University of Marburg was founded in 1978. The scope for clinical and research work was initially very narrow and resources were scarce. The early years were dominated by our efforts to establish neurosurgery in Marburg as a fully fledged clinical discipline, with regard both to our clinical work and to research and academic teaching. After a 6-year "pioneer period," the move into the new university hospital division on the Lahnberge was a great step forward. Neurosurgical wards comprising 30 beds, two operating theaters, research laboratories, and our own intensive care unit now enabled effective work. As the experience of our medical staff increased, the range of surgery performed could be extended, and now comprises about 900 operations per year.

We have had three scientific priorities: research on the glycosphingolipid composition of gliomatous tumors, neuroendoscopy, and clinical risk research. In addition, we have also been interested in neurosurgery of metastases and algotherapy.

In science, what is true today does not necessarily hold true tomorrow. The topics for the 44th Annual Congress were chosen in consideration of the theoretical and practical aspects of surgical strategy and microsurgery.

Cerebellar infarctions are not a nosological entity. Many questions of classification and pathophysiology have not as yet been conclusively answered. This is also the case for the optimal therapeutic procedure – regarding the indication for surgery, and the choice of surgical method, and its optimal timing.

This is not the first time that the effort has been made to introduce endoscopy into practical neurosurgery. Such methods have become of topical importance for neurosurgery as a result of the rapid development in what we prefer to term minimally invasive endoscopic neurosurgery. Great attention was paid to these developments very early in the lay press, which reflects the wishes of patients. In view of this, we should welcome all investigations which also consider the adverse consequences of such treatments. Neuroendoscopic methods remain controversial and a source of unresolved problems for neurosurgeons. Technical advances concerning minaturized endoscopes, flexible and maneuverable as well as rigid endoscopes, and advances in microchip camera technology have led to the development of an improved range of instruments. Nevertheless, this does not solve all the prob-

---

[1] Neurochirurgische Universitätsklinik, Baldingerstr., 35033 Marburg, Germany.

Advances in Neurosurgery, Vol. 22
B. L. Bauer, M. Brock, M. Klinger (Eds.)

lems that occur in the treatment of pathological lesions of the cerebral midline, the base of the skull, or the brainstem.

Minimally invasive endoscopic neurosurgery does indeed offer exciting prospects in some fields of neurosurgery; however, it does not yet meet the safety standards established in current microneurosurgery. The history of minimally invasive endoscopic neurosurgery has taught us a great deal about the problems in bridging the gap between future requirements and present realities of endoneurosurgery. These problems are a major focus of interest today not only on the part of the patients and their surgeons but also in the field of health policy and medical ethics. The neurosurgeon bears a special responsibility both as a technical expert and as the guardian of patients' interests. He must justify the confidence placed in him, above all in the recommendation of new strategies of treatment. Especially in this respect it is, in my opinion, very important to discuss minimally invasive endoscopic neurosurgery with experienced colleagues from Europe and overseas.

Space-occupying midline lesions in the central nervous system give rise to complex clinical symptoms. Their multivarious pathological nature and their accessibility to surgical operations differs. The corresponding diversity in the routes of approach and surgical strategies require thoroughgoing discussion.

There has been increasing public interest in the work of European and American physicians in recent years. Legislative and economic constraints will have a crucial effect on the work of physicians in the coming decades. This is also of substantial importance with regard to the undergraduate and postgraduate training of the next generation of neurosurgeons. In Germany, the new law for reforming the provision of health care drastically limits material resources, and I have no doubt that this will also have repercussions for neurosurgeons. One can expect the number of operations performed in Germany to fall in the coming years. This may mean that current training programs can no longer be completed as envisaged within 6 years, which is of particular importance for those wishing to acquire additional qualifications after the completion of their training, for example, in special neurosurgical intensive care medicine, endoneurosurgery, and stereotactic surgery.

When Sir Victor Horsley (encouraged by a group of neurologists headed by Sir Hughlins Jackson) first approached a problem case by operating on the putative brain tumor, he saw the patient die under his surgeon's knife. Years later, some unknown person wrote "murderer" on his grave stone. When Wilder Penfield was buried a generation later, however, no one would have considered doing so in his case. Along this long road, William McEwen, Harvey Cushing, Walter E. Dandy, Percival Bailey, Herbert Olivecrona, Wilhelm Tönnis, Otfrid Foerster, Fedor Krause, Hugo Krayenbühl, and my own teacher Hans Werner Pia were only some of the many who have passed on the baton. We are their successors and disciples.

I hope that the 44th Annual Meeting of the German Neurosurgical Society will expose some errors and reveal some truths. Nevertheless, the brain, the fragile repository of the soul, will continue to remain a mystery.

Cerebellar Infarct

Microsurgical Anatomy and Territories of Perfusion of the Superior Cerebellar Artery

S. Hussein[1], D. Woischneck[1], and S. Schulze[1]

Introduction

The first descriptions of neurological symptoms in vascular diseases of the cerebellum and brainstem were based on detailed anatomic work [6, 7, 9, 11, 12]. With the progress in neuroradiology and microsurgery, the anatomic variability of these areas became of interest again, especially the vascular supply. We therefore examined in an anatomic study the route of the superior cerebellar artery (SCA) and the territories supplied.

Materials and Methods

We examined 30 brains 6–24 h postmortem. The patients died at ages between 25 and 90 years. Both SCAs were selectively cannuled and perfused with a physiological solution of NaCl. Then, a mixture of gelatin and gray ink was injected. Afterwards, the preparations were fixed in a formalin solution (2%).

We prepared and examined the brains under the operation microscope. For analysis of the vascular supply we performed stereotactically oriented slices. The brains were embedded in acryl, and ventriculography was performed. After definition of the Ca-Cp line, we made 5-mm slices parallel to the descent of this line in a frontal orientation (Fig. 4). These slices were prepared in agreement with the stereotactic results of Schaltenbrand and Warren [8]. The areas supplied by SCA were identified by a color detector and quantified on a six-point color scale.

Results

In all brains the SCA was present on both sides. In 44 of 60 hemispheres (73%) the artery showed one major stem and in 14 (23%) two major stems. In one hemisphere the artery was doubled at its origin, and in one we found three branches originating from the basilar artery as the SCA. The length of the basilar artery averaged 29.8 mm (24.3–41.9 mm) from the beginning to the division into the two SCA. The distance between the SCA and the posterior cerebellar artery (PCA) was

[1] Neurochirurgische Klinik, Medizinische Hochschule Hannover, Konstanty-Gutschow-Str. 13, 30623 Hannover, Germany.

Advances in Neurosurgery, Vol. 22
B. L. Bauer, M. Brock, M. Klinger (Eds.)

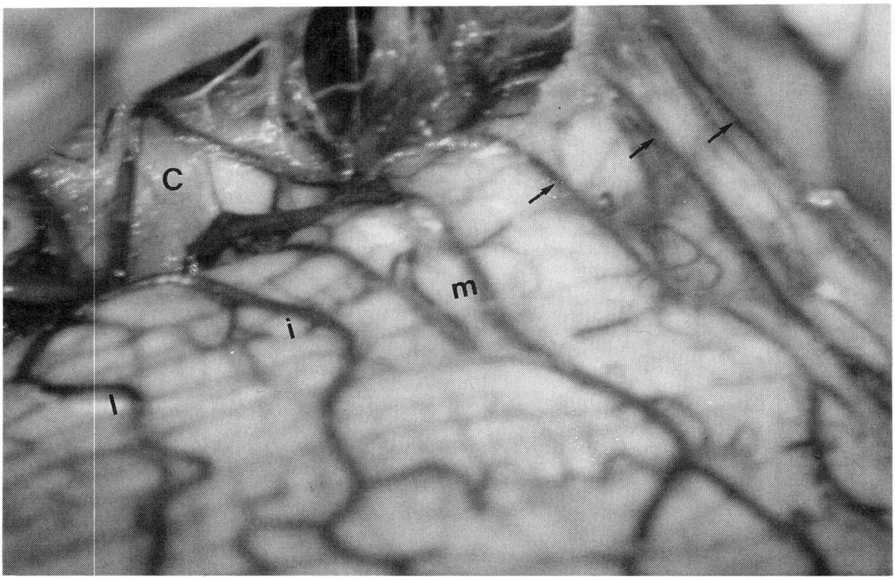

Fig. 1. Dorsolateral view on the cerebellar surface: branches of the SCA. *C*, Cisterna cerebellomesencephalica; *m*, medial branch; *i*, intermedial branch; *l*, lateral branch of aa hemisphericae; *arrows*, aa vermes of the PCA

1.71 mm on average (0.5–5.8 mm). In five hemispheres we found an extreme caudal origin of the SCA at a distance of 3.3–5.8 mm to the PCA. In 15 hemispheres (25%) anastomotic branches between the SCA and the P1 segment of the PCA were detected with a radius of 0.7–1.0 mm. In 16 cases (26%) anastomoses to the anterior inferior cerebellar artery as pial vessels in the area of the trigeminal root were found. In at least 25 cases (41%) we saw anastomoses even to the posterior inferior cerebellar artery.

The SCA takes its route rostrally (cisterna interpeduncularis), laterally, and infratentorially into the cisterna pontocerebellaris. In 98% of our material, inside this cistern the artery divided into a rostral and a caudal trunk. This bifurcation was found 20.8 mm (11.6–45.4 mm) after the SCA origin. At least the rostral and caudal trunks were detected in all hemispheres as a consequence of the division of the SCA or because of a doubling of the vessel (Fig. 1).

The diameter of the SCA at its origin was 1.78 mm (1.2–2.6 mm) at the rostral trunk 1.2 mm (0.8–1.6 mm) and at the caudal trunk 1.25 mm (0.7–1.4 mm). The first significant branch of the SCA is the a marginalis, which was found at the proximal SCA in 35 hemispheres; in two cases it originated from the caudal branch. We divided the cortical branches of the SCA into two groups, according to Hardy et al. [3]: (a) The aa vermes, coming from the rostral trunk of the SCA, took a craniocaudal direction to vermis superior. There were two in 33 cases, one in 26 cases, and three in one case (Fig. 2). (b) The aa hemisphericae, coming from both

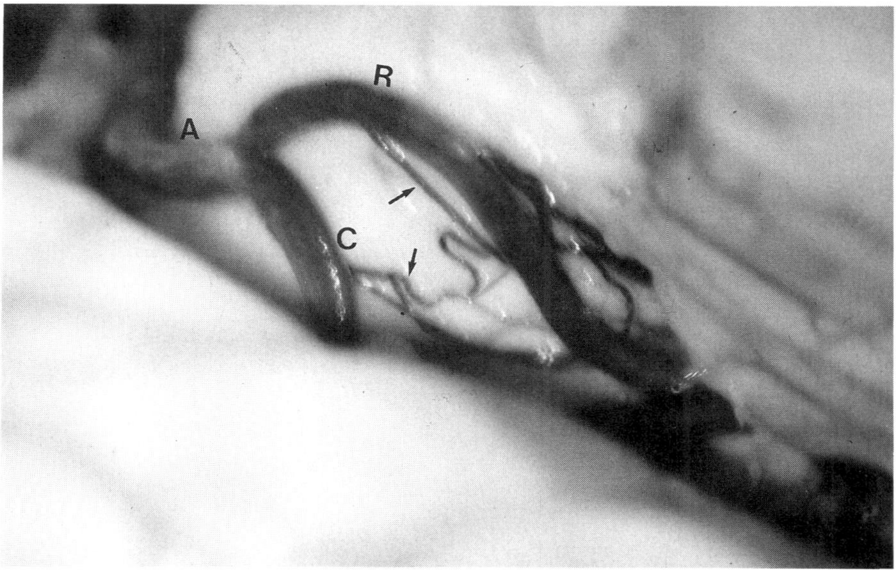

Fig. 2. Lateral view of the cisterna cerebellomesencephalica: exploration of the SCA bifurcation *(A)*. *R*, rostral branch; *C*, caudal branch; *arrows*, small branches to mesencephalon

main trunks of the SCA went craniocaudally to the cerebellar surface. In 33 cases (55%) we found three of these (Fig. 2) and in seven cases even four.

In the literature, the topographic relationship to the nervi oculomotorius et trochlearis is described exactly, and we can therefore omit this here. Of further interest for the neurosurgeon is, of course, the relationship of the SCA to the trigeminal nerve (Fig. 3). In five cases we found a close contact between nerve and artery. In three cases the proximal stem of the SCA and in two cases the caudal branch seemed to compress the trigeminal nerve. In the other cases, we saw a distance of 1–4 mm between the trigeminal root and the SCA.

Figure 4 presents the orientation of the slices that we performed to analyze the areas of vascular supply of the SCA. Vascular supply by the SCA starts on slice 0.5, which is at the level of brachium conjunctivum. This structure in 85% of the cases is supplied mainly by the SCA. In the next slices we analyzed the lemniscus medialis (in 68% supplied by the SCA), colliculus inferior (14.6%), and locus coeruleus (16.7%). The mesencephalic structure was thus dependent on the SCA while the pontine structures never showed a supply from this artery. On the other hand, the dominant area of the SCA is the cerebellar cortex, especially the lobulus quadrangularis (supplied by the SCA in all cases) and lobulus simplex (on average, 73% of the area supplied by the SCA). The rostral part of the lobus semilunaris was perfused by the SCA in 45%–55% of cases and by the lobulus paramedianus and lobus biventer in only 5%–10%. The upper vermal structures (such as lobus centralis, lingula, culmen, declive) were supplied by the SCA in 70%–100%.

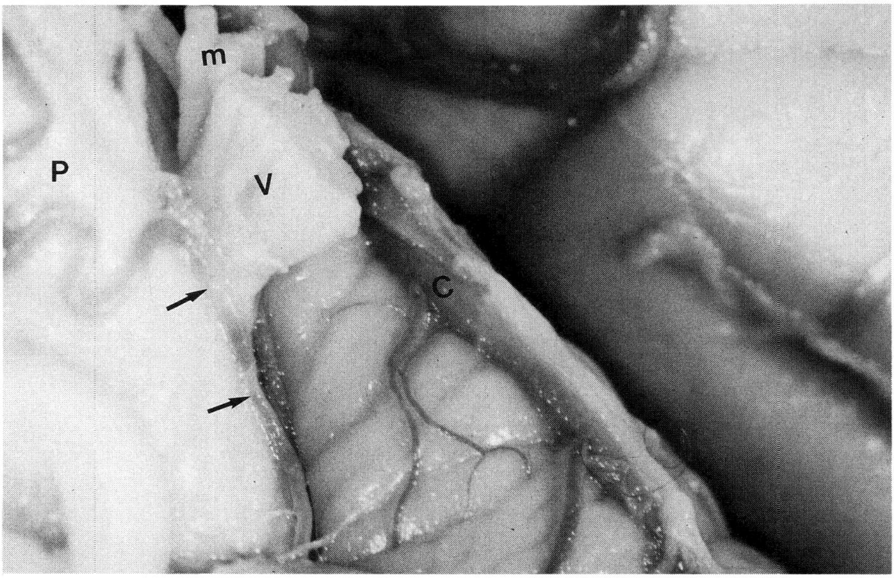

Fig. 3. Relationship between the SCA and the trigeminal nerve. *C*, caudal branch of SCA; *m*, radix motoria nervi trigemini; *arrows*, anastomosis between SCA and anterior inferior cerebellar artery

Middle and lower vermal structures were not reached by the artery. The nucleus dentatus and rostral parts of the substantia medullare superius were supplied by the SCA in 100% while the nucleus emboliformis, globosus, and fastigii were reached by it in only 50% of our cases.

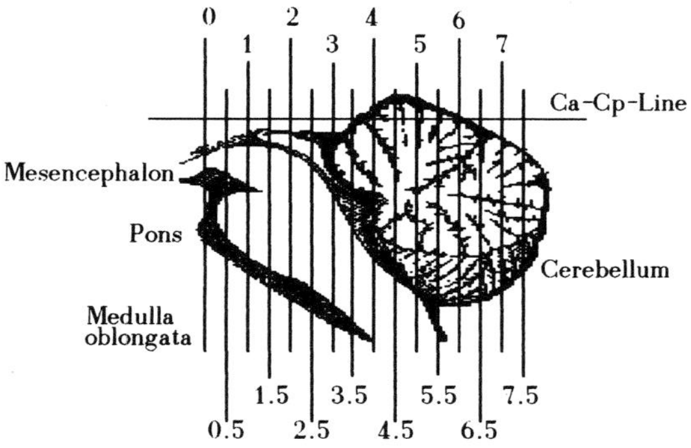

Fig. 4. Stereotactically oriented slices of cerebellum and brainstem in correlation to the Ca-Cp-line (thickness of slices, 0.5 mm)

Discussion

We considered the SCA from a microsurgical point of view and therefore favor the scheme of Hardy et al. [3]: The anterior segment of the artery, lying ponto-mesencephalically is reached by a pterional or subtemporal approach. The lateral (mesencephalic) segment can be explored subtemporally or suboccipitally. The cerebellomesencephalic parts of the artery and the cortical segment are explored by a suboccipital, medial, or lateral approach.

Our results on the number and diameter of the SCA at origin are in agreement with other findings [1]. Also the anastomoses to the PCA and the other cerebellar arteries are well known. The relationship between the SCA and the trochlear nerve has been reported by Hardy et al. [3] and Janetta [5]. Under discussion is whether this nerve compression may lead to idiopathic trochlear paresis. The relationship to the trigeminal nerve root has been described principally by Hardy et al. [3] and Janetta [5], as the cause of trigeminal neuralgia, who states that in 80% of the cases the neuralgia is caused by compression of the SCA and its branches. In our material the SCA is only seldom in close contact to the trigeminal nerve.

Stopford [10] has described a clinical syndrome caused by closure of the SCA, which was first suspected by Mills [7]. In the beginning the patient shows vomiting, disorientation, and vertigo. In the nucleus dendatus is involved, there is a certain intention tremor. Ischemia of symphatetic fibers along the oculomotorius nerve can lead to Horner's syndrome. In some cases even the tractus spinothalamicus and quintothalamicus may be damaged, with the consequence of contralateral loss of pain and temperature sensitivity. Our findings show that the fasciculus longitudinalis and lemniscus lateralis also may be affected. This may lead to nystagmus or contralateral hypoacusis. As we have shown, the pontine structures never take part in such ischemia: the prognosis therefore remains good.

Conclusions

According to Hardy [3], the SCA is divided into three segments: an anterior part, reached by a pterional or subtemporal approach, a mesencephalic part, reached subtemporally or suboccipitally, and a cerebellomesencephalic segment, reached by a suboccipital craniotomy. The artery is suspected for nerve compression syndromes, especially of the trochlearis and trigeminus. In contrast to the literature, the latter is in our material in contact with the SCA in only 5% of cases. The areas supplied by the SCA (detected by stereotactic slices after selective injection) include mesencephalic and cerebellar structures. In contrast to the views of others, the SCA does not to contribute to the pontine structures, which is of clinical significance in ischemic situations.

References

1. Cavatortio P (1905) Di una variazoni arterio della base dellencefalo homo. Monit Zool Ital 12:294–315
2. Davison C, Goodhardt SP, Savitzky N (1935) The syndrome of the superior cerebellar artery and its branches. Arch Neurol Psychiatr 33:1143–1174
3. Hardy DG, Peace DA, Rhoton AL (1980) Microsurgical anatomy of the superior cerebellar artery. Neurosurgery 6:10–28
4. Janetta PJ (1967) Arterial compression of the trigeminal nerve at the pons in patients with trigeminal neuralgia. J Neurosurg 26:159–162
5. Janetta PJ (1976) Microsurgical approach to trigeminal nerve for tic douloureux. Neurol Surg 7:180–200
6. Obersteiner L (1912) Anleitung des Baus der nervösen Zentralorgane, 5th edn. Berlin
7. Mills CL (1908) Hemianesthesia to pain and temperature and loss of emotional expression on the right side with ataxia of upper limb on the left. J Nerv Dis 35:331–332
8. Schaltenbrand G, Warren W (1977) Atlas for stereotaxy of the human brain. Thieme, Stuttgart
9. Senator H (1881) Apoplektische Bulbärparalyse mit wechselseitiger Empfindungsstörung. Arch Psychiatr 11:713–726
10. Stopford JSB (1966) The arteries of pons and medulla oblongata. J Anat Physiol 50:131–164
11. Wallenberg A (1895) Akute Bulbäraffektion. Arch Psychiatr 27:504–540
12. Whitaker JR (1921) Anatomy of the brain. Edinburgh

Neuropathology of Cerebellar Infarction: Its Morphology in Comparison to Selective Postmortem Angiography of Cerebellar Arteries

C. Roßberg[1], N. Mai[1], W. Müller-Forell[2], P. Stoeter[2], and M. Schumacher[3]

Introduction

A typology of infarctions [11, 20] is established for the cerebral hemispheres and has recently also been used, chiefly in neuroradiological diagnosis, for cerebellar infarctions [2–5, 8, 10, 16]. Detailed clinical [12] and microangiographic [7, 9, 13, 15, 17] investigations of the vascularization of the posterior cranial fossa can be referred to in this context. With the aid of selective postmortem angiograms we examined the territories of the superior cerebellar artery (SCA), anterior inferior cerebellar artery (AICA), and posterior inferior cerebellar artery (PICA) on serial sections in the three planes of projection. The sagittal plane offers decisive advantages for assigning cerebellar infarctions to the vascular territories. The results were compared with the findings of computed tomography and magnetic resonance imaging of cerebellar infarctions.

Materials and Methods

For postmortem angiographies a cannula was inserted in the origin of the SCA, and AICA, PICA of 27 freshly isolated brains, and about 1 ml of a Micropaque gelatine mixture (3:1, 25% gelatine) was injected. After fixing in formalin the cerebellum and brainstem were sliced into frontal, horizontal, or sagittal sections about 4 mm thick. The horizontal sections deviate from the canthomeatal plane, and the frontal sections deviate from the plane perpendicular to the Frankfort horizontal by about 15° each. For schematic reproduction of the vascular territories, photographs and photographic enlargements of microangiographic images (Definix Médical, 20 kV, 3 mA, 3 min) of all the cerebellar sections were superimposed on a projector by means of marks.

The infarction study includes 53 cases with 78 cerebellar infarctions at least 5 mm in size from autopsy material (19 cases) as well as from clinical material (34 cases) with high-resolution computed tomography and/or magnetic resonance imaging studies (Table 1). Isolated infarctions in the brainstem were not taken into account. The pathological findings were correlated with the postmortem angiograms with the aid of anatomic reference planes. The sagittal sections were

[1] Department of Neuropathology, University of Marburg, Marburg, Germany.
[2] Department of Neuroradiology, University of Mainz, Mainz, Germany.
[3] Department of Neuroradiology, University of Freiburg, Freiburg, Germany.

Advances in Neurosurgery, Vol. 22
B. L. Bauer, M. Brock, M. Klinger (Eds.)

Table 1. Distribution of infarctions from the neuroradiological and neuropathological material on the basis of their topography and classified according to infarction typology by postmortem angiography

Infarction	SCA		AICA		PICA		Total ($n = 78$)	
	n	%	n	%	n	%	n	%
Total	3	4	–	–	4	5	7	9
Partial	23	29	4	5	35	45	62	79
Boundary	2[a]	3	–	–	7[b]	9	9	12

[a] SCA/PICA.
[b] Medial/lateral PICA.

8 mm apart, cutting through the midline (vermis), the dentate nucleus, corpus medullare, and folia. The horizontal sections were situated in the mesencephalon, the fourth ventricle, and the medulla oblongata. The five coronal sections were taken from the brainstem, fourth ventricle, dentate nuclei, corpus medullare, and folia. The infarctions were classified according to Zülch [20] and Kautzky [11] into total, partial, and boundary infarctions. Lacunae and isolated brainstem infarctions were not taken into account.

Results

Vascularization Areas. Postmortem angiograms and vascularized structures were correlated for the three cerebellar arteries on section sequences in the three planes of projections (Fig. 1). The sagittal plane was the best projection for an accurate differentiation of the vascular territories. There was no agreement between the boundaries of the vascularization areas of the SCA, AICA, and PICA and the classical anatomic outlines of cerebellar lobules.

The SCA runs over the upper surface of the cerebellum and supplies the cranial parts of the vermis and hemispheres above the horizontal fissure, including the upper cerebellar peduncle, the dentate nucleus and the upper part of the roof of the fourth ventricle. The PICA is situated on the lower surface and supplies the caudal parts of the vermis, hemispheres below the horizontal fissure, and lower part of the roof of the fourth ventricle. The AICA contributes little to the supply of the midline structures of the cerebellum but vascularizes mainly the nodulus and flocculus within the cerebellar-pontine angle, the middle cerebellar peduncle, and the anterolateral parts of the cerebellar hemispheres around the horizontal fissure but does not reach the dorsal circumference. We also found the well-known variations of a vicarious supply mainly between the AICA and PICA territories. In addition, there were numerous anastomoses between the ipsi- and contralateral arteries (Fig. 2), which explains the wide overlapping of the vacularization areas.

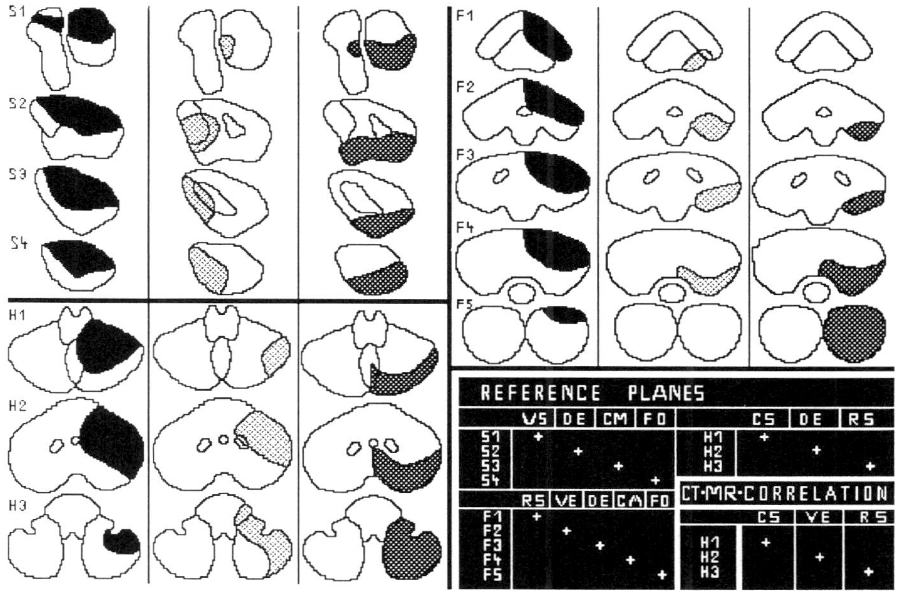

Fig. 1. Vascularization territories of the SCA *(left column, black)*, PICA *(right column, dark gray)*, and AICA *(middle column, light gray)* on sagittal (S1–S4 from medial to lateral), horizontal (H1–H3, from caudal to cranial), and frontal (F1–F5, from rostral to dorsal) serial sections. Separation into an upper portion supplied by the SCA, which also includes the nucleus dentatus, and a lower portion supplied by the PICA is detectable on all sagittal sections. The interposed territory of the AICA is seen mainly on the paramedian and lateral sections. In the horizontal and frontal planes, the identification of the vascular territories is more complex. The anatomical reference planes are indicated (*CM*, corpus medullare; *CS*, caudal brainstem; *DE*, nucleus dentatus; *f*, frontal; *FO*, folia; *h*, horizontal; *RS*, rostral brainstem; *S*, sagittal; *VE*, ventricle; *VS*, vermis)

Infarctions. The topographic correlation of 78 infarcts to the vascular territories are shown in Table 1. In three of seven total infarctions, the SCA was involved with the brainstem and with increased intracranial pressure in two cases. Three infarctions of the PICA (one total and two partial infarctions) extended to the contralateral side (Fig. 3 a, b). All partial infarctions of the AICA also affected the middle cerebellar peduncle and pons (Fig. 4). There were no preferred locations for the partial infarction. In three cases, bilateral symmetric infarctions between the medial and lateral branches of the PICA and an additional unilateral one in the same area were classified as boundary infarctions. Two other lesions in the dorsal part of the hemispheres between the SCA and PICA territories were also classified as boundary infarctions (Fig. 3 d). Hemorrhagic infarctions were found preferentially in the folia (Fig. 3 c). Nine lesions could not be classified.

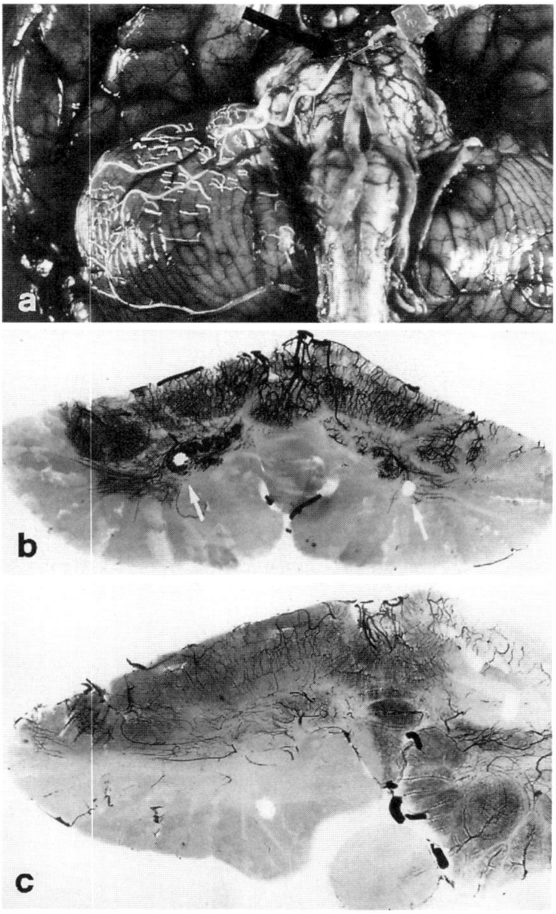

Fig. 2 a–c. Injected specimen. **a** Cannula inserted into the origin of the SCA *(arrow)* and anastomotic filling of the ipsilateral PICA. **b** Postmortem angiography (horizontal section) after filling of both SCA; *white arrows*, projection marks. **c** Postmortem angiography (frontal section) after injection of the left SCA with collateral filling of the contralateral PICA

Discussion

In the postmortem study as well as in clinical imaging, the cerebellar infarctions could be correlated with the vascular areas [9, 13] and classified into the various types [11, 20], most accurately in the sagittal plane. According to their craniocaudal arrangement, the arterial territories could be separated into a superior (SCA) and an inferior (PICA) area on the median and an additionally interposed (AICA) segment on paramedian and midsagittal sections.

In our studies, only 7 of 78 lesions were total infarctions. In two of the three SCA infarctions, the brainstem was also involved, possibly because of increased intracranial pressure due to additional severe supratentorial infarctions. In accordance with the observation of Kase [10], there seems to be a protective effect of the blood supply from the anterior circulation, and an additional lesion in the

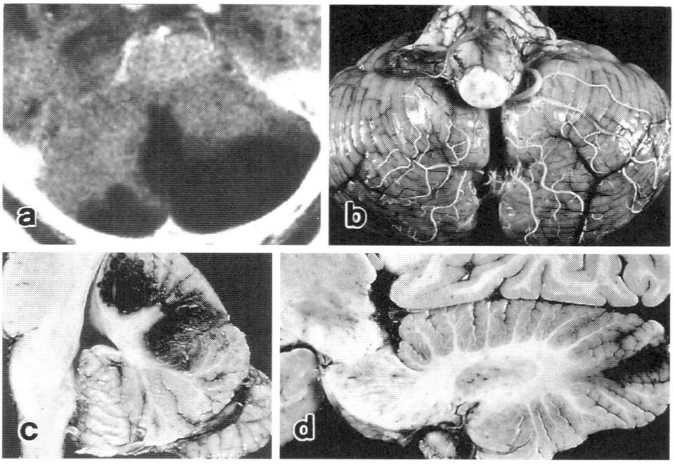

Fig. 3 a–d. Different types of cerebellar infarctions. **a** Computed tomography of total PICA infarction with contralateral extension. **b** Injected specimen shows variation of PICA with corresponding supply of contralateral paramedian territory. **c** SCA partial infarction with predominant involvement of folia on midsagittal section. **d** Boundary infarction between SCA and PICA territories on sagittal section

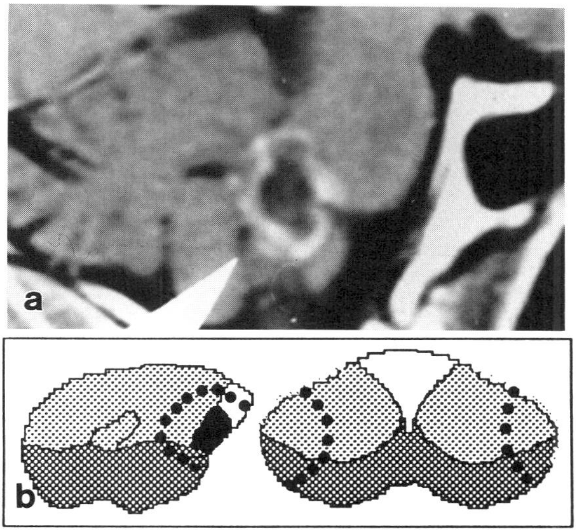

Fig. 4. a Magnetic resonance imaging of hemorrhagic partial AICA infarction (sagittal section). **b** Schematic drawing of the territories of SCA *(light gray)*, PICA *(dark gray)*, and AICA *(surrounded by points)* showing the absence of overlapping of the AICA territory in the sagittal section *(black)*

carotid territory may be necessary in some cases to produce brainstem ischemia. The four other total infarctions were in the PICA territory. All other infarctions were partial ones of a highly variable distribution [15]. This may be due to abundant ipsi- and contralateral anastomoses [8, 9, 13, 14] between the cerebellar arteries, which we showed by postmortem angiography (Fig. 2, 3 b).

The partial infarctions in the region of the medial branches of the PICA, which had the known triangular shape [1], extended to the contralateral region in three cases. This can be explained by the bilateral distribution of one PICA territory, whereas in most cases, the paramedian region is protected by anastomoses crossing the midline over the cerebellar surface [9, 14, 17]. We regularly found a bilateral filling of the branches of the PICA by postmortal angiography (Fig. 3 b).

Infarctions of the AICA are rare [5] and only partial. In our material mainly the lateral area of the pons is affected [2, 16], which is supplied by perforating terminal branches [5, 9] and does not benefit from the anastomotic network of the cerebellar surface [7]. This observation, on the other hand, may be also explained by the fact that the lateral pontine area is the only region in which the PICA territory does not overlap with those of other cerebellar arteries and can therefore be identified without difficulty.

In our material, boundary zone infarctions [3, 5, 15, 16] were localized mainly between the medial and lateral PICA branches and in only two cases between the SCA and PICA territories. A differentiation from other types of infarctions is possible only in the sagittal plane because of the difficult interpretation of the other projection planes [5, 18] in the case of a slight angular deviation [8].

Conclusion

The cerebellar infarctions could be correlated with the vascular territories and assigned to the infarction types [11, 20] most accurately on sagittal sections, which have been uncommon up to now [15, 18, 19] but have recently been used increasingly and have been included in neuroradiological analyses since the introduction of magnetic resonance imaging [5, 16]. Because of the abundant arterial anastomoses on the cerebellar surface [7, 9, 13, 14] total infarctions are rare, and partial infarctions show a variable distribution [15]. Boundary infarctions are difficult to classify and are found mainly between the medial and lateral PICA branches. The orientation of the vascular territories in the sagittal plane has some similarity to the functional organization [6, 14] of the cerebellum.

References

1. Amarenco P, Roullet E, Hommel M, Chaine P, Marteau R (1990) Infarction in the territory of the medial branch of the posterior inferior cerebellar artery. J Neurol Neurosurg Psychiatry 53:731–735

2. Amarenco P, Roullet E, Goujon C, Chéron F, Hauw J-J, Bousser M-G (1991) Infarction in the anterior rostral cerebellum (the territory of the lateral branch of the superior cerebellar artery). Neurology 41:253–258
3. Amarenco P, Kase CS, Rosengart A, Pessin MS, Bousser M-G, Caplan LR (1993) Very small (border zone) cerebellar infarcts. Brain 116:161–186
4. Amarenco P (1991) The spectrum of cerebellar infarctions. Neurology 41:973–979
5. Cormier PJ, Long ER, Russell EJ (1992) MR Imaging of posterior fossa infarctions: vascular territories and clinical correlates. Radiographics 12:1079–1096
6. Dichgans J (1984) Clinical symptoms of cerebellar dysfunction and their topodiagnostical significance. Human Neurobiol 2:269–279
7. Dor P, Salamon G (1970) The arterioles and capillaries of the brainstem and cerebellum: a microangiographic study. Neuroradiology 1:27–29
8. Hinshaw DB, Thompson JR, Hasso AN, Casselman ES (1980) Infarctions of the brainstem and cerebellum: a correlation of computed tomography and angiography. Radiology 137:105–112
9. Hoffman HB, Margolis MT, Newton TH (1974) The superior cerebellar artery. In: Newton TH, Potts DG (eds) Radiology of the skull and brain. Mosby, St. Louis, pp 1809–1830
10. Kase CS, White JL, Joslyn JN, Williams JP, Mohr JP. Cerebellar infarction in the superior cerebellar artery distribution. Neurology 35:705–711
11. Kautzky R, Zülch K-J, Wende S, Tänzer A (1982) Neuroradiology. A neuropathological approach. Springer, Berlin Heidelberg New York
12. Lang J (1991) Clinical anatomy of the posterior cranial fossa and its foramina. Thieme, Stuttgart
13. Lazorthes G, Gouazé A, Salamon G (1976) Vascularisation et circulation de l'encéphale. Masson, Paris
14. Mayr R (1979) Makroskopische Anatomie des Kleinhirns, Cerebellum. Die Architektonik des Kleinhirns. In: Ferner H, Staubesand J (eds) (Lehrbuch der Anatomie des Menschen, vol 3). Nervensystem, Haut und Sinnesorgane. Urban and Schwarzenberg, Munich, pp 61–71, 192–217
15. Rodda R (1971) The vascular lesions associated with cerebellar infarcts. Proc Aust Assoc Neurol 8:101–109
16. Savoiardo M, Bracchi M, Passerini P, Visciani A (1987) The vascular territories in the cerebellum and brainstem: CT and MR study. AJNR 8:199–209
17. Scialfa G, Bank W, Megret M, Corbaz JM, Salamon G (1976) The arteries of the roof of the fourth ventricle. Neuroradiology 11:67–71
18. Stevens JM, Kendall BE (1985) Aspects of the anatomy of the cerebellum on computed tomography. Neuroradiology 27:390–398
19. Tschernyscheff A, Grigorowsky I (1930) Über die arterielle Versorgung des Kleinhirns. Arch Psychiatr Nervenkr 92:8–85
20. Zürich K-J (1985) The cerebral infarct. Pathology, pathogenesis, and computed tomography. Springer, Berlin Heidelberg New York

Surgical Aspects in Treatment of Cerebellar Infarction

R. Laumer[1], F. Erbguth[2], and P. Nomikos[1]

Introduction

Supratentorial cerebral infarction is usually treated medically, but in some cases ventricular drainage is necessary. Regarding infratentorial cerebellar infarction a more aggressive treatment including decompression of the posterior fossa is currently under discussion. There have been a number of case reports suggesting surgical decompression as the treatment of choice in cerebellar infarction [1, 3, 5, 6]. The advantage of early operative treatment was first described in the 1950s [4, 8]; however, recent investigations seem to overestimate the benefit of aggressive therapy, based on isolated case reports with lack of new information. The main problem in evaluating the benefit of surgical decompression arises primarily from patient selection and timing of the surgical procedure. The case reports presented here demonstrate that so far there is no standard therapy for optimal treatment of cerebellar infarction. Outcome was assessed in terms of the modified Rankin scale [9] (the original Rankin scale did not include grades 0 and 6):

Grade 0: *No symptoms at all*
Grade 1: *No significant disability despite symptoms*: able to carry out usual duties and activities
Grade 2: *Slight disability*: unable to carry out all previous activities but able to look after own affairs without assistance
Grade 3: *Moderate disability*: requiring some help but able to walk without assistance
Grade 4: *Moderately severe disability*: unable to walk without assistance and unable to attend to own bodily needs without assistance
Grade 5: *Severe disability*: bedridden, incontinent, and requiring constant nursing care and attention
Grade 6: *Died*

[1] Neurochirurgische Klinik, Universität Erlangen-Nürnberg, Schwabachanlage 6, 91054 Erlangen, Germany.
[2] Neurologische Klinik, Universität Erlangen-Nürnberg, Schwabachanlage 6, 91054 Erlangen, Germany.

Advances in Neurosurgery, Vol. 22
B. L. Bauer, M. Brock, M. Klinger (Eds.)

Case Reports

Case 1. A 52-year-old woman with acute onset of headache 1 day prior to admission presented with lack of orientation and additional cerebellar symptoms. Cranial computed tomography (CT) revealed a right-sided cerebellar infarction and hydrocephalus (Fig. 1). A ventricular drainage was placed immediately. The

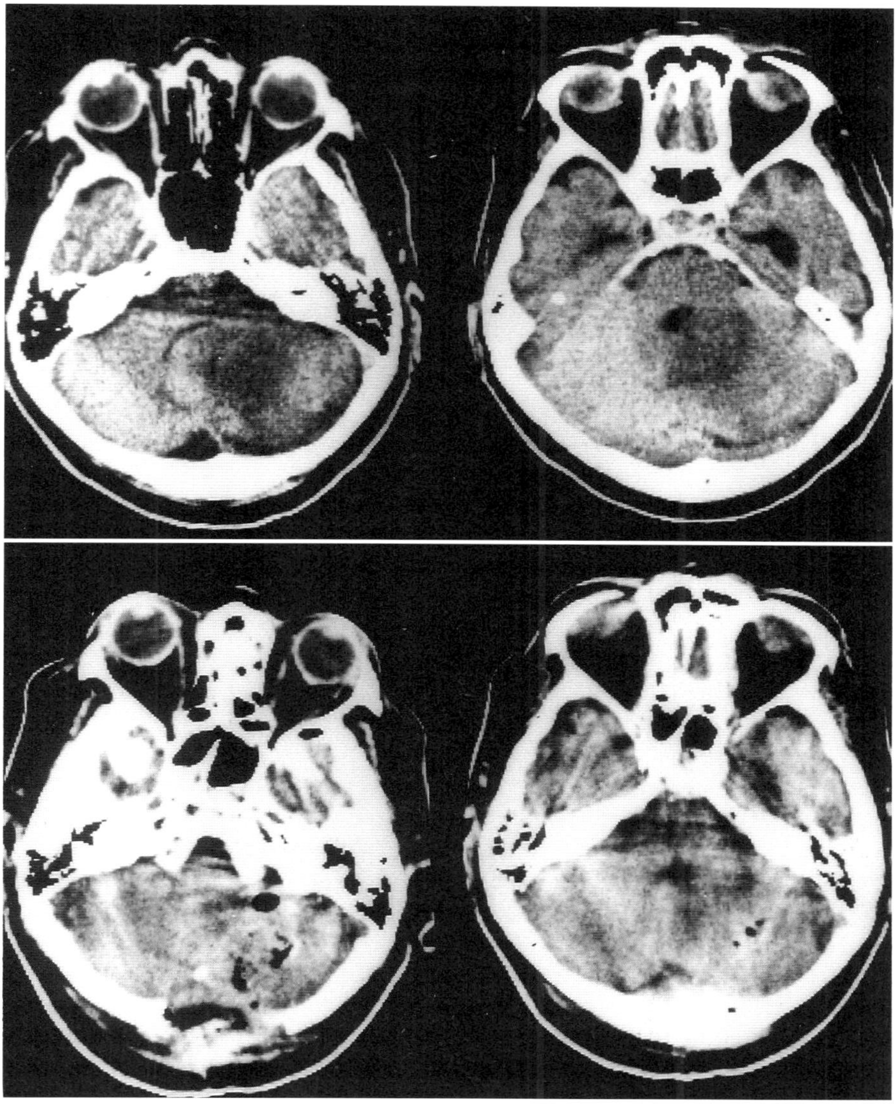

Fig. 1. Case report 1. CT scan of a right-sided cerebellar infarction at admission *(above)* and after decompression of the posterior fossa *(below)*

clinical condition initially improved but deteriorated again 24 h later. We performed a suboccipital craniectomy and decompression of the posterior fossa. The patient improved within a few weeks (outcome Rankin 2).

Case 2. A 74-year-old woman was admitted to a regional hospital with sudden onset of headache and nausea. Her condition deteriorated 5 days later, and she became unconscious. After admission to our Department cranial CT revealed a left-sided cerebellar infarction (Fig. 2). We performed ventricular drainage. There

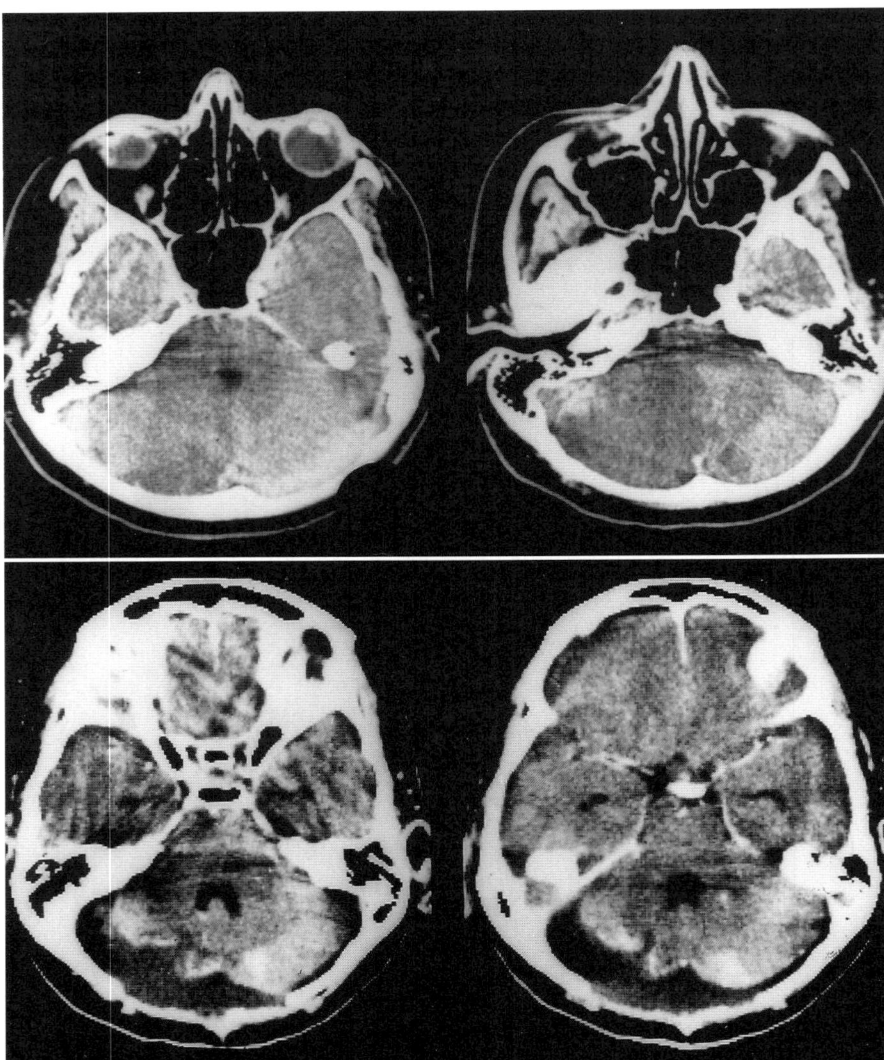

Fig. 2. Case report 2. CT scan of a left-sided cerebellar infarction at admission *(above)* and after decompression of the posterior fossa *(below)*

was no improvement in the following hours, and we performed suboccipital craniectomy and decompression of the posterior fossa. The patient recovered well and needed only little help after discharge (outcome Rankin 3).

Case 3. A 72-year-old man suffering from sudden onset of vertigo, nausea, and vomiting became lethargic the day before admission. On admission he demonstrated hemiplegia, dysarthria, and a positive Babinski sign; cranial CT

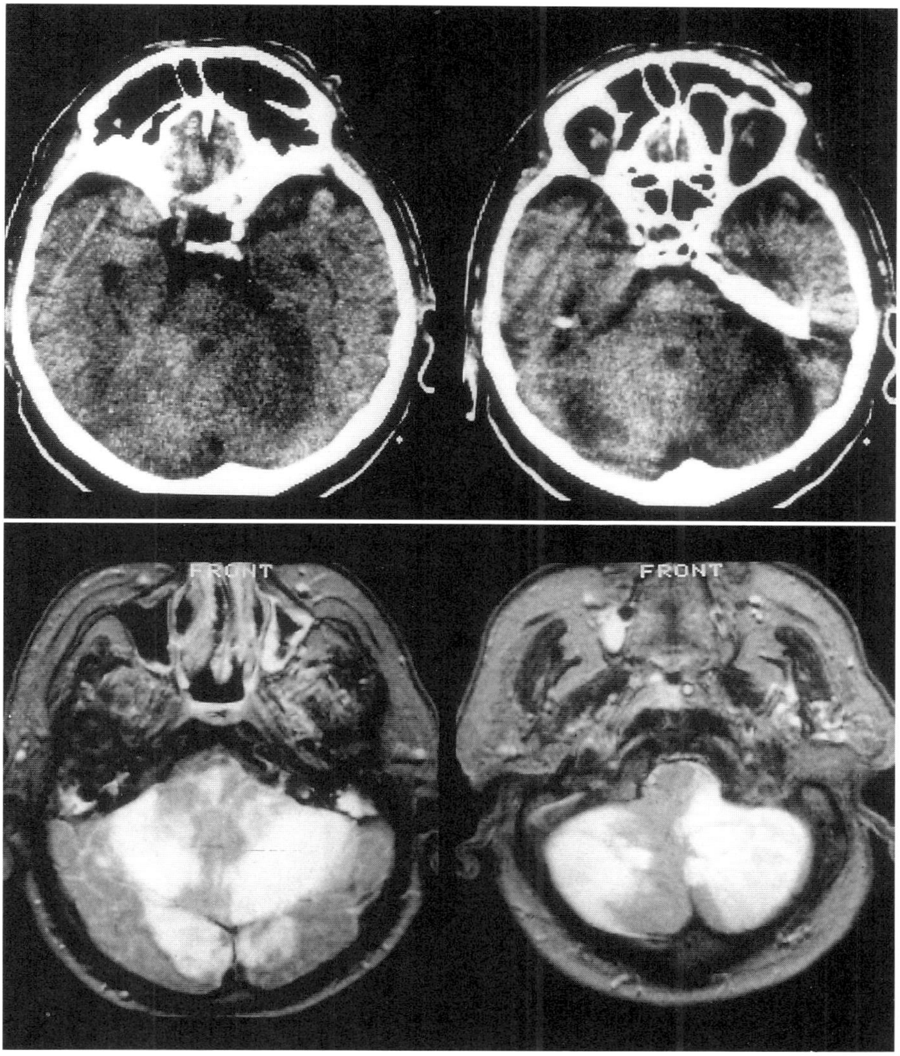

Fig. 3. Case report 3. CT scan of a right- and left-sided cerebellar infarction at admission *(above)* and magnetic resonance imaging demonstrating additional brainstem infarction *(below)*

demonstrated a right-sided cerebellar infarction with possible affection of the brainstem (Fig. 3). We performed ventricular drainage, but the patient remained comatose. He was observed in the intensive care unit and treated with supportive medical modalities. There was no clinical improvement. Magnetic resonance imaging – performed 24 h later – demonstrated brainstem infarction. In this case we saw no indication for a decompression of the posterior fossa. The patient died 3 days later (outcome Rankin 6).

Case 4. A 70-year-old man with acute onset of headache and vertigo was first seen in our Department 5 days later. He showed ataxia and bulbar speech. Cranial CT revealed a left-sided cerebellar infarction. Because of the good condition of the patient on day 5 after onset we performed no operation. He recovered completely (outcome Rankin 0).

Conclusion

The most important parameter in considering appropriate therapy in cerebellar infarction seems to be the neurological status of the patient, with special reference to the level of consciousness. In many cases of nearly asymptomatic infarction, conscious patients do not need any operative treatment. On the other hand, a frontal burrhole for emergency ventriculostomy should be considered [2]. In unconscious patients ventriculostomy seems appropriate in any case. However, instead of uncontrollable CSF drainage a continuous monitoring of intracranial pressure should be performed. In cases of CT-confirmed compression of the brainstem the indication for an aggressive operative therapy should be seen more widely. Patients with secondary deterioration or lack of improvement after ventriculostomy seem to benefit from early decompression of the posterior fossa. In cases with additional infarction of the brainstem, easily detected by magnetic resonance imaging, aggressive surgical treatment seems to be of no benefit for the patient. These results point out the importance of the multicenter study GASCIS initiated in 1992 [7].

References

1. Amarenco P, Hauw JJ (1990) Cerebellar infarction in the territory of the anterior and inferior cerebellar artery. A clinopathological study in 20 cases. Brain 113 (1):139–155
2. Bertalaffny H, de Vries J (1992) Management of cerebellar infarction with associated occlusive hydrocephalus. Clin Neurol Neurosurg 94 (1):19–23
3. Chen HJ, Lee TC, Wei CP (1992) Treatment of cerebellar infarction by decompressive suboccipital craniectomy. Stroke 23 (7):957–961
4. Fairburn B, Oliver LC (1956) Cerebellar softening. A surgical emergency. Br Med J 1:1335–1336
5. Heros RC (1992) Surgical treatment of cerebellar infarction. Stroke 23 (7):937–938
6. Kase CS, Norring B, Levine SR et al. (1993) Cerebellar infarction. Clinical and anatomic observations in 66 cases. Stroke 24 (1):76–83

7. Krieger D, Busse O, Schramm J, Febert A (1992) German-Austrian Space Occupying Cerebellar Infarction Study (GASCIS): study, design, methods, patient characteristics. The steering and Protocol Commission. J Neurol 239 (4):183–185
8. Lindgren SO (1956) Infarctions simulating brain tumours in the posterior fossa. J Neurosurg 13:575–581
9. Van Swieten et al. (1988) Assessment of handicap after stroke. Stroke 603–608

Operative Management of Space-Occupying Cerebellar Infarctions: 12 Years of Experience

D. S. Rust[1], H. Ebel[1], and A. Laun[1]

Introduction

With the reports of Fairburn and Oliver [6] and Lindgren [16] on the surgical treatment of cerebellar infarction by suboccipital craniectomy, the operative management of space-occupying cerebellar infarctions is still under discussion today. Apart from the question of whether surgical intervention can improve the clinical course, the method, extent, and timing of surgery remain controversial. Concerning the indications for surgical intervention no reliable multicenter study results are available [14]. This retrospective study reports our experiences in the surgical treatment of patients with space-occupying cerebellar infarctions, especially suboccipital craniectomy, with special consideration of the long-term outcome.

Patients and Methods

Data collected from all patients with space-occupying cerebellar infarctions treated surgically in the Department of Neurosurgery of the University of Giessen from 1981 to 1992 were reviewed retrospectively. Clinical features that were analyzed included especially the level of consciousness as determined by the Glasgow Coma Scale, imaging studies with computed tomography, operative and intraoperative findings, pre- and postoperative course, and outcome at discharge from our institution as measured by Glasgow Outcome Scale (GOS). A follow-up was also carried out to determine the long-term functional outcome.

Results

A total of 25 patients with space-occupying cerebellar infarctions (9 women and 16 men) with a mean age of 59.4 years (range 38–72 years) underwent surgical treatment in our institution from 1981 to 1992. Investigation of stroke risk factors had shown that most of the patients were multimorbid. Eighteen patients (72%) had hypertension, 13 (52%) diabetes mellitus, and 14 (56%) cardiac disease. Only four

[1] Neurochirurgische Klinik, Justus-Liebig-Universität Giessen, Klinikstr. 29,
35385 Giessen, Germany.

Advances in Neurosurgery, Vol. 22
B. L. Bauer, M. Brock, M. Klinger (Eds.)

patients (16%) had a past history of cerebral ischemia and three (12%) were current or former cigarette smokers.

The decision for surgical intervention was made on the basis of the CT neurological symptoms on admission and clinical course. In 23 patients progressive deterioration of consciousness with or without development of brainstem symptoms led to the operation. In two patients the indication for surgery was the development of brainstem symptoms without deterioration of consciousness. In 23 patients CT showed signs of an expanding infratentorial mass lesion with shift or compression of the fourth ventricle and/or with constriction or obliteration of the basal cisterns. In 19 cases secondary supratentorial occlusive hydrocephalus had occurred.

Whereas initially such unspecific symptoms as dizziness (68%), nausea and vomiting (64%), and headache (44%) and cerebellar symptoms such as ataxia (48%) were frequent, preoperatively brainstem symptoms such as central respiratory disturbance (44%), positive Babinski's sign (44%), hemiparesis (32%), and pupil abnormalities (32%) were predominant in addition to the progressive deterioration of consciousness. An initially appearing disturbance of consciousness was generally transient, but preoperatively 13 patients (52%) were comatose, 10 (40%) had a progressive deterioration of consciousness, and only 2 (8%) were awake. The deterioration of consciousness began 1–4 days (mean 2.6 days) and the onset of coma 1–5 days (mean 2.8 days) after the appearance of the first symptoms.

The surgery was performed between the first and sixth days after occurrence of the first neurological deficit (mean 3.5 days). In 19 patients (72%) the operation was carried out between the third and fifth days. In 17 patients (68%) a suboccipital craniectomy with resection of the ischemic tissue for acute decompression was carried out after implantation of an external ventricular drainage frontal or occipital. In six patients (24%) a suboccipital craniectomy without ventricular drainage was performed, and in two (8%) only a temporary ventricular drainage was implanted for relief of the occlusive hydrocephalus.

The cerebellar infarctions were located on the left side in 17 patients (68%) and on the right in 7 (28%). In one patient there were infarctions in both cerebellar hemispheres. In 21 patients (84%) the territory of the posterior inferior cerebellar artery (PICA) was affected. An infarction in the territory of the superior cerebellar artery (SCA) was seen in one patient, and in three several territories were affected. We classified the cerebellar territories according to Amarenco [1] and Hinshaw [12]. Intraoperatively we found hermorrhagic infarctions in 19 patients (82.6%) and ischemic infarctions without any hematoma in 4 (27.3%). In 19 patients treated with suboccipital craniectomy a massive swelling in the posterior fossa with raised intracranial pressure was found, leading to an axial herniation into the foramen magnum in 13 patients. In 12 of these patients a resection of the ipsilateral cerebellar tonsil was carried out.

Compared to the preoperative clinical status a significant improvement ($p = 0.002$) of the level of consciousness within the first 24 h resulted postoperatively in 18 patients (72%). Six patients (24%) were unchanged, and only one (4%) deteriorated. Immediately after the operation 61% of the preoperative comatose patients improved to an awake or at least somnolent level of consciousness.

The mean duration of stay in our Department was 14.5 days, ranging from 3 to 55 days. At discharge 21 patients (84%) were alert, and only one patient was comatose. Three patients died during the period of inpatient treatment 5, 7, and 55 days after the operation, in two cases of septic complications and in one of progressive brainstem infarction. At discharge the surviving patients generally presented symptoms of an isolated cerebellar dysfunction.

At discharge 13 patients (52%) were severely disabled (GOS 3). Nine (36%) presented slight or no disability. At the same time a significantly worse outcome was shown for patients who had been comatose preoperatively ($p < 0.001$). Of the preoperatively noncomatose patients 73% were not or were only slightly disabled (GOS 4, 5); in contrast, 91% of the preoperatively comatose patients presented a severe disability (GOS 3) at discharge.

A retrospective follow-up was carried out in the surviving 22 patients (84%). The mean duration of follow-up was 5 years, ranging from 39 days to 11.2 years. In the period of follow-up six patients (27%) died, in three cases of myocardial infarction, in two of cerebral infarction, and in one patient the cause of death was unknown. The duration of survival after the operation ranged from 2.3 to 7.7 years with a mean value of 4.8 years for these patients. Four who survived the period of follow-up had suffered a myocardial or cerebral infarction. At the time of follow-up seven patients (44%) presented a complete recovery or a slight neurological deficit which did not result in any disability. Four (25%) had a moderate disability requiring some help. Five (31%) were severely disabled and dependent on permanent care. In terms of long-term outcome there was no significant difference between preoperatively comatose and noncomatose patients. Of the surviving preoperatively comatose patients 78% and of the noncomatose patients 57% showed a good outcome, i.e., slight or no disability at the time of the follow-up. Due to the small number of patients the statistical analysis of the results showed no significant difference between outcome and age, the method or extent of operation, or the intraoperative findings.

Discussion

The operative management of space-occupying cerebellar infarctions remains a matter of debate. Several authors reject surgical treatment with primary use of suboccipital craniectomy and recommend a graduated management with anti-edemic medical treatment and single use of temporary ventricular drainage for relief of secondary occlusive hydrocephalus [8, 12, 13, 17].

In accordance with previous reports [2–4, 6, 15, 20] we can report encouraging results of the surgical treatment, mostly by primary decompressive suboccipital craniectomy, in patients with space-occupying cerebellar infarctions. Although more than 50% of patients were preoperatively comatose and 92% of all patients showed deterioration of consciousness, the operative treatment led to a significant improvement within the first 24 h in 72% of all patients and in 61% of the preoperatively comatose patients.

In addition, suboccipital craniectomy proved a relatively safe procedure, with a low rate of complications even in multimorbid and older patients. In contrast to the high surgical mortality of 28% reported by Feely [7] there was no intraoperative mortality among our patients. Postoperative mortality within the first 30 days was 8% and was independent of complications caused by surgical treatment. The mortality of patients with space-occupying cerebellar infarctions without any treatment has been estimated at 80% [18].

Although primary suboccipital craniectomy for acute decompression with or without external ventricular drainage is an aggressive procedure, there seem to be several advantages compared to the use of a single temporary ventricular drainage. Acute decompression by suboccipital craniectomy with resection of the ischemic tissue directly removes the pressure on the brainstem produced by the expanding brain edema and permits sufficient circulation of the cerebrospinal fluid [2]. If the hydrocephalus is relieved only by single ventricular drainage, there is an increasing risk of upward transtentorial herniation [5, 9, 19, 20] and postoperative infection caused by the inevitable long duration of the drainage [4]. Combined with decompressive craniectomy temporary ventricular drainage can be removed on the second or third day after operation. We have operated on six patients by suboccipital craniectomy without any ventricular drainage and have observed no significant difference in outcome to patients treated with decompressive craniectomy and ventricular drainage. The rapid postoperative improvement in our patients indicates that decompression can reduce the duration of artificial respiration and inevitable intensive care especially in preoperative comatose patients. This can lessen the risk of postoperative complications.

Another point of controversy is the correct timing of surgery. Several reports appear to suggest "that surgery should be considered only as a lifesaving last resort when all medical means fail and death appears imminent" [11]. We agree with Heros that decompressive suboccipital craniectomy is a low-risk procedure, and that there is no reason to wait until the patient deteriorates to coma and develops midbrain symptoms. In our opinion, it is important to save time in the urgent decompression of the brainstem since the interval between onset of coma and operation is an important criterion for survival [2, 10, 18].

The results of this retrospective study show that patients who were operated before the onset of coma have a significantly better outcome at discharge than preoperatively comatose patients. This can reduce the duration of inpatient treatment and result in an earlier and easier reintegration into social life. On the other hand, our experiences are favorable with decompressive craniectomy in older patients and in patients who develop midbrain symptoms or signs of severe brainstem compression with deep coma [3, 15]. We have found no correlation between age and outcome or between the preoperative level of consciousness and long-term outcome determined in the follow-up. Considering our experiences, we cannot agree with others who restrict the indication for surgery to younger patients with a generally satisfactory clinical state [2, 8]. The indication for surgery should be extensive.

Conclusions

The prognosis of patients with space-occupying cerebellar infarctions is surprisingly good if surgical intervention is performed quickly. Early suboccipital craniectomy with resection of the ischemic tissue for acute decompression is a life-saving, low-risk procedure which can significantly decrease mortality in patients with space-occupying cerebellar infarctions. Most of our patients (69%) had a good long-term outcome with complete recovery or minimal neurological deficit. The duration of survival following the operation is not dependent on complications caused by the operation but is limited by the progression of the preexisting cardiovascular disease.

References

1. Amarenco P (1991) The spectrum of cerebellar infarctions. Neurology 41:973–979
2. Auer LM, Auer T, Sayama I (1986) Indications for surgical treatment of cerebellar haemorrhage and infarction. Acta Neurochir 79:74–79
3. Busse O, Laun A, Agnoli AL (1984) Verschlußhydrozephalus bei Kleinhirninfarkten. Fortschr Neurol Psychiatr 52:164–171
4. Che HJ, Lee TC, Wei CP (1992) Treatment of cerebellar infarction by decompressive suboccipital craniectomy. Stroke 23:957–961
5. Cunes RA, Caronna TJ, Winestock PP (1979) Upward transtentorial herniation. Arch Neurol 36:618–623
6. Fairburn D, Oliver LC (1956) Cerebellar softening: a surgical emergency. Br Med J 1:1335–1336
7. Feely MP (1979) Cerebellar infarction. Neurosurgery 4:7–11
8. Greenberg J, Shubick D, Shenkin H (1979) Acute hydrocephalus in cerebellar infarct and hemorrhage. Neurology 29:409–413
9. Heros RC (1979) Cerebellar infarction resulting from traumatic occlusion of a vertebral artery. J Neurosurg 51:111–113
10. Heros RC (1982) Cerebellar hemorrhage and infarction. Stroke 13:106–109
11. Heros RC (1992) Surgical treatment of cerebellar infarction. Stroke 23:937–938
12. Hinshaw DB, Thompson JR, Hasso AN, Casselman ES (1980) Infarctions of the brainstem and cerebellum: a correlation of computed tomography and angiography. Radiology 137:105–112
13. Khan M, Polyzoidis KS, Adegbite ABO, McQueen JD (1983) Massive cerebellar infarction: "conservative" management. Stroke 14:745–750
14. Krieger D, Busse O, Schramm J, Ferbert A (1992) German-Austrian scape occupying cerebellar infarction study (GASCIS): study design, methods, patient characteristics. J Neurol 239:183–185
15. Laun A, Busse O, Calatayud V, Klug N (1984) Cerebellar infarcts in the area of the supply of the PICA and their surgical treatment. Acta Neurochir 71:295–306
16. Lindgren SO (1956) Infarctions simulating brain tumors in posterior fossa. J Neurosurg 13:575–581
17. Shenkin HA, Zavala M (1982) Cerebellar strokes: mortality, surgical indications, and results of ventricular drainage. Lancet 429–431
18. Sypert GW, Alvord EC Jr (1975) Cerebellar infarction. A clinicopathological study. Arch Neurol 32:357–363

19. Scotti G, Spinnler H, Sterzk R, Vallar G (1980) Cerebellar softening. Ann Neurol 8:133–140
20. Taneda M, Okazi K, Wakayama A, Yagi K, Kaneda H, Irino T (1982) Cerebellar infarction with obstructive hydrocephalus. J Neurosurg 57:83–91

Local Intra-arterial Fibrinolytic Therapy in Vertebrobasilar Occlusion

M. Schumacher[1], R. Siekmann[1], W. Radü[2], and A. K. Wakhloo[1]

Introduction

Approximately 15% of strokes involve the vertebrobasilar circulation. Acute bilateral vertebral artery or basilar artery thrombosis is considered one of the most important life-threatening emergencies. The prognosis in untreated basilar occlusion is known to be poor, and it is rarely survived [1,4]. Anticoagulation as well as intravenous systemic thrombolysis with recombinant tissue plasminogen activator (rTPA) have shown unsatisfactory results [5]. Local intra-arterial fibrinolysis is currently regarded as the method of choice in vertebrobasilar occlusion [3].

Materials and Methods

Intra-arterial local fibrinolysis was performed in 29 patients (22 men and 7 women; aged 22–80 years, mean 52.2). Cerebral infarction on hemorrhage visible on computed tography, a previous operation or severe trauma, nontreatable disorder of coagulative system, coma for more than 6 h and loss of brainstem reflexes, and other signs of decerebration were exclusion criteria. In addition, occlusions of the midbasilar artery with good retrograde circulation from the carotid artery and patency of the posterior and anterior cerebellar arteries were not considered for treatment. Two groups were defined: group 1, patients with mild brainstem and/or cerebellar symptoms and still conscious ($n = 20$, 69%); and, group 2, patients with acute onset of severe neurological deficits with coma and/or tetraplegia present for up to 6 h ($n = 9$, 31%). Clinical outcome after treatment was classified into five grades: grade I, no neurological deficit; grade II, minimal neurological deficit; grade III, moderate neurological defecit; grade IV, severe neurological deficit; and grade V, death.

Fibrinolysis was undertaken once the diagnosis of a basilar occlusion was confirmed by Doppler sonography; this latter diagnostic modality was omitted if the clinically suspected diagnosis was reasonably certain, or a rapid progression of the severe neurological deficits (group 2) occurred. Angiography and thrombolysis was started without obtaining an Doppler sonography if more than 6 h had elapsed.

---

[1] Section of Neuradiology, University of Freiburg, Hauptstr. 5, 79104 Freiburg, Germany.
[2] Department of Neuradiology, Kantonsspital Basel, Petersgraben 4, 4031 Basel, Switzerland.

Advances in Neurosurgery, Vol. 22
B. L. Bauer, M. Brock, M. Klinger (Eds.)

After complete diagnostic angiography a microcatheter (Tracker 18) was placed distally, bypassing the thrombus. Thrombolysis was started, and the microcatheter was retreated gradually into the thrombus. If this was not feasible, the tip of the catheter was placed into the thrombus proximally or as close as possible to the thrombus. After an initial intravenous bolus of 5000 U heparin, 200 000 U urokinase was injected manually within 15 min. Subsequently up to 1 x 10^6 U urokinase was infused until a recanalization was detected angiographically. A continuation of thrombolysis with a total of 1.5 x 10^6 U urokinase was required in three patients because fragmented primary thrombi of the basilar artery were flushed into the posterior circulation.

The duration of the fibrinolysis was limited to 2 h. After the procedure heparin was administered at twice the partial thromboplastin time for an average of 2 days. During this time the femoral sheath was left in place to avoid local bleeding.

Results

Findings on the efficacy of fibrinolysis are summarized in Fig. 1. The recanalization was technically successful in 65.5% of cases. Patients in group 1 showed higher incidence of nearly a fourfold recanalization than patients in group 2. Outcome was related to clinical condition at admission: 55% of those in group 1 and only 22.2% of those in group 2 had a grade I or II outcome (Fig. 2). The frequency of minimal deficits (grades I, II) was similar to that of severe deficits (grades IV, V). In a subgroup of eight patients with clinical outcome grade I or II, magnetic resonance imaging was performed 4 days–3 months after treatment. This revealed ischemic lesions in all patients, although results of the initial computed tomography had been normal. There were circumscribed (1 mm–1 cm) pontine, mesen-

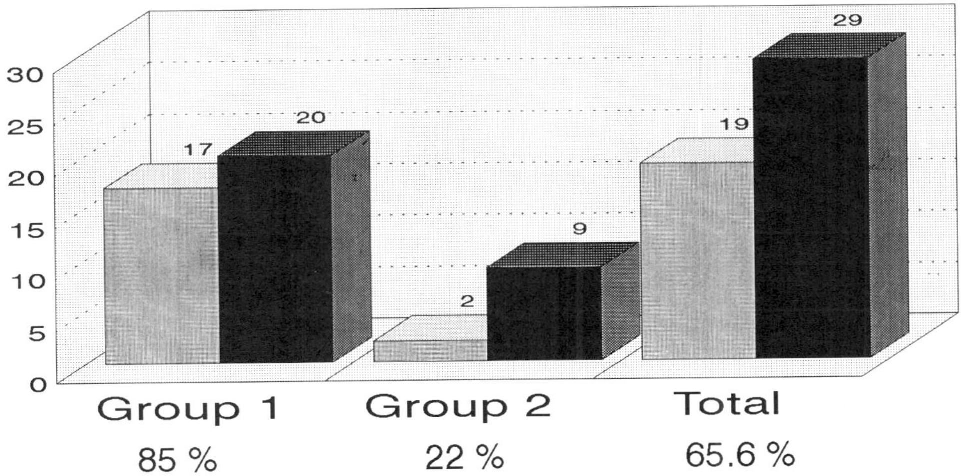

Fig. 1. Recanalization after fibrinolysis ($n = 29$). *Light column*, successful recanalization; *dark column*, total number of treated patients

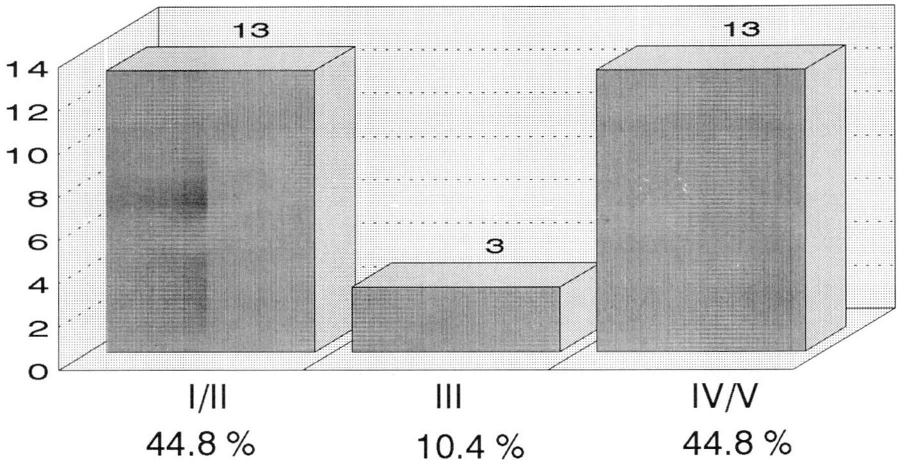

Fig. 2. Clinical outcome after fibrinolysis ($n = 29$). *I*, No deficit; *II*, minimal deficit; *III*, moderate deficit; *IV*, severe deficit or death

cephalic, and/or thalamic lesions. Hemorrhagic transformation of a missed stroke or secondary hemorrhage resulting from thrombolysis did not occur in any of the patients.

Discussion

Acute thrombolic or embolic basilar or bilateral vertebral artery occlusion is being increasingly diagnosed at an early stage, and immediate endovascular therapy is being performed more frequently. This has reduced the mortality of the disease conservatively treated from over 90% [6] to about 40% if selective thrombolysis is performed. Unlike the carotid circulation, where the time delay prior to intra-arterial fibrinolysis seems to be the most important factor, the clinical condition of the patient at the initiation of the therapy determines the outcome in vertebrobasilar occlusion. Previously reported observations in 138 cases support our findings. Nearly 30% of treated patients have had good clinical outcome [3]. The frequency of recanalization and good clinical outcome was significantly more favorable in groups 1 and 2 than among patients with severe neurological deficit and/or markedly impaired consciousness at admission. To improve the results of endovascular therapy, angiography should be performed earlier and more frequently in suspected basilar artery thrombosis. Only about one-third of all patients develop a coma initially [1], whereas a progressive stroke is apparent in 75% of all cases [2]. Approximately 50% of patients present with an unequivocal prodomal stage with vertigo, nausea, and headache. Since nearly all vertebrobasilar occlusions lead to progressive stroke within a few hours, fibrinolysis must be performed immediately. Observation and the policy of wait-and-see is not justified in most cases.

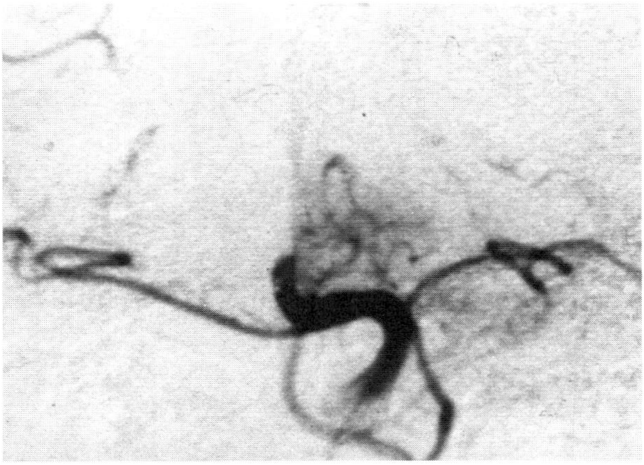

Fig. 3. Left vertebral angiogram shows occlusion of the middle portion of the basilar artery. The anterior inferior cerebellar artery is still visualized, but a good cerebellar collateralization is not seen

Comparative studies between intravenous systemic fibrinolysis [5] and local intra-arterial treatment [4, 6] have revealed many advantages of local administration of the drug. A higher efficacy of rTPA compared to urokinase has not been verified. Neither a higher frequency of recanalization nor a significantly shorter throm-

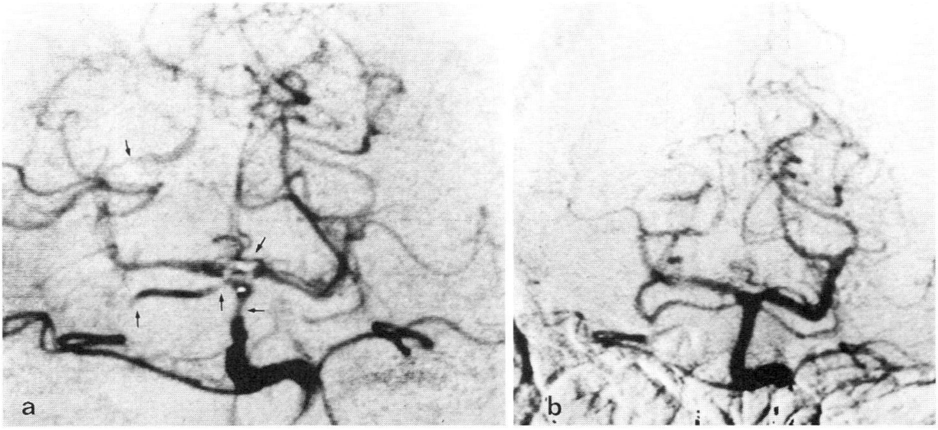

Fig. 4 a, b. Control angiogram shows partial recanalization. **a** Thrombotic fragments are seen in the superior and posterior cerebellar arteries bilaterally and in the top of basilar artery *(arrows)*. Continued fibrinolysis up to 1.5 x 10^6 U urokinase led to complete resolution of the basilar artery thrombus. **b** Good perfusion of the superior cerebellar artery bilaterally and of the posterior cerebellar artery on the left is observed. Note the residual embolus in the right posterior cerebellar artery bolysis time could be shown [7]. Thus, at present there is no justification for replacing urokinase with the substantially more expensive rTPA. Fragmentation of an embolus with occlusion of the more distal circulation during fibrinolysis (Figs. 3, 4) requires continued heparinization even after successful recanalization. Heparinization improves the prognosis in such cases by avoiding a reocclusion. Further, during heparinization autonomous fibrinolysis, which is slower and sets in later, can support the fibrinolysis induced by rTPA.

Our study supports the current opinion that local intra-arterial fibrinolysis is the most effective therapy in an acute vertebrobasilar occlusion. It improves the frequency of recanalization as well as the clinical outcome. Patients with severe brainstem symptoms benefit from the treatment only if thrombolysis is initiated up to 6 h after the onset of symptoms. In cases with milder or exclusive cerebellar symptoms more time is available for starting the treatment without increased risk of complications.

References

1. Archer CR, Horenstein S (1977) Basilar artery occlusion. Clinical and radiological correlation. Stroke 8:383–390
2. Ferbert A, Brückmann H, Drummen R (1990) Clinical features of proven basilar artery occlusion. Stroke 21:1135–1142
3. Hacke W, Hirschberg M (1992) Zerebrovaskuläre Verschlüsse. Indikation zur Thrombolysetherapie. Internist 33:241–246
4. Hacke W, Zeumer H, Ferbert A, Brückmann H, del Zoppo GJ (1988) Intraarterial thrombolytic therapy improves outcome in patients with acute vertebrobasilar occlusive disease. Stroke 19:1216–1222
5. Von Kummer R, Forsting M, Sartor K, Hacke W (1991) Intravenous plasminogen activator in acute stroke. In: Hacke W, del Zoppo GJ, Hirschberg M (eds) Thrombolytic therapy in acute ischemic stroke. Springer, Berlin Heidelberg New York
6. Zeumer H (1992) Fibrinolysis in cerebrovascular diseases of the central nervous system. In: Vinuela F, van Halbach B, Dion JE (eds) Interventional neuroradiology: endovascular therapy of the central nervous system. Raven, New York, pp 141–151
7. Zeumer H, Freitag HJ, Zanella F, Thie A, Arning C (1993) Local intra-arterial fibrinolytic therapy in patients with stroke: urokinase versus recombinant tissue plasminogen activator (r-TPA). Neuroradiology 35:159–162

Midline Tumors

Postoperative Results and Complications of Supratentorial, Intraventricular Tumors

J. Schramm[1], C. Cedzich[1], and K. Bingham[1]

Introduction

Intraventricular tumors are rare. No reports of exact incidence have been published. For ventricular papillomas Norlen [11] reported an incidence of 0.4%, and for meningiomas an incidence between 0.5% and 4.5% has been published [4–6]. The most commonly reported clinical features include symptoms of elevated intracranial pressure, and the duration of symptoms prior to hospitalization vary widely [6]. In a total series of 62 supratentorial, intraventricular processes we compared the preoperative status of patients with postoperative morbidity in terms of tumor localization, histology, radicality of surgical procedure, and the surgery itself.

Patients and Results

We evaluated 62 patients with primarily supratentorial, intraventricular tumors operated upon between 1983 and 1993 (62% women, 38% men). Histological examination of the tumors showed 19 gliomas (30.6%), 12 meningiomas (19.3%), 10 colloid cysts (16.1%), 10 tumors arising from the ependyma and plexus (16.1%), 3 pineocytomas/pineoblastomas (4.8%), and 8 others (angiomas, craniopharyngeomas, metastases; 12.9%). Preoperative clinical symptoms were caused mainly by elevated intracranial pressure, such as headache, vomiting, ataxia, and disturbance of consciousness, but focal neurological symptoms were also seen due to the specific localization of the intraventricular tumor. Most common were visual disturbances, such as visual field defects (22.5%), decreased visual acuity (24.2%), memory deficits (21%), and hemiparesis (13%). Other focal symptoms, such as gaze paresis and endocrinological disturbances, were rare (Table 1). There were 28 tumors localized in the lateral ventricles, 5 in the lateral ventricles plus third ventricle, 15 in the anterior part of the third ventricle, and 14 in the posterior part of the third ventricle.

The operative approach to the anterior part of the third ventricle was exclusively transcortical-transventricular; the approach to the posterior part of the third ventricle was transcallosal in 6 cases and infratentorial-supracerebellar in 8. The

[1] Neurochirurgische Klinik, Friedrich-Wilhelm-Universität Bonn, Sigmund-Freud-Str. 25, 53127 Bonn, Germany.

Advances in Neurosurgery, Vol. 22
B. L. Bauer, M. Brock, M. Klinger (Eds.)

Table 1. Preoperative symptoms ($n = 62$)

ICP-related symptoms	
Headache	37
Vomiting	15
Ataxia	9
Disturbance of consciousness	6
Focal symptoms	
Decreased visual acuity	15
Visual field defects	14
Hemiparesis	8
Gaze paresis	6
Memory loss	13
Endocrinological disturbances	2
Hydrocephalus	3

ICP, Intracranial pressure.

tumors of the lateral ventricles were reached by lateral temporoparietal approaches in 9 cases, by occipito-parietal in 5, by frontal transcortical-transventricular in 13, and frontal transcallosal in 1. To remove large tumors lying within the lateral ventricles plus the third ventricle frontal, transcortical-transventricular approaches were used in 4 patients and in 1 patient a lateral temporoparietal approach was performed. Total tumor removal was possible in 48 patients (77.4%), subtotal tumor removal in 12 (19.4%), and only a tumor biopsy was performed in 2 patients (3.2%). In 33 patients treatment was required for hydrocephalus occlusus prior to the tumor surgery. In 22 patients a permanent shunt system was implanted, and in 11 external CSF drainage systems were implanted (Table 2). Complications of these hydrocephalus treatments included a high percentage of CSF infections (54.5%), especially in those patients who were treated by a permanent shunt system (42.4%) (Table 2).

The mortality rate after tumor surgery was 6.45% ($n = 4$). Two of these patients died of sepsis with multiple organ system failure, one of intraventricular hemorrhage, and one of a malignant brain edema with transtentorial herniation. The mor-

Table 2. Treatment of pre- and postoperative hydrocephalus ($n = 62$)

Primary treatment	*n*	Permanent shunts	No shunt	CSF infections
Permanent shunt	22	20	2	14
External CSF drainage	11	2	9	4
No drainage or shunt necessary	29	0	29	2

Table 3. Postoperative morbidity by localization ($n = 62$)

	Lateral ventricle	Lateral ventricle + third ventricle	Anterior third ventricle	Posterior third ventricle	Total
Psychosyndrome		1			1
Memory loss		1			1
Hemiparesis	5				5
Gyrus angularis syndrome	1				1
Gaze paresis				3	3
Visual acuity			1		1
Seizures	1				1
Dysphasia	2				2
Incontinence	1				1
Hemiballism			1		1
Sepsis	1[a]				1
Hemorrhage	2[a]				2
Herniation	1[a]				1

[a] Patient death

bidity rate was 27.4%, i.e., 17 patients showed new postoperative neurological symptoms, especially hemiparesis (8%) and gaze paresis (4.8%) (Table 3).

Discussion

While both the histological diagnosis and the prognosis of intraventricular tumors are varied, the clinical symptoms are caused mostly by elevated intracranial pressure [4–6], i.e., headache, vomiting, ataxia, and disturbances of consciousness. In our series these symptoms were observed in 53.2%. Therefore the treatment of hydrocephalus was necessary prior to the tumor surgery in 33 patients. The high infection rate after an initial permanent shunt implantation induced a new management in the treatment of hydrocephalus; all patients with symptoms of increased intracranial pressure were treated by external CSF drainage systems, as described previously [4]. Apuzzo [2] has reported many different approaches to the ventricular system. We used only few approaches for tumor removal in this series. The choice of the specific approach depended on the tumor size and localization, radicality of extirpation, suspected histology, preoperative neurological deficits, and the patient's condition.

The mortality rate after intraventricular tumor surgery is reported at 0% for meningiomas by Criscuolo et al. [6], 20.7% for craniopharyngeomas by Konovalov and Gorelyshev [10], 16.9% for tumors of the lateral ventricles by Fornari et al. [7], 13.3% for tumors of the posterior part of the third ventricle by Sambasivan [12], and 22% for tumors of ventricles I–III by Goldmann and Niebeling [8]. The morbidity rate is described at 10.8% by Stein [13], 33.3% by Criscuolo et al. [6], 42% by Antunes et al. [1] and Guidetti et al. [9], and 71% by Boyd et al. [3]. Our mortality rate of 6.4% and morbidity rate of 27.4% thus represent good results and demonstrate the possibility of intraventricular tumor surgery. Only certain approaches of the wide variety possible seem necessary for tumor removal. To reduce postoperative complications by infection the initial treatment of hydrocephalus should be the implantation of an external CSF drainage system.

References

1. Antunes JL, Muraszko K, Quest DO, Carmel PW (1982) Surgical strategies in the management of tumors of the anterior third ventricle. In: Brock M (ed) Modern neurosurgery, vol 1. Springer, Berlin Heidelberg New York, pp 215–224
2. Apuzzo MLJ, Giannotta SL (1987) Transcallosal interforniceal approach. In: Apuzzo MLJ (ed) Surgery of the third ventricle. Williams and Wilkins, Baltimore, pp 354–380
3. Boyd M, Steinbok P (1987) Choroid plexus tumors: problems in diagnosis and management. J Neurosurg 66:800–805
4. Cedzich C, Kaden B, Schramm J (1992) Pre- and postoperative hydrocephalus in supratentorial intraventricular tumors. Acta Neurochir (Wien) 114:33–35
5. Cedzich C, Schramm J, Bingham K Intraventrikuläre Tumore der supratentoriellen Ventrikelabschnitte. Zentralbl Neurochir (submitted)
6. Criscuolo GR, Symon L (1986) Intraventricular meningioma. Acta Neurochir (Wien) 83:83–91
7. Fornari M, Savoiardo M, Morello G, Solero CL (1981) Meningiomas of the lateral ventricles: neuroradiological and surgical considerations in 18 cases. J Neurosurg 54:64–74
8. Goldhahn WE, Niebeling HG (1985) Die operative Behandlung von Tumoren der Ventrikel I–III nach Erfahrungen aus den Jahren 1953–1983. Zentralbl Neurochir 46:99–102
9. Guidetti B, Delfini R, Gagliardi FM, Vagnozzi R (1985) Meningiomas of the lateral ventricle. Surg Neurol 24:364–370
10. Konovalov AN, Gorelyshev SK (1992) Surgical treatment of anterior third ventricle tumors. Acta Neurochir (Wien) 118:33–39
11. Norlen G (1949) Papillomas of the choroid plexus: with report of a successfully removed tumor of the lateral ventricle in a 7 month old child. Acta Chir Scand 98:273–279
12. Sambasivan M (1982) Posterior third ventricular tumors. In: Brock M (ed) Modern neurosurgery, vol 1. Springer, Berlin Heidelberg New York, pp 225–231
13. Stein BM (1982) Transcallosal approach to third ventricle tumors. In: Schmideck HH, Sweet WH (eds) Operative neurosurgical techniques: indications, methods and results. Grune and Stratton, Paris, pp 575–584

The Interhemispheric Approach for Ventricular and Periventricular Lesions

B. Meyer[1], K. Schaller[2], V. Rohde[2], and W. E. Hassler[2]

Introduction

Since the introduction [4, 5] of the two basic surgical principles for lesions affecting the supratentorial ventricular system – the transcortical and interhemispheric transcallosal approaches – there has been argument about the better of the two alternatives. The literature describes numerous approaches and variations on these two principles for any part of the third or lateral ventricles. Authors claim to have better results with their preferred approach, but a comparative study does not exist. Our own study is also purely descriptive and updates our recent experiences with the interhemispheric transcallosal approach.

Patients and Methods

A total of 33 patients (18 women, 15 men; mean age 38.7 years) were operated on between January 1991 and November 1992 at our institution for the following pathologies: 24 intra-periventricular and 9 deep-seated midline lesions. Histo-

Table 1. Histology of 24 intra-/periventricular and 9 deep midline lesions

Histology	Ventricular	Midline
Neurocytoma	8	
Astrocytoma	5	
Plexuspapilloma	2	
Oligodendroglioma	2	
Epidermoid	2	
Meningioma	2	4
Vascular malformation	2	5
Ependymoma	1	
Total	24	9

[1] Department of Neurosurgery, University of Bonn, Sigmund-Freud-Str. 25, 53127 Bonn, Germany.
[2] Department of Neurosurgery, Klinikum Kalkweg, Zu den Rehwiesen 9, 47055 Duisburg, Germany.

Advances in Neurosurgery, Vol. 22
B. L. Bauer, M. Brock, M. Klinger (Eds.)

logical findings were heterogeneous (Table 1). The latter group served as a control regarding technical aspects of interhemispheric preparation without callosotomy.

The former group presented preoperatively as follows: 4 (16.7%) focal sensorimotor deficits, 5 (20,8%) mild hydrocephalic signs, 11 (45.8%) psychoorganic deficits, and 4 (16.7%) acute unconsciousness.

In addition to routine preoperative preparation, we consider angiography mandatory for planning the operative strategy. Depending on the anatomy of the bridging veins the trepanation is kept variable. A shunt was placed only when unavoidable. All operations were performed microscopically by the senior author (W. E. H.). After a large midline trepanation wide and thorough interhemispheric preparation was performed with special attention to adhesions in the anterior region. The corpus callosum was partially split 14 times in the anterior/middle and 10 times in the posterior region. The splenium itself, however, was always spared.

Intraventricular tumor surgery was performed according to the localization and type of the lesion. An external ventricular drainage was always placed intraoperatively and left for several days. Mean postoperative follow-up was 7 months to establish long-term results.

Results

In the control group of nine patients with deep-seated midline lesions and pure interhemispheric preparation both the operative mortality and the transient and permanent morbidity was 0%. In our group of 24 patients with intra-periventricular pathologies operated on via the interhemispheric transcallosal approach operative mortality was also 0%. Minor, asymptomatic local bleedings were observed in four patients (16.7%) but required no reoperation. In four (16.7%) subdural hygromas were seen, of which two required permanent shunting. One patient (4.2%) with an epidural hematoma underwent reoperation. In spite of perioperative external ventricular drainage three patients (12.5%) needed permanent shunting (Table 2). The overall *transient* operative morbidity of 62.5% ($n = 15$) included the following new or accentuated deficits: 4 (16.7%) focal sensorimotor deficits, 13 (54.2%) psycho-

Table 2. Operative complications in 24 cases of interhemispheric transcallosal approaches for ventricular lesions

Complication	*n*	%
Local bleeding	4	16.7
Subdural hygroma	4	16.7
Epidural hematoma	1	4.2
Permanent shunt (postoperative)	3	12.5
Total	12	50.0

Table 3. Transient operative morbidity in 24 cases after transcallosal operation

Symptom	*n*	%
Focal sensorimotor deficit	4	16.7
Psycho-organic deficit	13	54.2
Combination	2	8.2
Total	15	62.5

organic deficits, and 2 (8.4%) combinations of these (Table 3). Recovery in these cases was slow and lasted up to 8 weeks.

Results at late follow-up (mean 7 months) were as follows: 15 patients (62.5%) were graded as better and 7 (29.1%) as equal to their preoperative status. Two focal motor deficits accounted for the *permanent* operative morbidity of 8.4%. There was no correlation between postoperative deficit and operative strategy or site of callosotomy (anterior versus posterior etc.). The strongest correlation to postoperative deficits was seen with preoperative clinical status.

Discussion

With careful preoperative planning and delicate microsurgical technique, the interhemispheric preparation of the corpus callosum is a safe and unproblematic procedure, yet time consuming in comparison to the transcortical operation. Problems such as large bridging veins, interhemispheric adhesions, and arterial anomalies [1, 3, 6, 10] must be recognized preoperatively and can then be overcome [2, 6]. This experience is underlined by the results obtained in our own control series of nine patients, in whom we encountered no operative complications and therefore no postoperative morbidity and mortality.

One of the most frequent and strongest arguments against the transcallosal approach is the occurrence of disconnection syndromes. However, commisural fibers are also cut in the transcortical procedure [6, 8]. Futhermore, the overwhelming opinion is that of a multifactorial etiology for postoperative neuropsychological deficits, such as mutism or other impairment in crossed integration [1–3, 6–9]. The only region of the corpus callosum to be spared is the splenium [1, 2, 6–8], which can be achieved even in the posterior transcallosal approach to the trigonum [2, 6]. All recent series report a considerable transient operative morbidity [1–3, 6–9], namely psychoorganic syndromes, which are, however, unrelated to the site of callosotomy [7, 8] but are strongly related to preoperative clinical status and other factors such as tumor size, histology, localization, and duration of symptoms [1–3, 6–9]. All reports also state that the recovery is often slow. At long-term follow-up, the remaining neuropsychological consequences are almost never detectable by routine neurological examinations and are not recognized by the patient himself or by relatives [1, 2, 6, 8, 9]. However, subtle neuropsychological tests do detect permanent "occult" deficits which are not unequivocally attributed to partial callosotomy [1, 2, 8, 9]. Our own results in the 24 cases of operated intra-/periventricular lesions confirm these opinions expressed in the literature in all points.

Conclusion

We therefore conclude that with a strict preoperative and microsurgical rationale the interhemispheric preparation itself poses no problem. Despite a high incidence of transient postoperative morbidity and an often slow recovery, the long-term results of the interhemispheric transcallosal approach are very good. The outcome is closely related to preoperative status, tumor size, localization, and histology, but not to the site of callosotomy.

References

1. Apuzzo MLJ, Oleg KC, Gott PS, Teng EL, Zee CS, Giannotta SL, Weiss MH (1982) Transcallosal, interfornicial approaches for lesions affecting the third ventricle: surgical considerations and consequences. Neurosurgery 10:547–554
2. Bellotti C, Pappada G, Sani R, Oliveri G, Stangalino C (1991) The transcallosal approach for lesions affecting the lateral and third ventricle: surgical considerations and results in a series of 42 cases. Acta Neurochir (Wien) 111:103–107
3. Benes V (1990) Advantages and disadvantages of the transcallosal approach to the III ventricle. Childs Nerv Syst 6:437–439
4. Bush, E (1944) A new approach for the removal of tumors of the third ventricle. Acta Psychiatr Scand 19:57–60
5. Dandy WE (1922) Diagnosis, localization and removal of tumors of the third ventricle. Johns Hopkins Hosp Bull 33:188–189
6. Gilsbach JA, Eggert HR, Hassler W (1985) Possibilities and limits of the midline interhemispheric approach. Acta Neurochir (Wien) [Suppl] 35:85–88
7. Nakasu Y, Isozumi T, Nioka H, Handa J (1991) Mechanisms of mutisms following the transcallosal approach to the ventricles. Acta Neurochir (Wien) 110:146–153
8. Oepen G, Schulz-Weiling R, Birg W, Straesser S, Gilsbach J (1988) Neuropsychological assessment of the transcallosal approach. Eur Arch Psychiatr Neurol Sci 237:365–375
9. Petrucci RJ, Bucheit WA, Woodruff GC, Karian JM, Defillipp GJ (1987) Transcallosal parafornicial approach for third ventricle tumors: neuropsychological consequences. Neurosurgery 20:457–464
10. Rhoton AL, Yamamoto I, Peace DA (1981) Microsurgery of the third ventricle, part 2. Operative approaches. Neurosurgery 8:357–373

Tumors of the Lateral and Third Ventricles: Follow-up Postoperative Morbidity and Mortality

W. E. K. Braunsdorf[1], H. M. Mehdorn[1], and G. Fritsch[1]

Introduction

Tumors of the lateral and third ventricles are deeply seated central lesions which always require careful treatment planning. Considering the close relationships to vital neural and vascular structures, each operative approach is challenging, especially in the light of new developments such as neuroendoscopy, stereotactically guided microsurgery or biopsy, and gamma-knife surgery. In our opinion the tumor's exact location must be determined as *decision making* is influenced mainly by the expected surgical anatomy and less by the expected histology. We present the evidence of our experience over a 10-year period in which neuroimaging was available.

Materials and Methods

We have investigated 55 surgically treated patients with tumors of the lateral or third ventricle since 1980. Patients with congenital malformations, craniopharyngeomas, sellar region or pineal region tumors are excluded. Clinical symptoms and the value of diagnostic investigations were evaluated; in all cases computed tomography and, since 1988, magnetic resonance imaging were performed. Our surgical steps were revised, and a careful follow-up with analysis of the results in relation to the anatomical localization and chosen surgical approach was carried out. According to Kaplan and Meier [6], the cumulative survival rate was calculated in relation to direct approaches versus solely shunting procedures, complete versus incomplete resections, tumors of lateral ventricle versus third ventricular tumors, and early versus late mortality. To assess performance status a modification of the Karnofsky Index was used with the following grades: A, normal daily activity, only mild neurological disturbances; B, disabled living at home, moderate/severe neurological disturbances; C, no independence, severe neurological disturbances, living in a nursing home.

---

[1] Klinik für Neurochirurgie, Christian-Albrecht-Universität, Weimarer Str. 8, 24106 Kiel, Germany.

Advances in Neurosurgery, Vol. 22
B. L. Bauer, M. Brock, M. Klinger (Eds.)

Results

Since 1980, we have operated on 55 patients, 38 with lateral ventricle tumors and 17 with third ventricle tumors. There was no particular difference in the number of men and women. Younger ages were more frequent among the group with third ventricular tumors, and there was a significantly higher percentage in children. The median age of patients with lateral ventricular tumors was 32 years and that among patients with third ventricular tumors 23 years. Most of the lateral ventricular tumors were located in the anterior horn and at the foramen of Monro (22 /38); nine were located in the cella media, six in the trigone, and only one in the posterior horn. The number of third ventricular tumors is too small to distinguish between anterior or posterior parts. Nearly one-half of all tumors had infiltrated surrounding structures such as thalamus, basal ganglia, and corpus callosum.

In terms of histopathological distribution, we observed a wide variety of tumor types (Table 1). There was a majority of low-malignant or benign tumors. Lateral ventricular tumors were often of astrocytic origin. Clinically, signs of raised intracranial pressure were dominant. All third ventricular tumors were associated with hydrocephalus but only 76% of ventricular tumors. These were generally large, had grown slowly within the ventricles, and caused symptoms only in the early stage, if the foramen of Monro was occluded. The expected clinical symptoms due to the anatomic localization were seldom observed (Fig. 1).

We performed 67 surgical procedures in 55 patients. In 15 cases with lateral ventricular tumors a complete resection by a direct approach was carried out. In 12 cases a subtotal resection was performed, and in nine an additional shunt was implanted. In these cases a transcortical-transventricular approach was used 15 times. Tumors of the trigone were approached from a parieto-occipital transcortical-trans-

Table 1. Histology of the tumors of the lateral ventricle ($n = 38$) or third ventricle ($n = 17$)

Histology	Third ventricle	Lateral ventricle
Glioblastoma	3	2
Mixed glioma II/III	–	2
Pilocytic astrocytoma	5	7
Giant cell astrocytoma	–	2
Oligodendroglioma	1	–
Ependymoma/-blastoma	–	3
Ganglioglioma	–	1
Plexus papilloma	–	2
Lymphoma	–	1
PNET	2	–
Schwannoma	–	1
Germinoma	1	–
Meningioma	1	4
Colloid cyst	2	7
Histology unknown	2	6

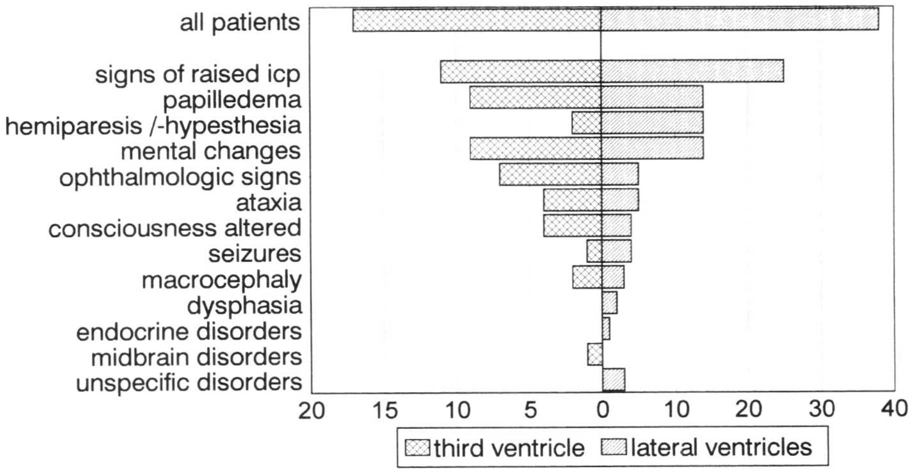

Fig. 1. Symptoms in patients with tumors of the third ventricle ($n = 17$) or lateral ventricle ($n = 38$)

ventricular route. Eleven patients were treated solely by a shunt. Six of these were diagnosed for extensive infiltration of the thalamus and basal ganglia, in three cases there was restricted operability due to a reduced general condition, and in two cases of colloid cyst of the foramen of Monro family members refused a direct exploration. Ten patients had to be operated on twice. Postoperative complications led to a reoperation in two cases. The decision for a direct approach was mostly in third ventricular and anterior horn and foramen of Monro tumors. Third ventricular tumors were operated on primarily by an interhemispheric-transcallosal approach; in some cases the transcortical-transventricular or supracerebellar-infratentorial ac-

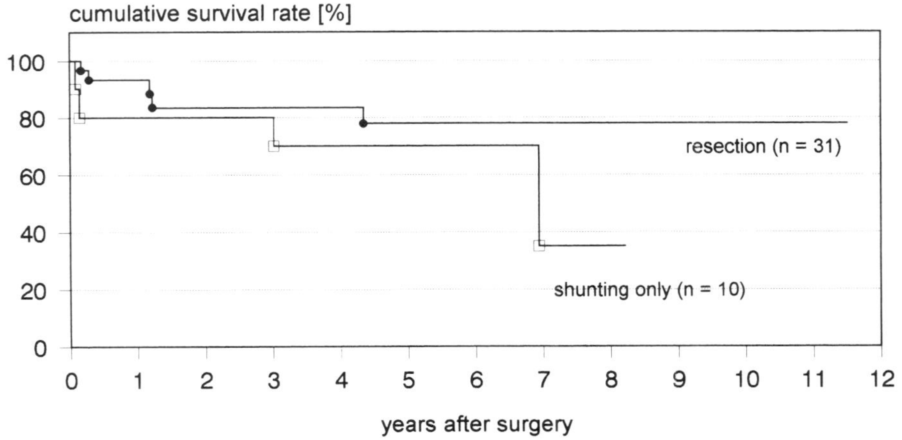

Fig. 2. Cumulative survival rate in all patients with surgery for tumors of the third ventricle or lateral ventricle (excluding postoperative mortality), treated with resection ($n = 31$) or palliative shunting only ($n = 10$)

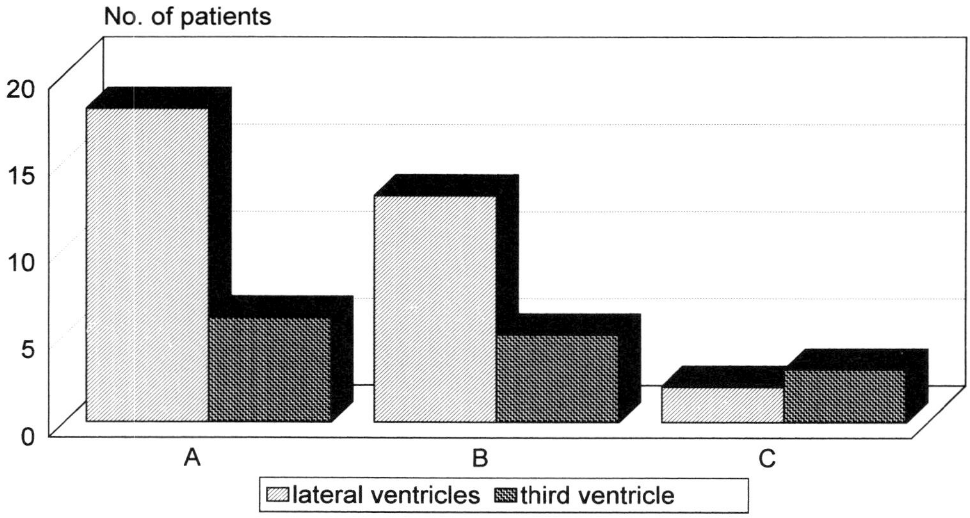

Fig. 3. Postoperative Karnofsky performance score *(A, B, C)* of patients with surgery of tumors of the third ventricle or lateral ventricle

cess was used. Complete resection was performed in five cases and a subtotal in nine. Three received shunts. In all, ten patients were additionally irradiated.

Kaplan-Meier life-time tables were calculated. Two-thirds of all patients recovered, without a relationship to tumor localization. Early mortality was about 20% and overall mortality about 30%, with a marked decrease in the last 5 years. (Since 1987 only one patient has died!) The cumulative survival rate was not influenced by localization or histology, but there was a significantly better prognosis for patients with direct resection than for the solely shunted patients (Fig. 2). The overall cumulative survival rate for all patients showed an initial decrease, and more of 50% are still alive after 11 years. Postoperative complications consisted of hypothalamic dysregulations in nearly 20%. Outcome in terms of performance status demonstrates an independence on the part of 20 patients, while 9 were disabled and 4 needed continuous nursing care (Fig. 3). Concerning this parameter there was also a significant decrease in the last 5 years.

Discussion

The results in treating patients with ventricular tumors must be reviewed in the light of new surgical tools. The overall mortality has decreased over the past 10 years, particularly during the past 5 years. These results are due to carefully planned surgical treatments with magnetic resonance imaging in advance, allowing a precise microneurosurgical-anatomical approach. Various surgical approaches share several features, and the choice must be made in each individual case [1, 7, 10, 11]. From the surgical point of view these tumors should be evacuated

piecemeal to minimize further lesions of the already demyelinized white matter due to chronically raised intracerebral pressure. Therefore self-retractors should be avoided if possible. An injury of the choroidal arteries must be avoided.
Most of these tumors in younger patients are of low malignancy [8, 9], grow slowly, and therefore offer a chance for curative surgical treatment. As others have mentioned [9], a general prognosis cannot be established due to the highly variable histological nature. Our results indicate that direct and complete resection is the other dominant factor influencing the prognosis (Fig. 3). There is an initial decrease in operative complications, but the long-term follow-up confirms the better prognosis in the treatment group. The rather high incidence of patients receiving only shunts is due to a temporarily more restrictive attitude in the early 1980s, as the decision not to operate directly was made if unresectable tumors were suspected, or patients refused or were in bad general condition. Nowadays shunt implantation should be perfomed if signs of severely raised intracranial pressure indicate a hazard to the patient to gain time for further diagnostic investigations. The other indication is the dominant localization of the tumor mass within the thalamus, basal ganglia, or corpus callosum.

Colloid cysts can be stereotactically punctured and evacuated or endoscopically unloaded, but in our own experience and that of others [2] nowadays with magnetic resonance imaging cysts that must be operated on can be reliably distinguished. Among our patients there was a young woman with a suspected colloid cyst which was in fact an astrocytoma. Histological examination is mandatory. Two patients with malignant lymphoma who received shunts and irradiation did not benefit for a longer period. Irradiation without confirmed histology should be abandoned [1].

Conclusion

Tumors of the lateral and third ventricle are generally benign or of low-malignant character. A long follow-up of 11 years with acceptable morbidity and mortality is possible if precise surgical therapy is offered. CSF shunting, with minimal mortality offers no advantage in long-time follow-up. Magnetic resonance imaging (or further neuromagnetic imaging) is the main diagnostic tool and permits adequate planning of a microneuroanatomical approach [11]. New technology such as neuroendoscopy and real-time stereotaxic navigational microsurgery together with visualization computers should improve the results within the near future.

References

1. Apuzo MLJ (ed) (1987) Surgery of the third ventricle. Williams and Wilkins, Baltimore
2. Camacho A, Chad DA, Kelly PJ, Laws ER (1989) Colloid cysts: experience with the management of 84 cases since the introduction of computed tomography. Neurosurgery 24:693–700

3. Fornari M, Savoiardo M, Morello G et al. (1981) Meningiomas of the lateral ventricles: neuroradiological and surgical considerations in 18 cases. J Neurosurg 54:64
4. Geffen G, Walsh A, Simpson D et al. (1980) Comparison of the effects of transcortical and transventricular removal of intraventricular tumors. Brain 103:773
5. Jun LJ, Nutik SL (1988) Surgical approaches to intraventricular meningiomas of the trigone. In: Schmiedek HH, Sweet WH (eds) Operative neurosurgical techniques, indications and results. Grune and Stratton, New York, pp 597–600
6. Kaplan EL, Meier P (1958) Nonparametric estimation from noncomplete observations. J Am Stat Assoc 53:457–481
7. Kemple LG, Blaylock R (1976) Lateral-trigonal intraventricular tumors. A new operative approach. Acta Neurochir (Wien) 35:233–242
8. Lapras C, Deruty R, Bret P (1984) Tumors of the lateral ventricles. In: Symon L, Calliauw L, Cohadon F et al. (eds) Advances and technical standards in neurosurgery, vol 11. Springer, Berlin Heidelberg New York, p 103
9. Spencer DD, Collins W, Kimberlee JS (1988) Surgical management of lateral intraventricular tumors. In: Schmiedek HH, Sweet WH (eds) Operative neurosurgical techniques, indications and results. Grune and Stratton, New York, pp 583–596
10. Stein BM (1988) Transcallosal approach to third ventricle tumors. In: Schmiedek HH, Sweet WH (eds) Operative neurosurgical techniques, indications and results. Grune and Stratton, New York, pp 381–388
11. Timurkanyak E, Rhoton AL, Barry M (1986) Microsurgical anatomy and operative approaches to lateral ventricles. Neurosurgery 8:357–373

Postoperative Visual Outcome of Meningiomas Located in the Sellar Region

J. Meixensberger[1], M. Janka[1], J. Sold[2], K.-A. Bushe[1], and K. Roosen[1]

Introduction

Meningiomas of the sellar region represent approximately 4%–10% of all intracranial meningiomas [3, 7, 9], involving the tuberculum sellae, anterior clinoid processes, diaphragma sellae, and planum sphenoidale. Because of their association with important vascular and functional regions their treatment causes some major problems. Besides endocrinological disturbances, headaches, seizures, and mental disorders, visual loss and bitemporal hemianopsia are common symptoms. Operative mortality and mobidity have been improved by microsurgical methods and progress in neuroanesthesia and intensive care [10]. The postoperative visual outcome is an important problem for the patient and may worsen the prognosis of these tumors. In this study 40 tumors of the sellar region presenting visual symptoms were reviewed to evaluate the postoperative course of visual disturbances and prognostic criteria.

Patients and Methods

Between 1985 and 1992, 40 patients with meningiomas of the supra- and parasellar region were operated on at the Department of Neurosurgery, University of Würzburg. There were 30 women (75%) and 10 men (25%) with a mean age of 58 years (range 17–81). Diagnosis was confirmed by histopathological examination. Almost all tumors (classified as atypical meningiomas) were benign meningiomas (24 endotheliomatous), 10 transitional, 4 fibrous, and 2 atypical). On admission all patients had preoperative visual disturbances. The duration of symptoms and the visual status were documented by a detailed ophthalmological examination. In the postoperative follow-up visual function after 6 months was used to evaluate prognostic criteria. The size of the tumors and the extent of surgery was determined by computed tomography and magnetic resonance imaging pre- and postoperatively. Additional operative complications were noted.

[1] Neurochirurgische Klinik und Poliklinik, Universität Würzburg, Josef-Schneider-Str. 11, 97080 Würzburg, Germany.
[2] Klinik und Poliklinik für Augenheilkunde, Universität Würzburg, Josef-Schneider-Str. 11, 97080 Würzburg, Germany.

Advances in Neurosurgery, Vol. 22
B. L. Bauer, M. Brock, M. Klinger (Eds.)

Results

Extent of Tumor Removal, Mortality and Morbidity Rates

Using a frontopterional (90% of cases) or a transcallosal (10%) approach 32 of the tumors (80%) were totally removed. In 8 patients (20%) a subtotal tumor resection was achieved using microsurgical operation techniques. In these cases the extent of tumor removal was limited by infiltrative meningioma growth into the cavernosus sinus, pituitary stalk, and hypothalamus. There was 0% mortality during the first 6 months postoperatively. Postoperative complications were as follows: temporary hemiparesis, 3 (7.5%); single seizures, 6 (15%); permanent seizures 2 (5%; pituitary-hypothalamic insufficiency, 0. There was low permanent morbidity (5%) in addition to the visual disturbances. Only the two patients with postoperative seizures required anticonvulsive drugs.

Visual Outcome

Preoperative Visual Loss. Monocular visual disturbances were found in 27 (67.5%) of the patients, according to the morphological unilateral extent of the meningioma on computed tomography or magnetic resonance imaging, and 13 (32.5%) showed binocular visual symptoms. Table 1 summarizes the preoperative visual symptoms. In addition to the impairment of visual acuity, additional visual field defects were observed in 23 patients. The duration of preoperative visual symptoms is shown in Fig. 1. Most of the patients (70%) were operated on within 6 months after the onset of visual symptoms.

Postoperative Visual Outcome. Visual function was improved in 8 cases (20%), remained constant in 18 (45%), and worsened in 14 (35%) 6 months after surgery (Fig. 2). Vision usually improved rapidly within the first 3–4 weeks after operation. After 6 months improvement of visual function was rare. Figure 3 summarizes the pre- and postoperative values for visual acuity in the group with improved

Table 1. Preoperative extent of visual loss ($n = 40$)

	n	%
Monocular visual symptoms	27	67.5
Binocular visual symptoms	13	32.5
Papillatrophy	9	22.5
Ophthalmologically verified visual loss	17	42.5
Finger counting hand movement	17	42.5
Light perception	3	7.5
Blindness	3	7.5
Visual field defects (quadrantenanopsia, hemianopsia)	23	57.5

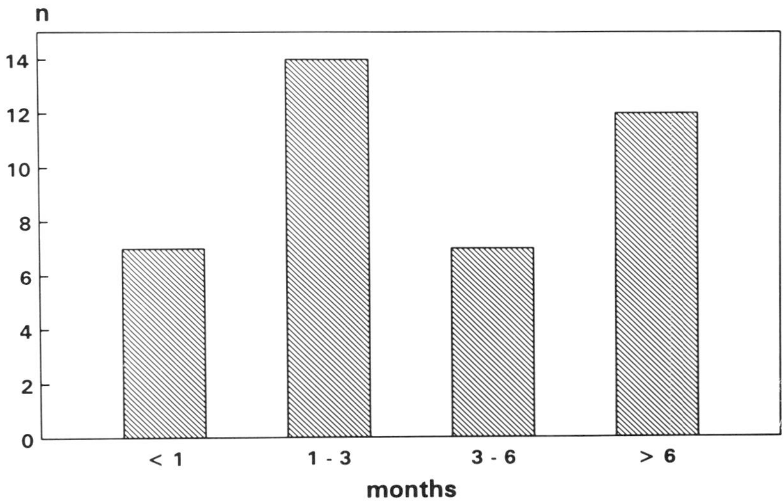

Fig. 1. Duration of preoperative disturbance of vision

and worsened visual outcome. In both groups the mean visual acuity was 0.5 and improved to 0.7 or worsened to 0.2. Among those with improved visual acuity no patient had papillatrophy; 75% of the cases were operated within 3 months after onset of symptoms, and in 75% of the cases the tumor size was smaller than 25 mm. In those with worsened visual outcome 36% were found to have papillatrophy (total number of patients with preoperative papillatrophy), and in most the duration of symptoms was longer than 3 months (71% of cases). As additional

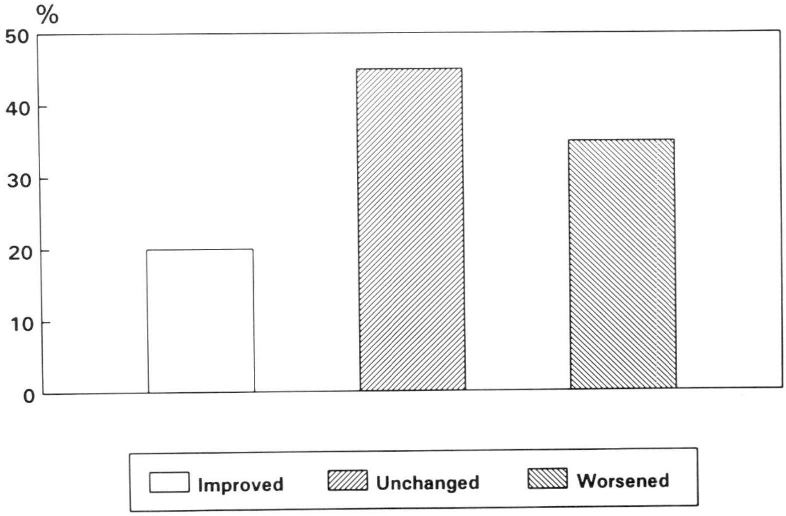

Fig. 2. Overall visual outcome 6 months after operation

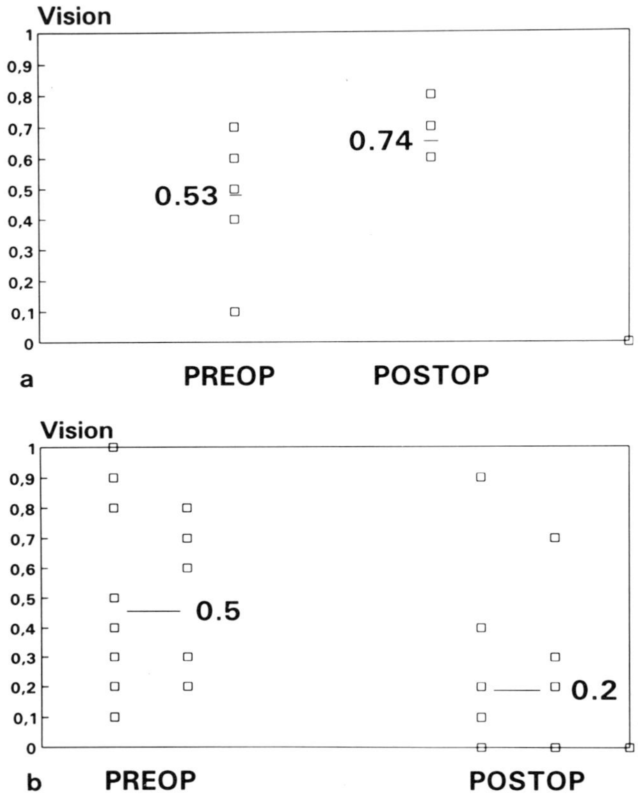

Fig. 3 a, b. Preoperative and postoperative values of visual acuity (6 months after craniotomy). **a** Group with improved visual function ($n = 8$). **b** Group with worsened visual function ($n = 14$). *Asterisk*, mean

factors influencing visual outcome there was a worsening of preoperative visual acuity below 0.5 (65% of cases) and a tumor size larger than 25 mm (86%). In the group with improved and worsened visual outcome we detected no significant difference in terms of age or sex. In 23 patients (57.5%) we diagnosed an additional monocular (52%) or binocular (48%) visual field defect. Half of the patients ($n = 11$, 48%) were improved independently of monocular or binocular disturbances 6 months after surgery. Usually the visual field defects improved with visual acuity.

Discussion

In the literature reports on the operative mortality for excision of suprasellar meningiomas range from 10% to 67% [1]. Injury to major vessels is one of the causes for high operative mortality. Another important factor is tumor size. Jane and McKissock [5] reported 44% mortality in their series ($n = 32$) with a tumor size of 30 mm or more. New neuroradiological imaging techniques and surgical and anesthesiological advances have improved the operative results. Andrews and Wilson [2] reported in their series of 38 suprasellar meningiomas a mortality rate of 2.6%, and Symon and Rosenblum [10] a 3% versus 7.4% mortality rate in a group of microsurgically versus nonmicrosurgically treated suprasellar meningiomas. In our series no death occurred; this is due to modern-day surgical techniques and the effect of microsurgery, which makes midline surgery generally safer. Despite these advances the postoperative functional improvement in visual disturbances varies in the different series [2, 4–6, 8]. Jane and Kissock [5] reported in their series improvement of vision in 8 (44%) patients with large tumors (> 30 mm), worsening in 4 (22%), and no change in 6 (34%). In the group with small tumors (< 30 mm) 9 showed visual improvement and 8 were unchanged. Rosenstein and Symon [8] reported 101 cases and found visual outcome improved in 63.6%, no change in 12.1%, and worsening in 24.2%. Andrews and Wilson [2] reviewed 38 suprasellar meningiomas: 42% of patients had improved vision postoperatively, 30% were unchanged, and 28% were worse. Prognosis was generally affected by duration of symptoms, amount of preoperative visual loss, and tumor size. In our series of patients treated microsurgically in the past 8 years we found an overall visual outcome of 20% improved cases and 45% with unchanged visual function, but there were still 35% with worsening of vision. In agreement with others [4, 8, 10] we confirm the following prognostic criteria: duration of symptoms, optic disc status, preoperative visual signs, and tumor size. However, special vascular and nutritive conditions of the optic nerve may not be satisfactorily influenced by microsurgical operation techniques. These are responsible for the disappointing postoperative course of vision in some of our patients.

Conclusions

The results of this study confirm the safety of the microsurgical approach to midline tumors such as sellar meningiomas. However, despite decreased mortality and morbidity, functional improvement of vision is not sufficient in all patients. In addition to the prognostic criteria of duration of symptoms, optic disc status, amount of preoperative visual loss, and tumor size, special nutritive and vascular components are also important.

References

1. Al-Mefty O, Smith RR (1991) Tuberculum sellae meningiomas. In: Al Mefty O (ed) Meningiomas. Raven, New York, pp 395–411
2. Andrews BT, Wilson CB (1988) Suprasellar meningiomas: the effect of tumor location on postoperative visual outcome. J Neurosurg 69:523–528

3. Cushing H, Eisenhardt L (1938) Suprasellar meningiomas. In: Meningiomas: their classification, regional behaviour, life, history, and surgical end results. Thomas, Baltimore, pp 224–249
4. Gregorius FK, Hepler RS, Stern WE (1975) Loss and recovery of vision with suprasellar meningiomas. J Neurosurg 42:69–75
5. Jane JA, McKissock W (1962) Importance of failing vision in early diagnosis of suprasellar meningiomas. Br J Med 2:5–7
6. Kadis GN, Mount LA, Ganti SR (1979) The importance of early diagnosis and treatment of the meningiomas of the planum sphenoidale and tuberculum sellae: a retrospective study of 105 cases. Surg Neurol 12:367–371
7. Olivecrona H (1967) The suprasellar meningiomas. In: Olivecrona H, Tönnis W (eds) Handbuch der Neurochirurgie. Springer, Berlin Heidelberg New York, pp 167–172
8. Rosenstein J, Symon L (1984) Surgical management of suprasellar meningioma. II Prognosis for visual function following craniotomy. J Neurosurg 61:642–648
9. Solero CL, Giombini S, Morello G (1983) Suprasellar and olfactory meningiomas: report on a series of 153 personal cases. Acta Neurochir (Wien) 67:181–194
10. Symon L, Rosenstein J (1984) Surgical management of suprasellar meningiomas, part 1: the influence of tumor size, duration of symptoms, and microsurgery on surgical outcome in 101 consecutive cases. J Neurosurg 61:633–641

Optic Pathway Glioma: Management and Prognosis in 25 Surgically Treated Cases

J. M. Valdueza[1], F. Lohmann[1], C. Hagel[2], O. Dammann[3], J. Freitag[4], and H.-D. Herrmann[1]

Introduction

Gliomas of the optic pathway (OPG) are quite rare. These tumors arise intracranially and account for about 1% of all intracranial tumors. About 85% of OPG present in children under the age of 15. An association with neurofibromatosis 1 (NF1) is well known and occurs in about one-third of all patients with OPG [12]. A benign pilocytic astrocytoma (WHO grade I) is generally found to be associated with NF-1. OPG comprise a broad spectrum of tumor pattern and growth dynamics. They can involve the total length of the optic pathway, and show extreme variation in tumor shape and appearance. The tumor may be located intracranially or intraorbitally within the optic nerve structures (intrinsic growth). Sometimes they reveal a large extrachiasmatic portion compressing or infiltrating adjacent brain structures, especially the hypothalamic region (extrinsic growth). This great variety of findings has made the management of OPG controversial. Treatment modalities include different extents of surgery, [14], radiotherapy [18], and more recently chemotherapy [10]. Other investigators have found no benefit from any kind of treatment [6]. This report reviews of our cases in an attempt to clarify the management and to select relevant prognostic factors which may influence treatment strategies.

Patients and Methods

Since 1980, 25 consecutive patients presenting OPG have been treated surgically at our department. All patients were explored neurologically and ophtalmologically. Preoperative computed tomography scans ($n = 7$) or magnetic resonance imaging ($n = 18$) were evaluated carefully in regard to size and shape of the tumor, its relationship to the hypothalamus and third ventricle, and especially optic tract involvement. The radiological findings were used to divide the OGP into five groups

[1] Abteilung für Neurochirurgie, Universitätskrankenhaus Eppendorf, Martinistr. 52, 20251 Hamburg, Germany.
[2] Kinderklinik, Universitätskrankenhaus, Martinistr. 52, 20251 Hamburg, Germany.
[3] Abteilung für Neuropathologie, Universitätskrankenhaus, Martinistr. 52, 20251 Hamburg, Germany.
[4] Abteilung für Neuroradiologie, Universitätskrankenhaus, Martinistr. 52, 20251 Hamburg, Germany.

Advances in Neurosurgery, Vol. 22
B. L. Bauer, M. Brock, M. Klinger (Eds.)

Table 1. Classification of 25 optic pathway gliomas

Type	Extension and tumor shape	*n*
1	Tubular thickening of the optic nerve(s) and/or chiasm	2
2	Spindle-shaped tumor of the optic nerve(s)	1
3	Suprasellar chiasmatic tumor with contiguous optic tract expansion	6
4	Globular intrachiasmatic tumor (size < 2 cm)	2
5	Large suprasellar globular tumor with extension into the hypothalamus and/or third ventricle	14

(Table 1, Fig. 1), using a modified classification proposed by Fletcher and coworkers [3]. There were two major groups. Of 25 tumors 14 (56%) revealed a large globular suprasellar mass without affliction of the optic tracts (Fig. 2). In six cases (24%) a contiguous optic tract expansion was seen (Fig. 3). In 7 cases the tumor mass was less than 3 cm in size. In the remaining 18 cases the diameter of the lesion ranged between 3 and 6 cm.

There were 14 men and 11 women, with a median age of 15 years (range 12 months–66 years). The pediatric group comprised 80%. Seven children were aged under 5 years, five were 5–8 years old, and eight were 9–16 years old. Three

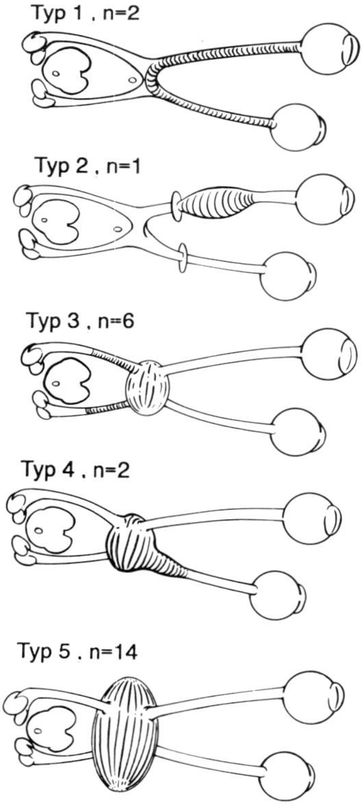

Fig. 1. Schematic presentation of the spectrum of optic pathway glioma

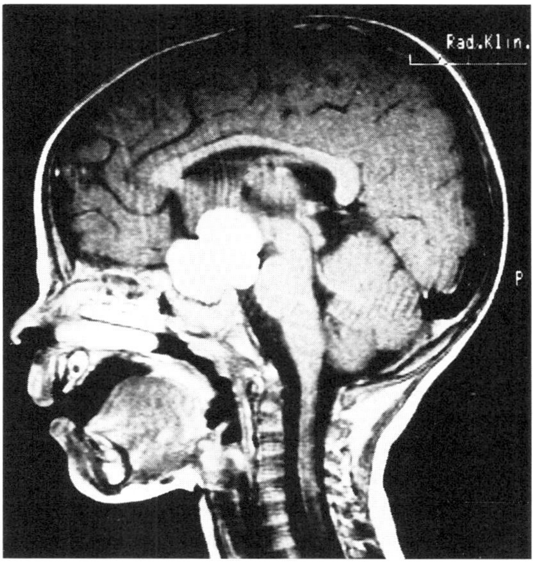

Fig. 2. Midsagittal T1-weighted magnetic resonance image with gadolinium-enhancement demonstrating a large suprasellar mass (type 5)

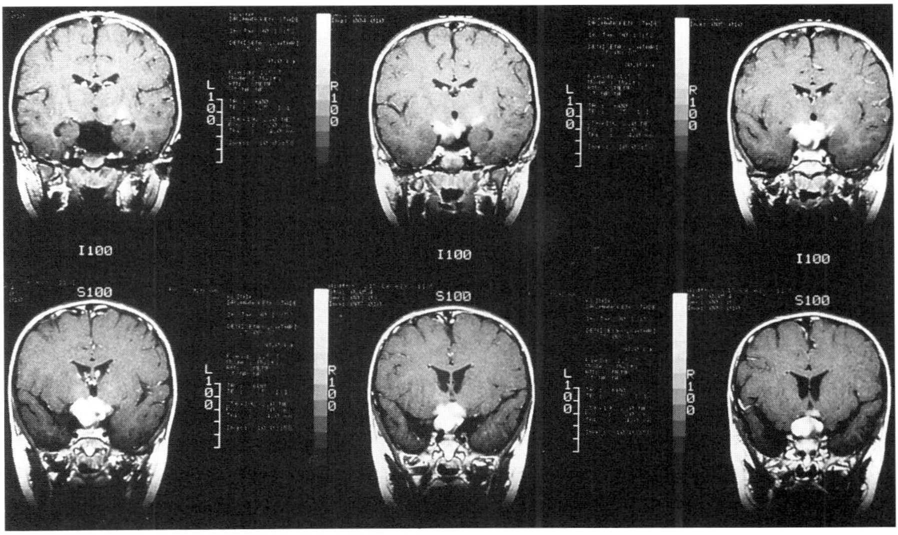

Fig. 3. Coronal T1-weighted magnetic resonance images with gadolinium enhancement revealing glioma with expansion into the optic tracts

patients were aged between 25 and 30 years. Two patients were 63 and 68 years old, respectively. Eight patients (32%) had clear evidence of NF-1.

The most common symptom was impaired vision, in 22 cases (88%). Endocrine/hypothalamic abnormalities were documented in 4 patients. The clinical findings are listed in Table 2.

Table 2. Symptoms and signs at presentation

	n	%
Decreased visual acuity	22	88
Visual field defects	14	56
Hydrocephalus	6	24
Nystagmus	4	16
Mental disorder	3	12
Sensorimotoric deficits	3	12
Precocious puberty	2	8
Growth hormone deficiency	1	4
Adipositas	1	4
Diencephalic syndrome	1	4

Results

Surgical Therapy. A total of 29 surgical approaches to the tumors were performed in 24 patients. All cases underwent a frontotemporal craniotomy. Subtotal resectioning (70%–90%) was possible in 12 cases. Ten patients underwent partial resectioning, and in seven cases surgery was limited to biopsy. Three patients, aged 2, 4, and 5 years upon admission, underwent second subtotal resectioning when there was tumor recurrence 1, 1.5, and 6 years later. In the second child a third tumor resectioning was performed after a further recurrence 2 years later. Three patients developed large tumor cysts which made drainage necessary. Four required shunts for treatment of hydrocephalus.

Histology. Of the 25 cases 24 were histologically verified. Twenty-one patients had juvenile pilocytic astrocytoma (WHO grade I). In one patient adult pilocytic astrocytoma (WHO grade II) was diagnosed, and two patients suffered from malignant glioma (WHO grade III).

Radiation Therapy. Conventional irradiation was performed in 11 patients. Radiation therapy was administered as part of the initial treatment after surgery in four patients and after tumor recurrence in three others. One child with progresssive enlargement received radiotherapy prior to surgery. Two patients underwent radiation therapy after the malignant glioma had been confirmed histologically. In one case radiation therapy was given prior to surgery because a large malignant glioma was assumed. Radiation therapy brought about radiographic improvement with reduction of the tumor in three patients. In four patients the tumor remained stable. Two tumors, one of which was malignant, progressed despite treatment.

Outcome. There were no deaths related to treatment. One patient with a malignant tumor died due to progression of the disease 6 months after biopsy and radiation therapy. Sixteen patients remained in stable condition. Eight revealed progression on neuroimaging. One patient suffered from hemiparesis and dysphasia related to a

Table 3. Outcome and morbidity

	Unchanged		Improved		Worsened		New	
	n	%	*n*	%	*n*	%	*n*	%
After surgery (*n* = 25)								
Visual acuity	13	52	6	24	6	24	0	
Endocrinology	21	84	0		0		4	16
Motor system	22	88	2	8	0		1	4
After irradiation (*n* = 11)								
Visual acuity	10	91	0		1	9	0	
Endocrinology	10	91	0		0		1	9

cerebral infarction after a subtotal resectioning of a type 5 tumor. In six patients (24%) visual acuity improved after surgery. Six patients (24%) suffered from visual deterioration postoperatively. This was not correlated with the extent of surgery. An endocrine dysfunction seemed to be related to surgery in four (16%) cases (two diabetes insipidus, two panhypopituitarism). In one case, precocious puberty appeared after surgery, but this seemed to be attributable to disease progression rather than to the surgical intervention. After radiation therapy one out of 11 cases (9%) experienced visual deterioration, and one patient suffered from growth hormone deficiency (Table 3).

Tumor Progression and Related Factors. Tumor progression, defined as an enlargement in tumor size, occurred in nine patients (36%). The median time for tumor progression was 18 months (range from 2 months–6 years). Within this group were both patients with malignant glioma and the patient with the adult type of pilocytic astrocytoma (WHO grade II). Of the remaining six patients four revealed prominent vascular features (proliferation of endothelial cells, angiomatous pattern, large sinusoidal vessels, rich vascularization) on histological examination. The other two cases revealed no striking features or signs of malignancy on histological examination. Neurofibromatosis was associated with a high recurrence rate. Four of eight patients (50%) suffered progression. Of the remaining 17 only 5 (30%) revealed progressive disease. The mean follow-up in the two groups was similar (3.7 and 3.4 years). Large globular chiasmatic/hypothalamic lesions without involvement of the optic tracts (type 5) presented a high number of recurrences. Six of 14 cases showed progression despite the high number of subtotal resections (64%). On the other hand, in the type 3 group with optic tract lesions in addition to globular suprasellar tumors, only one of six patients (17%) suffered a relapse, even though radical surgery had been limited to only one case (17%). The mean follow-up in the two groups was the same (Table 4).

Table 4. Tumor progression: relationship to type, extent of surgery, and NF-1

		Mean follow up (years)	Progression		Subtotal resection	
			n	%	*n*	%
Type 3	(*n* = 6)	3.7	1	17	1	17
Type 5	(*n* = 14)	3.9	6	43	9	64
NF-1	(*n* = 8)	3.7	4	50	–	–
Others	(*n* = 17)	3.4	5	30	–	–

Discussion

Management of OPG is controversial, and as yet no uniform therapeutic approach exists. This reflects some important problems in regard to these tumors: (a) their diversity in growth capacity, which ranges from a "hamartomatous" lesion to a highly proliferative glioma; and (b) their wide variety of tumor extension and size. There is also much disagreement in regard to the prognostic significance of specific factors such as tumor location and presence of NF-1.

Radical surgical resectioning, especially in the chiasmatic/hypothalamic region, was considered too hazardous in the past. The recent literature, however, presents increasing evidence that a surgical approach to this sensitive area can be carried out with favorable results and low morbidity in cases of hypothalamic gliomas [1, 5, 14]. Our patients underwent surgery with acceptable morbidity and no mortality. Morbidity was not correlated with the extent of resectioning (subtotal versus partial).

The role of radiation therapy in OPG is controversial. Some authors deny its usefulness [7] whereas others report significant improvement after such treatment regardless of histological confirmation [2, 15]. Others have rejected radiotherapy after observing a high incidence of intellectual impairment, especially in young infants [9]. In our study, radiation therapy was effective and safe. It led to a reduction in tumor size in three patients and to a stable disease in four others. This accounts for 64% of the irradiated patients. We believe that radiotherapy is necessary in malignant OPG and recurrent diseases, for example, after a second surgical approach. In the case of type 5 tumors with high vascularity irradiation should be discussed regardless of the extent of surgical resectioning.

Until now, the prognostic significance of the involvement of the optic tracts has not been debated in the literature. Our results indicate that lesions not involving the optic tracts (type 3) have a limited growth capacity (17%) whereas type 5 OPG without involvement of the optic tracts leads to a higher rate of recurrence (43%). This was not related to the extent of surgery. The significance of NF-1 as a prognostic factor in OPG has been discussed very controversially in the literature. Some authors believe that NF-1 patients with OPG have a better prognosis [11, 13] or the same prognosis [4, 7]. Others suggest a worse prognosis of OPG in association with NF-1, being, however, limited to intraorbital lesions [2]. In our series, 4 of 8 patients (50%) with NF-1 had progressive disease, compared to 5 of the remaining 17 patients (30%) who also suffered from a progressive tumor. The duration of follow-up, age, gender, and histological findings were very similar in the two groups. We conclude from our observations that NF-1 patients tend to exhibit a more aggressive course of disease.

Considering the prognostic significance of these data, we propose the following procedure in the management of OPG. Patients with an exophytic disease limited to the optic nerves (type 2) may be adequately managed by resectioning alone. In cases of tubular thickening of the optic nerve(s) and/or tract(s) (type 1 and partially type 3) the patients should be carefully observed. The radiological features are pathognomonic for OPG, so that bioptic confirmation is not required. In the more extensive suprasellar lesions without involvement of the optic tracts other neoplasms such as craniopharyngeoma, germinoma, and lymphoma must be excluded. In large chiasmatic/hypothalamic gliomas without affection of the optic tracts (type 5), extended surgery is possible with low morbidity and should be carried out as radically as possible. In the case of optic tract involvement (type 3) surgery should be limited to decompression and size reduction. In the presence of NF-1, or if a high vascularization is found histologically, radiotherapy should be considered after surgery, despite benign features.

Acknowledgements. We thank Mr. Freist for his photographic work, Mr. Davenport M.D. for the stylistic revision of the manuscript, and Mr. Schulz for the preparation of the figures.

References

1. Albright AL, Sclabassi RJ (1985) Cavitron ultrasonic surgical aspirator and visual evoked potential monitoring for chiasmal gliomas in children. Report of two cases. J Neurosurg 63:138–140
2. Alvord EC, Lofton S (1988) Gliomas of the optic nerve and chiasm. Outcome by patients age, tumor site, and treatment. J Neurosurg 68:85–98
3. Fletcher WA, Imes RK, Hoyt WF (1986) Chiasmal gliomas: appearence and long-term changes demonstrated by computerized tomography. J Neurosurg 65:154–159
4. Flickinger JC, Torres C, Deutsch M (1988) Management of low-grade gliomas of the optic nerve and chiasm. Cancer 61:635–642
5. Gillet GR, Symon L (1987) Hypothalamic glioma. Surg Neurol 28:291–300
6. Hoyt WF, Baghdassarian SA (1969) Optic glioma of childhood: natural history and rational for conservative management. Br J Ophtalmol 53:793–798
7. Imes RK, Hoyt WF (1986) Childhood chiasmal gliomes: update on the fate of patients in the 1969 San Francisco study. Br J Ophtalmol 70:179–182
8. Kovalic JJ, Grigsby PW, Shepard MJ, Fineberg BB, Thomas PR (1990) Radiation therapy for gliomas of the optic nerve and chiasm. Int J Radiat Oncol Biol Phys 18:927–932
9. Packer RJ, Sutton LN, Bilaniuk LT (1990) Treatment of chiasmatic/hypothalamic gliomas in childhood with chemotherapy: an updated report. Ann Neurol 23:79–85

10. Petronio J, Edwards MSB, Prados M, Freyberger S, Rabbitt J, Silver P, Levin VA (1991) Management of chiasmal and hypothalamic gliomas of infancy and childhood with chemotherapy. J Neurosurg 74:701–708
11. Rodriguez LA, Edwards MSB, Levin VA (1990) Management of hypothalamic gliomas in children: an analysis of 33 cases. Neurosurgery 26:242–247
12. Rubinstein L (1990) Pathologic features of optic gliomas. In: The National Neurofibromatosis Foundation (ed) Conference series, vol 2. Golden Tulip Barbizon, New York, pp 23–32
13. Rush JA, Younge BR, Campbell RJ, MacCarty CS (1982) Optic glioma: long-term follow-up of 85 histopathologically verified cases. Ophthalmol 89:1213–1219
14. Wisoff JH, Abbott R, Epstein F (1990) Surgical management of exophytic chiasmatic-hypothalamic tumors of childhood. J Neurosurg 73:661–667
15. Wong JYC, Uhl V, Wara WM, Sheline GE (1987) Optic gliomas. A reanalysis of the University of California, San Francisco experience. Cancer 60:1847–1855

Intra-axial Endophytic Brainstem Tumors: Postoperative Results in Childhood

J. Behnke[1], H.-J. Christen[2], F. Hanefeld[2], and E. Markakis[1]

Introduction

The only brainstem tumors that have been regarded as operable are those defined as focal, cystic, or exophytic or those located in the cervicomedullary junction [1, 3, 4]. Intra-axial endophytic brainstem tumors have traditionally been treated by irradiation, sometimes combined with chemotherapy, but with little success. This study shows that intra-axial endophytic brainstem tumors are also operable and carry a prognosis correlated to the histopathological finding, neurological state, and duration of clinical history.

Patients and Methods

Between July 1987 and January 1993 we operated upon 26 children (13 boys, 10 girls; 2–14 years old) and 15 adults suffering from intra-axial endophytic tumor of the brainstem. Only the 23 children operated on between July 1987 and January 1992 whose postoperative course could be assessed for a minimum of 1 year after operation are included in this study. All clinical examinations were performed by neuropediatricians and neurosurgeons together.

Tumors were localized in the pons or medulla oblongata and in some cases also in the thalamus or mesencephon. Excluded were other nonprimary endophytic tumors which invaded only the brainstem, or whose localization or major portion was mainly outside the brainstem. In two cases tumors affected the thalamus and in three the mesencephalon or quadrigeminal plate. In 16 of the 23 children tumor growth was seen in the pons (69%), in 10 the medulla oblongata (43%), and in 4 the upper part of the cervical myelon (17%). A lateral growth with infiltration of the peduncles was found in 9 cases (39%).

The operative approach chosen was a medial incision in the floor of the fourth ventricle in 13 of the 23 children (56%) and a lateral one in 7 (30%). The two thalamus gliomas were operated on with stereotactic guiding via the parietodorsal area. For preoperative assessment auditory evoked potentials, somatosensory auditory potentials, and magnetic stimulation were performed to document lesions of the

[1] Neurosurgical Department, University of Göttingen, Robert-Koch-Str. 40, 37075 Göttingen, Germany.
[2] Neuropediatric Department, University of Göttingen, Robert-Koch-Str. 40, 37075 Göttingen, Germany.

Advances in Neurosurgery, Vol. 22
B. L. Bauer, M. Brock, M. Klinger (Eds.)

sensory or motor and brainstem pathways. The operation began with incision of the superficial layers. The surgical procedure was followed by ultrasonic tumor aspiration, laser coagulation, or conventional tumor removal by coagulation and suction. The operation was defined as radical when the postoperative cranial computed tomography or magnetic resonance imaging showed a more than 70% resection, as partial after 50%–70% removal, and as biopsy when less than 50% was removed. Children suffering from grade III or IV tumors underwent postoperative radiation or a combination of radiation and chemotherapy.

Results

Depending on tumor localization and expansion a medial incision was performed in 13 of the 23 children (56%), a lateral one in 7 (30%); two of the three thalamus gliomas were approached with stereotactic guiding via the parietodorsal area and the third without guiding through the sylvian fissure. A radical operation was performed in 15 of the 23 children (65%), a partial resection in 5 (22%), and in 3 (13%) only small parts of the tumor could be removed. The most serious intraoperative complications during manipulation at the superficial layers of the pontomedullary region were hypertensive reactions up to 250–300 mmHg, bradycardia (30–40/min), or even short asystolic crises.

On histopathological examination the majority of tumors were astrocytomas (19/23, 83%), 5 of them grade I, 9 grade II, 3 grade III, and 2 grade IV. In the others we found two oligodendrogliomas, one ependymoma, and one angioma. We saw no cysts except for two tumors located in the low medulla oblongata and upper cervical myelon.

Six children suffering from grade III or IV tumors underwent postoperative radiation and four postoperative radiation and chemotherapy.

The most frequent preoperative symptoms were lesions of the pyramidal tract (91%) and ataxia (66%), followed by lesions of the cranial nerves such as the caudal nerve group (48%), the seventh (48%), the sixth (43%), and the eighth (22%), followed by nystagmus (22%) and gaze palsy (22%). Postoperatively, most of our patients showed some increase in the preoperative dificits, particularly of pyramidal, facial, or gaze palsy. This deterioration persisted for 2–3 months. The mean postoperative Karnofsky index (KI) was about 10% lower than the mean preoperative KI. The mean KI of the 13 children surviving more than 1 year was about 10% better than the preoperative mean. Seven children showed occurrence of first symptoms less than 3 months before diagnosis of the brainstem tumor; eight had a fatal course, dying within the first year after operation. Only two children who died within the first year had a longer history (7 months, 12 months).

Discussion

Several authors have pointed out that brainstem tumors are not a single entity and have described dorsally exophytic tumors, focal tumors, and tumors of the cervicomedullary junction as having a better prognosis [1–4]. In our series only intra-axial endophytic tumors were included, tumors which originated from and within the brainstem. All other nonprimary endophytic tumors which invaded only the brainstem, or whose localization or major portion was mainly outside the brainstem were excluded from this series. Using this definition, the so-called diffuse brainstem tumor as historical stereotype for brainstem neoplasm is the subject of this study. In contrast to reports in the literature these tumors were shown to be generally operable and that their histopathology is not mainly of high grade.

We thus consider brainstem tumors to be operable, even large and diffuse tumors. A history shorter than 3 months dramatically worsens the prognosis. We think that patients with advanced neurological deficits, especially respiratory disorders and progressive lesions of the caudal cranial nerves, should be excluded from operation. Not the size of the tumor but the preoperative symptoms should determine operative indication.

References

1. Epstein F, McClearly EL (1986) Intrinsic brain-stem tumors of childhood: surgical indications. J Neurosurg 64:11–15
2. Epstein F, Farmer JP (1993) Brain-stem glioma growth patterns. J Neurosurg 78:408–412
3. Stroink AR, Hoffman HJ, Hendrick EB, Humphreys RP, Davidson G (1987) Transependymal benign dorsally exophytic brain stem gliomas in childhood: diagnosis and treatment recommendations. Neurosurgery 20:439–444
4. Stoink AR, Hoffman HJ, Hendrick EB, Humphreys RP (1986) Diagnosis and management of pediatric brain-stem gliomas. J Neurosurg 65:745–750

Intraventricular and Intrapontine Vascular Malformations: Symptoms, Surgical Approach, and Postoperative Results

R. Verheggen[1] and E. Markakis[1]

Introduction

Comprehensive reviews by McCormick [4], Crawford et al. [1], and Ondra et al. [5] based on a histopathological classification in arteriovenous, venovenous, or cavernous angioma report a higher morbidity and mortality in patients with intracranial vascular malformations. Due to possible complications of neurosurgical intervention the advantages of an irradiation or interventional embolization have been analyzed critically [2]. Nevertheless, angiomas involving midline structures must be excluded from these alternative therapeutic procedures because of their blood supply, the small vessel diameter, and the deleterious consequences of an unselective embolization or radiotherapy. This retrospective analysis describes our preferred surgical approach and strategies and reports our postoperative results.

Patients and Methods

Between January 1987 and April 1993 a total of 15 patients with intraventricular, paraventricular, or intrapontine vascular malformations underwent direct supraselective surgery of the angiomas. Our group included nine men and six women aged 4–67 years (mean 29.5). In nearly all cases – except one – more than one intracerebral or infratentorial hemorrhage preceded the final diagnosis of a vascular malformation. However, the recurrence of bleeding was observed in some patients within a few days and in one case after 20 years. On hospitalization, patients suffering from intra- or paraventricular angiomas displayed hemiparesis, hemihypesthesia, jacksonian epilepsy, or short-term unconsciousness. In cases of brainstem angiomas ocular motility disturbances, paresis of ocular muscles, facial paresis, or cerebellar ataxia were observed.

Results

Histopathological findings revealed six para-/intraventricular and four intrapontine arteriovenous malformations (AVM) and two para-/intraventricular and three intrapontine cavernous angiomas. Diagnosis of AVM was confirmed in all cases by

---

[1] Neurochirurgische Klinik, Georg-August-Universität Göttingen, Robert-Koch-Str. 40, 37075 Göttingen, Germany.

Advances in Neurosurgery, Vol. 22
B. L. Bauer, M. Brock, M. Klinger (Eds.)

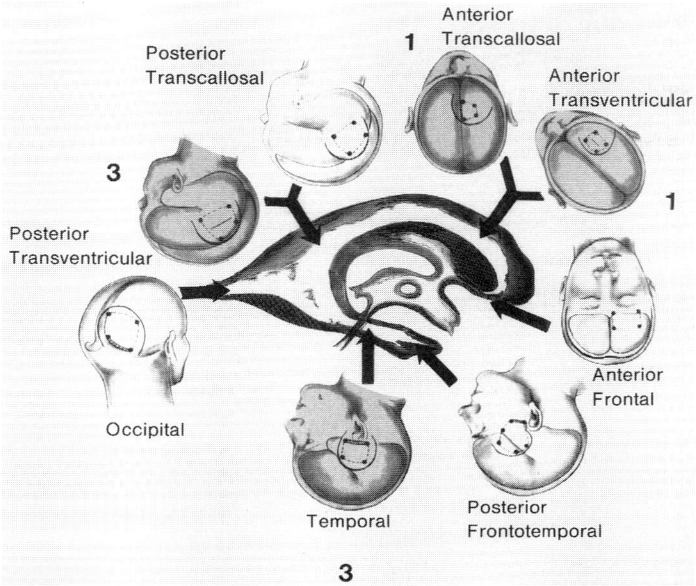

Fig. 1. The preferred surgical approaches to the vascular malformations

digital subtraction angiography and was further confirmed by magnetic resonance imaging in patients with cavernous angiomas. We achieved complete removal of the para-/intraventricular AVMs in controlled hypotension. In two cases the direct approach to the angioma was relieved by stereotactic guiding. We generally chose a transtemporal, transcallosal and intraventricular, or interhemispheric-transcallosal approach (Fig. 1).

As a representative case report, 13 years ago a now 27-year old woman sustained a subtotal extirpation of the cavernous angioma. Jacksonian seizures followed by mild hemiparesis required hospitalization. Computed tomography revealed a hyperdense area of 2.5 x 3 x 3 cm located in the vicinity of the precentral gyrus. The extension and the intraventricular portion of the cavernous angioma was especially stressed by T1-weighted coronal and transverse magnetic resonance images. The cavernoma including liquefied blood was totally removed via a transcortical route (Fig. 2).

To remove the brainstem angiomas we placed our patients in a sitting position and performed a suboccipital craniectomy. After splitting the vermis the rhomboid fossa was exposed to remove the AVMs. As demonstrated by radiological controls, AVMs of the fourth ventricle, even those involving the cerebellar peduncles, were totally extirpated with the exception of one patient with some residual malformation. After surgery the neurological condition of three inconspicuous patients remained unchanged whereas an improvement was observed in five cases. In a further six patients with minor neurological preoperative deficits no deterioration was detected. In only one case was the operation followed by a worsening of

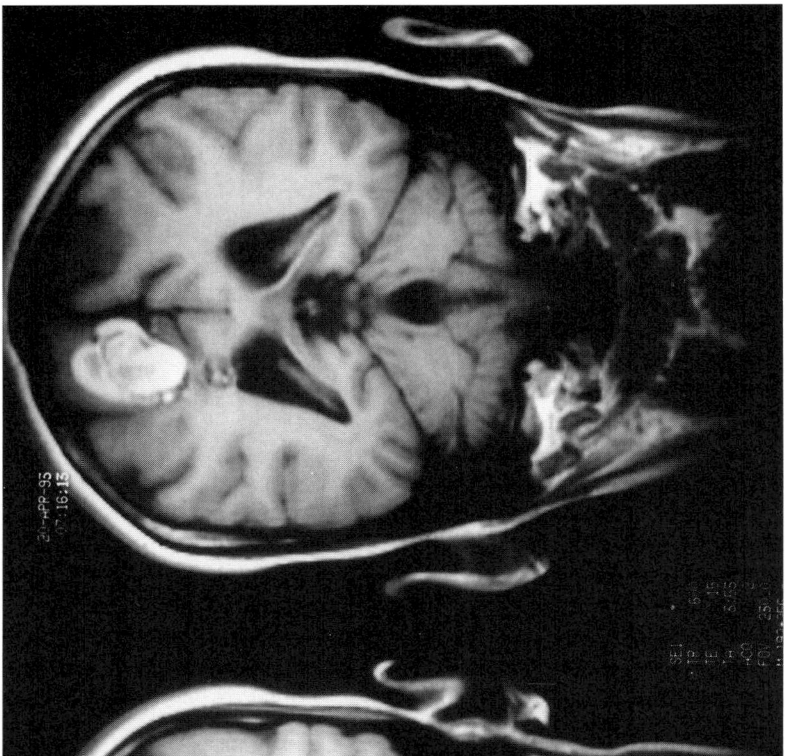

2 a

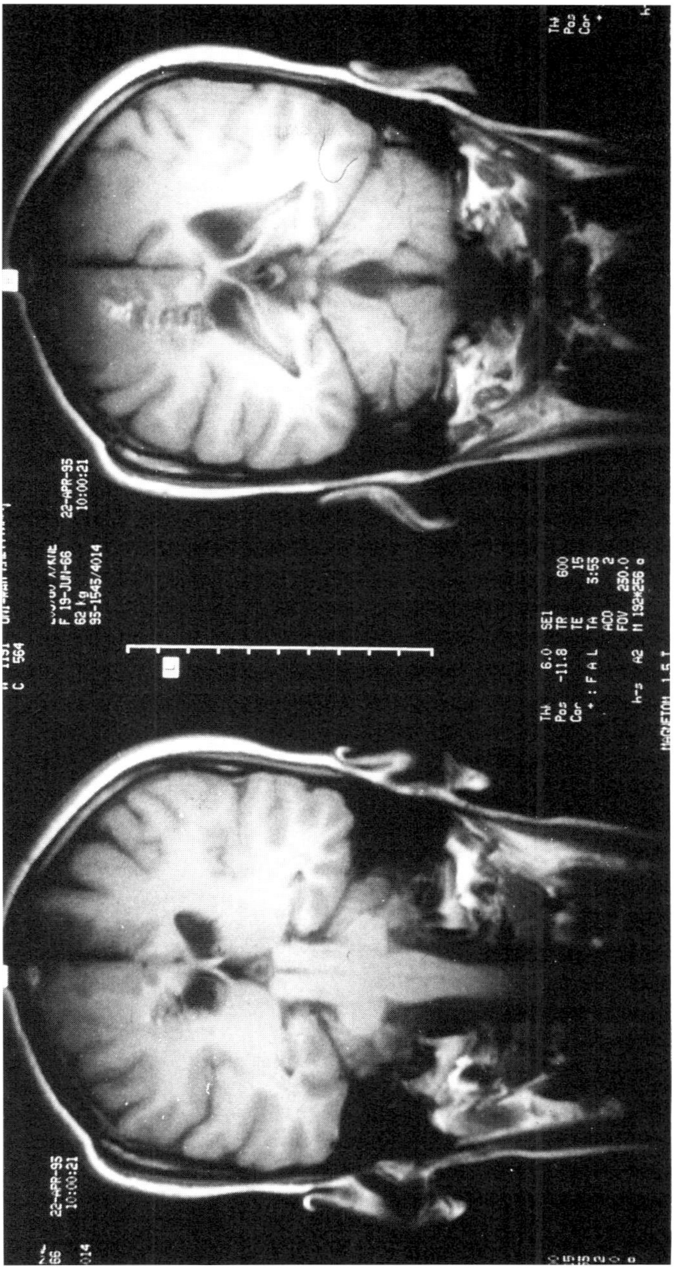

2 b

Fig. 2 a, b. Pre-and postoperative magnetic resonance images showing a thorough elimination of the cavernous malformation ocular muscle paresis while another patient died after sustaining at least five intracerebral and intraventricular hemorrhages prior to surgery of the AVM.

Discussion

The treatment of vascular malformations in the midline structures or the brainstem is a subject of controversy, and competing therapies such as gamma beam irradiation and selective immobilization have been recommended. However, radiotherapy rarely abolishes these malformations and subjects patients to the risk of radionecrosis and relapse to hemorrhages [7]. Embolization seldom eliminates these angiomas radically, and recurrent hemorrhages are reported in partially obliterated vascular malformations [3]. Provided the vascular malformation is totally eliminated, surgery can be considered unavoidable. In our experience, inspection of the ventricle is absolutely necessary in cases of paraventricular or callosal vascular malformations to ensure a thorough extirpation of an intraventricular portion of the angioma present in all our patients.

Patients who sustain hemorrhage from a brainstem malformation should be treated surgically if the angioma is favorably situated [8, 9]. Embolization in this area is hazardous, and radiotherapy, although effective, entails the risk of hemorrhages during the time required to shrink the malformation [6].

Our experience in the therapy of vascular malformations localized intra- or paraventricularly or in the brainstem supports the view that surgical obliteration of these angiomas is not only a feasible but a chosen form of treatment. Conservative methods leave the patient susceptible to recurrent hemorrhages which often result in devastating neurological deficiencies.

References

1. Crawford PM, West CR, Chadwick DW, Shaw MD (1986) Arteriovenous malformations of the brain: natural history in unoperated patients. J Neurol Neurosurg Psychiatry 49:1–10
2. Drake CG, Friedman AH, Peerless SJ (1986) Posterior fossa arteriovenous malformations. J Neurosurg 64:1–10
3. Luessenhop AJ, Presper JH (1975) Surgical immobilisation of cerebral arteriovenous malformations through internal carotid and vertebral arteries. J Neurosurg 42:443–451
4. McCormick WF (1984) Pathology of vascular malformations of the brain. In: Wilson CB, Stein BM (eds) Intracranial arteriovenous malformations. Baltimore; Williams and Wilkins, pp 44–63
5. Ondra SL, Troupp H, George ED, Schwab K (1990) The natural history of symptomatic arteriovenous malformations of the brain: a 24-year follow-up assessment. J Neurosurg 73:387–391
6. Solomon RA, Stein BM (1986) Management of arteriovenous malformation of the brain stem. J Neurosurg 64:857–864
7. Stein BM, Wolpert SM (1980) Arteriovenous malformations of the brain. Arch Neurol 37:69–75

8. Yamada S, Brauer FS, Knierim DS (1990) Direct approach to arteriovenous malformations in functional areas of the cerebral hemisphere. J Neurosurg 72:418–425
9. Zimmerman RS, Spetzler RF, Lee KS, Zabramski JM, Hargraves RW (1991) Cavernous malformations of the brain stem. J Neurosurg 75:32–39

Pre- and Intraoperative Transcranial Color-Coded Real-Time Sonography in Stereotactic Biospies of Midline Tumors

A. Krone[1], G. Becker[2], D. Koulis[2], A. Lindner[3], W. Roggendorf[3], U. Bogdahn[2], and E. Hofmann[4]

Introduction

Diffusely infiltrating tumors of midline structures (corpus callosum, basal ganglia, brainstem) are regarded to be difficult for surgical planning mainly because of poor differentiation between solid tumor tissue and peritumoral edema by computed tomography (CT) and magnetic resonance imaging (MRI). Encouraged by the positive results of transcranial color-coded real-time sonography (TCCS) in brain tumor localization [1, 2], we applied this technique to stereotactic biopsies pre- and intraoperatively to investigate its potential in preoperative planning and intraoperative real-time imaging monitoring.

Materials and Methods

In a prospective study TCCS was applied to 25 unselected consecutive patients preoperatively and to 15 patients intraoperatively. All patients underwent stereotactic biopsies of poorly delineated midline lesions. In all cases plain and contrast-enhanced CT as well as TCCS were performed prior to surgery. Additional MRI images with and without gadolinium-EDTA were obtained in all seven patients harboring nonenhancing lesions on CT. For TCCS examination a phased-array color-flow ultrasound system (Sonoline CF Siemens, Erlangen, Germany) was employed. A B-mode image was created by applying a 2.25-MHz probe through typical acoustic bone windows at the temporal region. The lesion was generally recorded from the contralateral side. Details of this technique have been described previously [1, 2]. CT-guided stereotactic serial biopsies were performed by applying a BRW guidance system (Radionics, Burlington, MA, USA).

In the 25 cases a total of 81 biopsy sites were evaluated. Histopathological findings (solid tumor, necrosis, normal brain tissue) were compared with CT (density,

[1] Neurochirurgische Klinik und Poliklinik, Universität Würzburg, Josef-Schneider-Str. 11, 97080 Würzburg, Germany.
[2] Neurologische Klinik und Poliklinik, Universität Würzburg, Josef-Schneider-Str. 11, 97080 Würzburg, Germany.
[3] Abteilung für Neuropathologie, Universität Würzburg, Josef-Schneider-Str. 11, 97080 Würzburg, Germany.
[4] Abteilung für Neuroradiologie, Universität Würzburg, Josef-Schneider-Str. 11, 97080 Würzburg, Germany.

Advances in Neurosurgery, Vol. 22
B. L. Bauer, M. Brock, M. Klinger (Eds.)

contrast enhancement) and TCCS data (echogenicity, echotexture) of each biopsy location separately. The accuracy of stereotactic biopsy sites was confirmed, and surgical complications were excluded by postoperative CT scans.

Results

Histological tumor diagnosis was established in 24 of the 25 cases by stereotactic biopsy and in one case by postmortem examination. In 24 of the 25 patients the tumor was clearly identified by TCCS because of its elevated echogenicity compared with normal brain tissue; in one patient TCCS failed to identify a frontal anaplastic astrocytoma. Histologically positive biopsies were obtained from three different sites of this tumor.

Contrast-enhancing lesions on CT appeared hyperechogenic on TCCS and generally contained solid tumor tissue (Fig. 1). In three cases intratumoral bleeding could not be differentiated because its hyperechogenic appearance on TCCS was indistinguishable from tumor tissue.

In hypo- and isodense non-contrast-enhancing areas on CT solid tumor tissue was obtained in all 26 locations which were hyperechogenic on TCCS. All seven hypoechogenic sites on TCCS turned out to be necrosis. Isoechogenic areas ($n = 15$) were identified either as normal brain tissue ($n = 13$) or tumor tissue (2 specimens from the anaplastic astrocytoma which were not detected by TCCS; Fig. 1). Figure 2a presents a typical example of a diffuse hypodense nonenhancing lesion on CT. Stereotactic serial biopsy confirmed that only a small hyperechogenic area within this lesion contained tumor tissue (Fig. 2 b, c). As in all other six hypodense or isodense nonenhancing lesions on CT, MRI provided no additional information regarding tumor size or location. In each of these lesions TCCS demon-

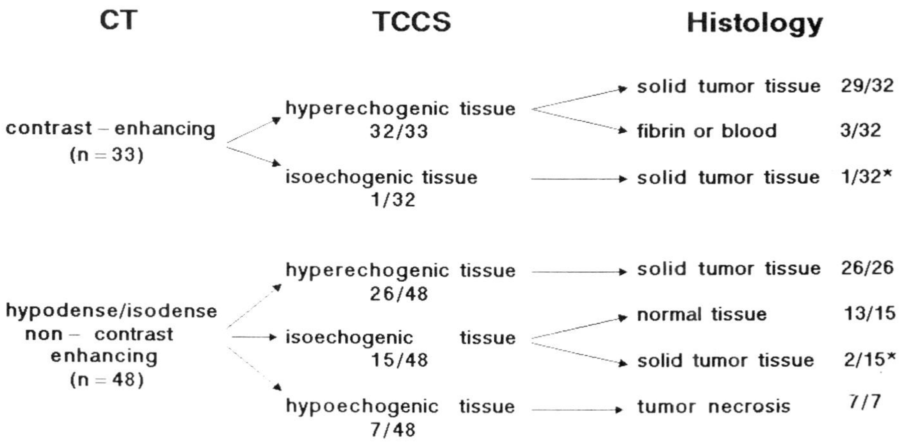

Fig. 1. Correlation among CT, TCCS, and histological findings at 81 stereotactic biopsy sites. *Asterisk*, TCCS-negative anaplastic astrocytoma

a 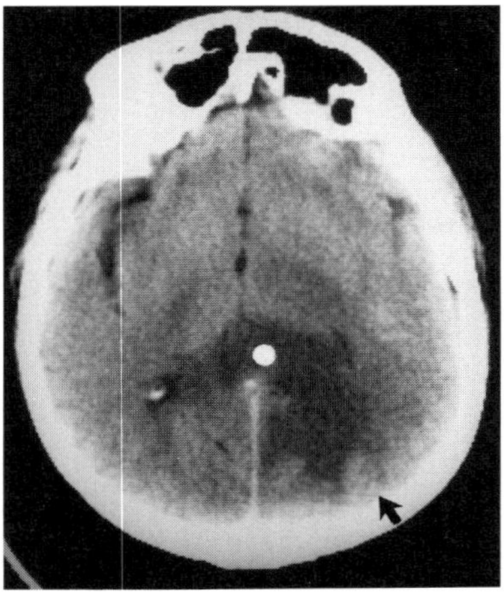

Fig. 2 a–c. Stereotactic biopsy: transoccipital approach. Target point within the splenium of the corpus callosum. Biopsy specimens obtained from the target point and target point –1 cm (tissue with regular echogenicity) revealed no viable tumor tissue. Biopsy specimens from target point –2 cm (hyperechogenic area in TCCS) contained solid tumor tissue. **a** Contrast-enhanced CT scan of a poorly defined hypodense midline lesion extending from the splenium of the corpus callosum into the left parieto-occipital paraventricular region. No contrast enhancement. *White spot*, target point of serial stereotactic biopsies; *arrow*, direction of stereotactic biopsy. **b** TCCS image: slightly hyperechogenic ellipsoid lesion within the occipital lobe. *Stars* marking an area of 2 x 4.4 cm. The frontal pole of the lesion is adjacent to the trigonum of the left lateral ventricle. **c** Schematic illustration of the TCCS image and the ultrasound scanning planes *1*, Brain tumor; *2*, 3rd ventricle; *3*, skull base; *4*, chorioid plexus of the lateral ventricle; *5*, thalamus; *6*, pineal gland; *7*, falx cerebri; *8*, middle cerebral artery; *9*, controlateral skull

strated a clearly defined hyperechogenic area within the CT hypodensity which corresponded well with the tumor extension, as was confirmed by serial biopsy.

Although the sensitivity of TCCS in tumor detection was inferior to that of CT and MRI (96% versus 100%), the specificity of CT was comparable with TCCS only for contrast-enhancing locations, which were generally hyperechogenic on TCCS (32/33, 97%) and contained tumor histologically (29/32, 91%). However, for hypodense lesions on CT tumor the result was only 63% (25/40) whereas all sonographically hyperechogenic areas within these lesions contained tumor tissue (23/23).

Intraoperative TCCS was able to visualize the biopsy needle in all 15 cases. In 14 cases correct probe placement within the hyperechogenic target area was demonstrated; one misplacement was detected. Significant intraoperative hemorrhage could be excluded in all cases. Clinically irrelevant hematomas of less than 1 cm in diameter cannot be differentiated by TCCS. The position of the needle in correlation to major vessels was well documented by applying color-coded Duplex sonography, which was superimposed on the B-mode image. Aspiration of three tumor cysts could be precisely monitored continuously.

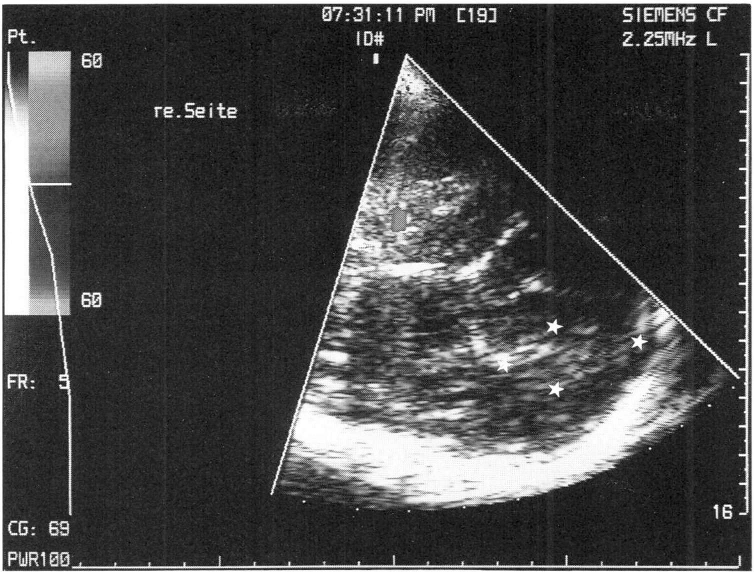

b

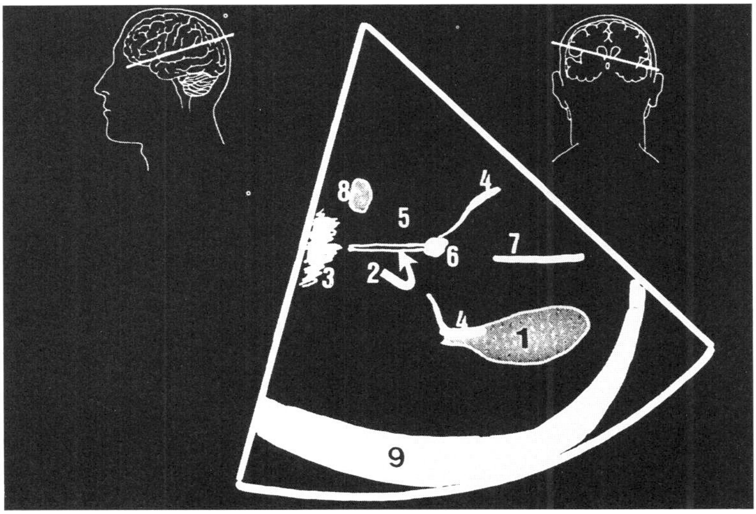

c

Discussion

Because of its clear delineation of tumor extension and characterization of tissue structures sonography has now become a routine method for intraoperative localization in microsurgery [3–5]. TCCS has recently been demonstrated to provide comparable information during the preoperative period [1, 2]. This experience suggests the use of TCCS in stereotactic brain tumor biopsies. By matching the neuroradiological, sonographic, and histological data for each of 81 biopsy locations in 25 brain tumors the specificity of both imaging modalities, CT (MRI) and TCCS, regarding the differentiation of tumor components was evaluated. In accordance with results from open biopsies [6] a strong correlation between hyperechogenicity on TCCS and solid tumor tissue (55/58) was demonstrated constantly, regardless of whether the lesion was contrast enhancing or hypodense and nonenhancing on CT. This finding may be due to the fact that sonography fails to visualize brain edema, which is indistinguishable from normal brain tissue. Sonography is therefore able to separate tumor tissue from edematous adjacent brain parenchyma. Our findings may indicate a superior specificity of TCCS compared to CT and MRI regarding identification of tumor tissue especially within diffuse nonenhancing hypodense CT lesions.

Conclusions

TCCS seems to be superior to CT and MRI in differentiating between solid tumor and edematous brain tissue. The information obtained by TCCS regarding tumor location, extension, and structure is helpful in planning stereotactic and nonstereotactic surgery especially for midline lesions, which are hypodense, diffuse, and nonenhancing on CT. As a noninvasive real-time method, TCCS offers a useful technique for intraoperative imaging monitoring.

References

1. Becker G, Perez J, Krone A, Demuth K, Lindner A, Hofmann E, Winkler J, Bogdahn U (1992) Transcranial color-coded real-time sonography in the evaluation of intracranial neoplasms and arteriovenous malformations. Neurosurgery 31:420–428
2. Bogdahn U, Becker G, Winkler J, Greiner K, Perez J, Meurers B (1990) Transcranial color-coded real-time sonography of adults. Stroke 21:1680–1688
3. Chandler WF, Knake JE, McGillicuddy JE, Lillehei KO, Silver TM (1982) Intraoperative use of real-time sonography in neurosurgery. J Neurosurg 57:157–163
4. Knake JE, Chandler WF, Gabrielsen TO, Latack JT, Gebarski SS (1984) Intraoperative sonographic delineation of low-grade brain neoplasms defined poorly by computed tomography. Radiology 151:735–739
5. LeRoux PD, Berger MS, Ojemann GA, Wang K, Mack LA (1989) Correlation of intraoperative ultrasound tumor volumes and margins with preoperative computerized tomography scans. J Neurosurg 71:691–698
6. McGahan JP, Ellis WG, Budenz RW, Walter JP, Boggan J (1986) Brain gliomas: sonographic characterisation. Radiology 159:485–492

Cerebral Gangliogliomas: A Study of 51 Cases

R. Kristof[1], J. Zentner[1], B. Ostertun[2], H. Wolf[3], M. Campos[1], and J. Schramm[1]

Introduction

Gangliogliomas are rather infrequent lesions of the central nervous system that account for 0.4%–1.3% of all brain tumors, with a higher incidence in infancy [13, 18]. The term ganglioglioma was originally proposed by Ewing in 1926 (cited in [16]). Due to their low frequency, most reports on these tumors are casuistic, and except for the study by Henry et al. [11], only a few minor series have been published [3, 5, 12, 18]. During the past 5 years we have operated on 51 patients with gangliogliomas and report on our findings here.

Patients and Methods

This study included 51 patients with gangliogliomas treated surgically during a 5-year period (January 1988 to January 1993) at the Department of Neurosurgery, University of Bonn. There were 29 men and 22 women. Ages ranged from 2 to 50 years with an average age of 25 years. The tumors were localized in the temporal lobe in 43 cases (84%), frontal lobe in 5 (10%), and occipital lobe in 1 (2%). In 2 cases (4%), the tumor was localized infratentorially, affecting pons and medulla oblongata.

Medical charts were reviewed retrospectively. Data evaluated included clinical signs and symptoms, duration of symptoms, diagnostic and therapeutic modalities, and the postoperative outcome. Preoperative computed tomography (CT) scans were available from 31 cases, 24 of them examined with and without contrast medium. Complete magnetic resonance imaging (MRI) data including T1-weighted images with and without gadolinium, proton-density, and T2-weighted images were obtained from 32 patients. Imaging data were reviewed by a neuroradiologist. Histopathological examination included the following stains and immunohistopathological reactions: hematoxilin and eosin, Nissl, glial fibrillary acid protein,

---

[1] Department of Neurosurgery, University of Bonn, Sigmund-Freud-Str. 25, 53105 Bonn, Germany.
[2] Department of Neuroradiology, University of Bonn, Sigmund-Freud-Str. 25, 53105 Bonn, Germany.
[3] Institute of Neuropathology, University of Bonn, Sigmund-Freud-Str. 25, 53105 Bonn, Germany.

Advances in Neurosurgery, Vol. 22
B. L. Bauer, M. Brock, M. Klinger (Eds.)

synaptophysin, neurofilament protein, and neuron-specific enolase. All glass slides were reviewed by two neuropathologists.

Results

The most common presenting symptom was epilepsy, observed in 47 patients (92%). Focal neurological deficits were found in 12 cases (24%). There were

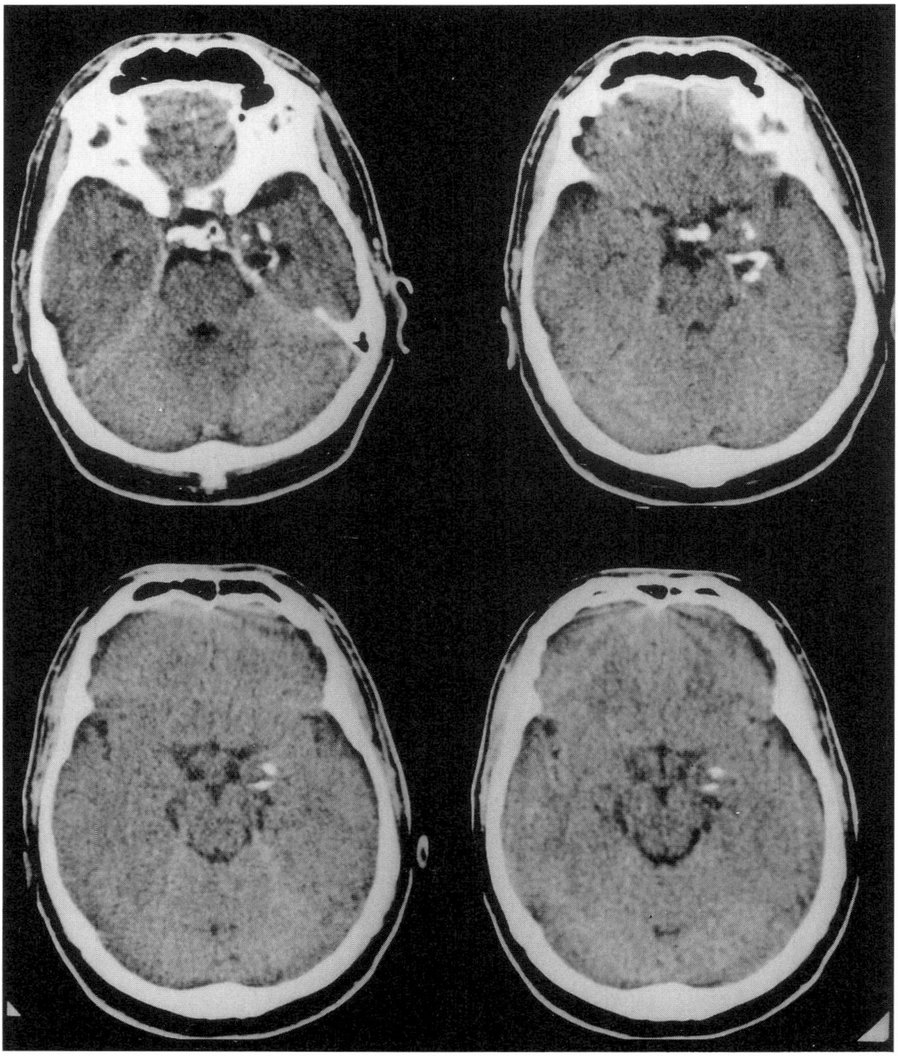

Fig. 1. Ganglioglioma (WHO grade I) of the left hippocampal formation in a 45-year-old patient. Native CT shows a hypodense lesion with distinct calcifications

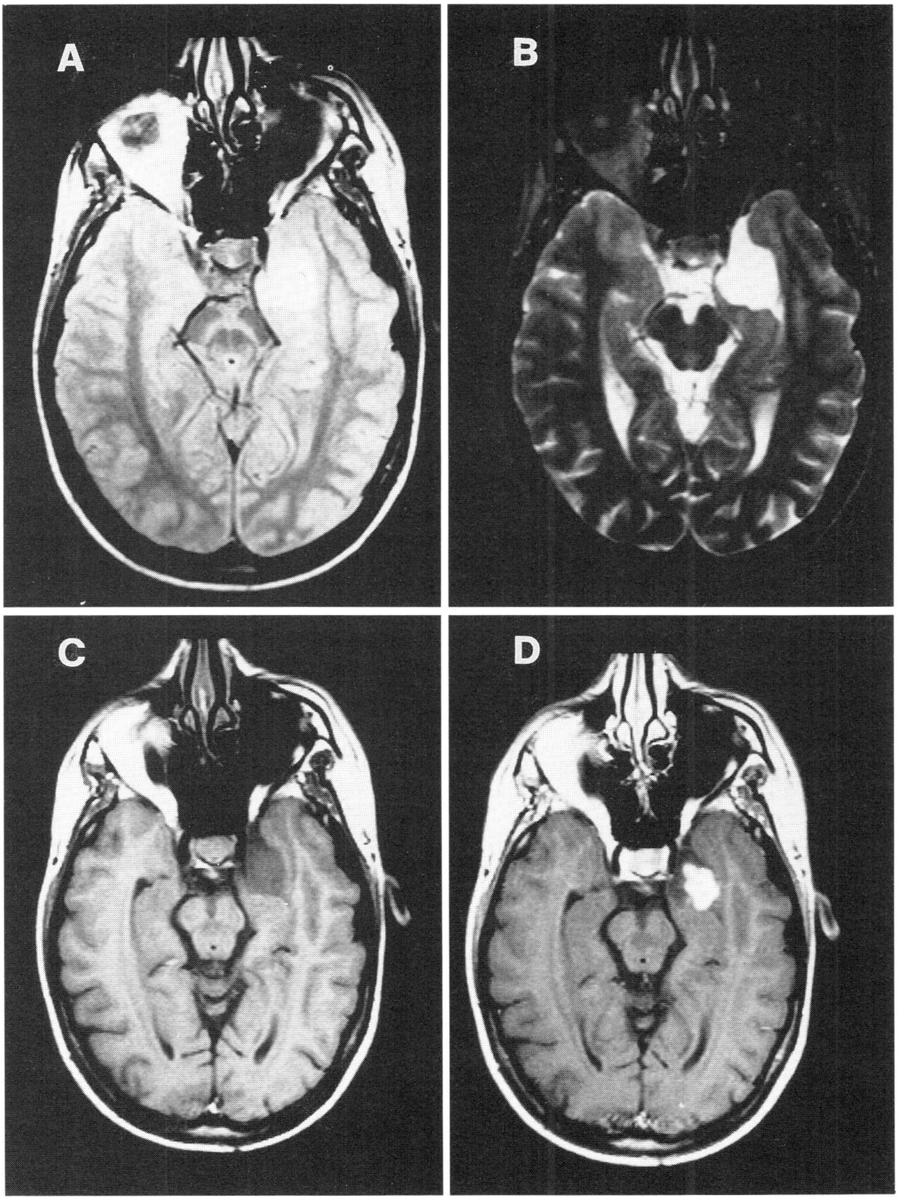

Fig. 2 A–D. Ganglioglioma (WHO grade I) of the left uncus in a 21-year-old patient. Proton-density (**A**) and T2-weighted (**B**) images show homogeneous signal increase. **C** T1-weighted image shows decreased signal. **D** Contrast-enhanced T1-weighted demonstrates inhomogenous enhancement

Table 1. MRI findings: signal intensity in 51 patients

Tumor Component	T1 native	Proton-density	T2
Solid	Isointense	Hyperintense	Hyperintense
Cystic	Hypointense	Hyperintense	Hyperintense
Calcified	Isointense	Hypointense	Hypointense

cranial nerve deficit in 7 (14%), motor deficit in 5 (10%), psychomotor retardation in 3 (6%), and increased intracranial pressure in 2 (4%). The duration of symptoms ranged from 3 months to 45 years and averaged 11 years.

Radiologically, most frequent CT appearance in two-thirds of the cases was a hypodense lesion with no or little mass effect. Contrast enhancement, usually inhomogeneous and eccentric, was found in parts of the tumor in about 40%. CT, the most sensitive method for detection of calcifications, was positive in this respect in half of the tumors (Fig. 1). MRI provided a more differentiated evaluation of various tumor components. In about 40% the tumor included enhancing areas characterized by strong hyperintensity on proton-density and moderate hyperintensity on T2-weighted images (Fig. 2). About half of the tumors also contained a nonenhancing cystic component that was hypointense on T1- and hyperintense on T2- and proton density-weighted images (Table 1). Calcifications were found in one-fourth of cases and thus were assessed with lower sensitivity by MRI than CT. In one-fifth of cases with positive MRI, enhanced CT yielded false-negative results.

Surgical treatment included complete tumor removal in 44 patients (86.3%) and partial resection in 7 (13.7%). Histological examination showed WHO grade I tumors in 43 cases (84.3%), grade II in 5 (9.8%), and grade III in 2 (3.9%). One patient (2.0%) died 2 weeks postoperatively after an uneventful primary course due to a pulmonary embolism. Temporary morbidity due to neurological complications was encountered in 7 patients (13.7%), related mainly to accentuation of a preexisting deficit. All these complications eventually resolved completely without further sequelae.

Discussion

The controversy regarding definition and nomenclature of ganglion cell tumors is reflected in several descriptive terminologies. The current terminology has been simplified to include only two major classifications. Tumors that are composed primarily of neuronal components are designated ganglioneuromas. The other type of tumor, which demonstrates primarily an obvious preponderance of glial cells is termed ganglioglioma [5, 17]. The existence of the ganglioglioma as a distinct clinicopathological entity is now widely recognized. These tumors may be found anywhere in the central nervous system [2, 7, 8, 9, 15]; however, the temporal lobe is the most common location [1, 3, 4]. In accordance with the literature, mainly young adults are affected. There is no sex preponderance, and most patients present with a long history of epileptic seizures, while focal neurological deficits are rather uncommon [6, 10, 12, 13, 19].

Essential CT findings include a hypodense lesion with intermingled calcifications [3, 6, 13, 14, 19]. However, in our series the tumor was missed on enhanced CT scans in one-fifth of cases. MRI has proven more sensitive than CT in identifying gangliogliomas. Increased signal on proton density- and T2-weighted images as well as decreased signal on T1-weighted images were most frequently observed. Similar MRI features have been observed by others [3, 4]; however, comprehensive data on this issue are almost lacking at this time.

Conclusions

Gangliogliomas are usually benign tumors which show a predeliction for the temporal lobe. Usually young adults are affected, and a long history of epileptic seizures seems to be the most striking clinical symptom. Although there is no typical singular radiological finding that is characteristic for gangliogliomas, the tentative diagnosis of such a lesion is possible with MRI showing enhancing and cystic tumor components. The additional finding of calcification, which more sensitively is provided by CT as compared to MRI, makes the diagnosis of a ganglioglioma much more probable. Complete tumor removal seems to be the treatment of choice. Further studies with long-term follow-up of more cases are necessary in order to clarify the biological behavior of these tumors.

References

1. Albright L, Byrd RP (1980) Ganglioglioma of the entire spinal cord. Childs Brain 6:274–280
2. Bevilacqua G, Sarnelli R (1979) Ganglioglioma of the spinal cord. A case with long survival. Acta Neuropathol (Berl) 48:239–242
3. Castillo M, Davis PC, Takei Y, Hoffmann JC (1990) Intracranial ganglioglioma: MR, CT, and clinical findings in 18 patients. AJR 154:607–612
4. Cheung YK, Fung CF, Chan FU, Leong LLY (1991) MRI features of spinal ganglioglioma. Clin Imag 15:109–112
5. Courville CB (1930) Ganglioglioma: tumors of the central nervous system; review of the literature and report of two cases. Arch Neurol Psychiatr 24:439–492
6. Dorne HL, O'Gorman AM, Melanson D (1986) Computed tomography of intracranial gangliogliomas. AJNR 7:281–285
7. Doyle JB, Kernohan JW (1931) Ganglioneuroma of the third ventricle with diabetes insipidus and hypopituitarism. J Nerv Ment Dis 73:55–61
8. Garcia CA, McGarry PA, Collada (1984) Ganglioglioma of the brain stem. Case report. J Neurosurg 60:431–434
9. Gritzman MCD, Snyckers FD, Proctor NSF (1983) Ganglioglioma of the optic nerve. A case report. S Afr Med J 63:863–865
10. Haddad SF, Moore SA, Menezes AH, Van Gilder JC (1992) Ganglioglioma: 13-years of experience. Neurosurgery 31:171–178
11. Henry JM, Heffner RR, Earle KM (1978) Gangliogliomas of the CNS: a clinicopathological study of 50 cases. J Neuropathol Exp Neurol 37:626 (abstract)

12. Johannsson JH, Rekate HL, Roessmann U (1981) Gangliogliomas: pathological and clinical correlation. J Neurosurg 54:58–63
13. Kalyan-Ramon UP, Olivero WC (1987) Ganglioglioma: a correlative clinicopathological and radiological study of ten surgically treated cases with follow-up. Neurosurgery 20:428–433
14. Katz MC, Kier EL, Schechter MM (1972) The radiology of gangliogliomas and glioneuromas of the central nervous system. Neuroradiology 4:69–73
15. Packen RJ, Sutton LN, Rosenstock JG et al. (1984) Pineal region tumors of childhood. Pediatrics 74:97–102
16. Perkins OC (1926) Ganglioglioma. Arch Pathol Lab Med 2:11
17. Russel DS, Rubinstein LJ (1977) Pathology of the tumors of the nervous system, 4th edn. William and Wilkins, Baltimore, pp 261–262
18. Silver JM, Rawlings CE, Rossitch E, Zeidman SM, Friedman AH (1991) Ganglioglioma: a clinical study with long-term follow-up. Surg Neurol 35:261–266
19. Sutton LN, Packer RJ, Rorke LB, Bruce DA, Shut L (1983) Cerebral gangliogliomas during childhood. Neurosurgery 13:124–128

Microembolization of Skull Base Tumors

M. Schumacher[1], F. D. Jüngling[1], W. Seeger[2], and A. K. Wakhloo[1]

Introduction

In spite of improved microsurgical techniques, the complex anatomical characteristics of skull base tumors remain a therapeutic challenge and require a multidisciplinary approach. The major drawbacks of surgery are the anatomical limitations, severe intraoperative blood loss and failure to preserve cranial nerve functions. Among all tumors, the surgery of clival and petroclival meningiomas still has the highest mortality and morbidity with up to 9%–17% and 50%, respectively [4, 6, 8, 11].

In the past 20 years technological developments have also improved neuroendovascular procedures. Superselective catheterization of the fragile vessels feeding skull base tumors and preoperative devascularization are well-established procedures. The decreased intraoperative blood loss after embolization improves the overall view during surgery significantly and reduces the operating time.

A previously described improved embolization technique for meningiomas [10] was implemented on different skull base tumors. The results using this technique are presented.

Material and Methods

Of a group of more than 200 cases treated for craniofacial extracerebral tumors, 31 patients (22 women and 9 men; mean age, 59; range, 37–81 years) harboring skull base tumors were preoperatively embolized. In three cases the tumor was located in the olfactory groove. Midskull base lesions included the sphenoorbital, the petroclival, and temporobasal regions, which were involved in 12, 10, and two patients, respectively. Posterior skull base mass was encountered in four cases.

The most common skull base tumors treated were meningiomas (19 cases) followed by juvenile angiofibromas (five cases), highly vascularized metastases (three cases), hemangiomas (two cases), and paragangliomas (two cases).

The embolization was performed using a microcatheter (Tracker 18 or 10, Target Therapeutics, Fremont, CA) for superselective catherization and injection of embolic agent. Embolization was undertaken using polyvinyl alcohol (PVA) par-

---

[1] Section of Neuroradiology, University of Freiburg, Hauptstr. 5, 79104 Freiburg, Germany.
[2] Department of Neurosurgery, University of Freiburg, Hugstetterstr. 55, 79106 Freiburg, Germany.

Advances in Neurosurgery, Vol. 22
B. L. Bauer, M. Brock, M. Klinger (Eds.)

ticles of 150–300 mm and 50–150 mm in three and 31 patients, respectively. The smaller-sized, highly diluted PVA particles (0.1 g/1000 ml) were injected extremely slowly (60–120 min for each tumor-feeding vessel).

In all but one of the patients the endovascular therapy was carried out through superselective catheterization either of the external or internal tumor-feeding carotid artery branches. The one patient presenting with a highly vascularized petroclival meningioma was embolized through tentorial branches of the internal carotid artery (ICA) after infraophthalmic temporary balloon occlusion of the vessel. Subsequently, small PVA particles were injected into the ICA proximal to the occlusion.

The efficacy of postembolization tumor necrosis was assessed utilizing contrast-enhanced magnetic resonance imaging (MRI), which was compared to intraoperative macroscopic and histologic findings. In addition, posttreatment tumor volume changes were calculated based on MRI data.

Results

Postembolization MRI depicted in all tumors embolized with smaller PVA particles an extensive necrosis of different degree (Table 1). Except in one patient with 20% tumor necrosis, posttreatment MRI in two patients showed no significant changes after injecting the larger PVA particles.

MRI volumetric measurements performed in meningiomas only revealed in one case a 10% increase of total tumor volume after the endovascular procedure. This may have caused the delayed transient oculomotor paresis after embolization. There were no other neurologic complications. Surgery was undertaken after 1 week following the embolization and clearly demarcated the devascularized and partly necrotic tumor tissue. The mean blood loss was approximately 300 ml. Since only a small group has been treated up to now, a statistical analysis seems not to be appropriate.

Table 1. Results after embolization with conventional ($n = 3$) and microembolization technique ($n = 28$)

	Conventional	Microembolization
Tumor necrosis		
51%–95%	0	9
30%–50%	1	9
< 30%	2	10
Average loss of blood	900	275 ml/patient
Average percentage of tumor necrosis[a]		39.3 per patient

[a] Necrosis only in one patient in conventional treatment group.

Reviewing the histologic specimens, embolic agent could be detected in 85% of all cases and was found in the precapillary bed in 80%.

Discussion

Preoperative embolization of craniofacial tumors, especially meningiomas, is a useful procedure for reducing tumor vascularity, which facilitates the surgical resection of these tumors. Several reports have been published attesting to the efficacy and safety of superselective preoperative particulate embolization [1, 3, 5, 7].

The initial tumor embolization centered on lesions located at the convexity, falx, and sphenoid wing. Advances in interventional technology and experience has promoted the endovascular therapy. Tumors of the skull base, including the cavernous region, supplied from the internal carotid (Fig. 1) and vertebral arteries are being more and more frequently treated [3, 9]. Those tumor-feeding branches may be embolized after superselective catheterization (feasible in eight of our treated patients). The injection of liquid or solid embolic agents into the internal carotid or vertebral arteries using the temporary balloon occlusion technique as

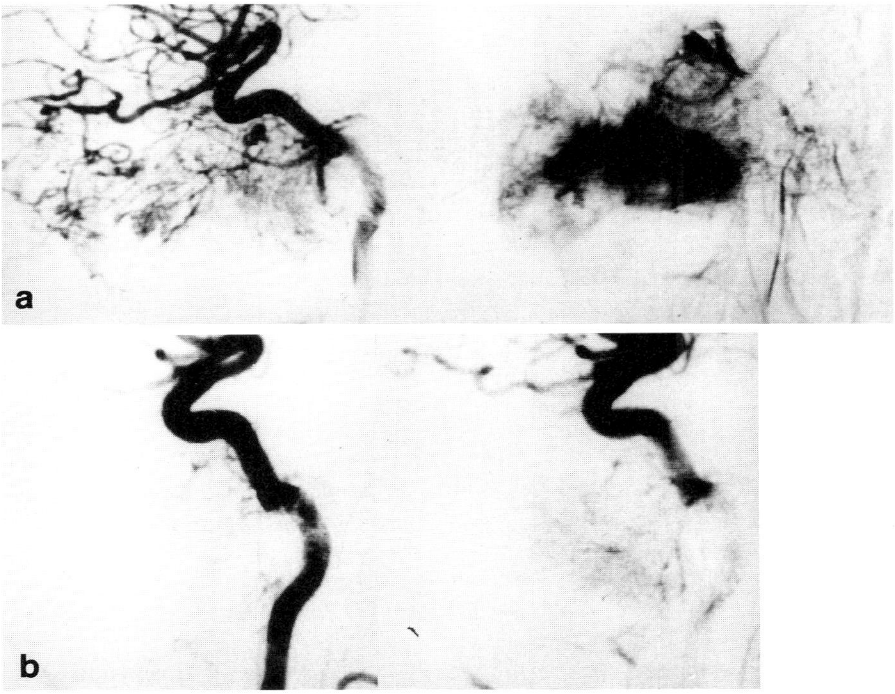

Fig. 1 a, b. Embolization of a juvenile angiofibroma. **a** Left lateral internal carotid angiogram delineates a high vascular mass involving the cavernous sinus. **b** Postembolization internal carotid angiogram shows almost complete devascularization of the tumor. After superselective catheterization of the tumor-feeding vessels, small PVA particles were injected

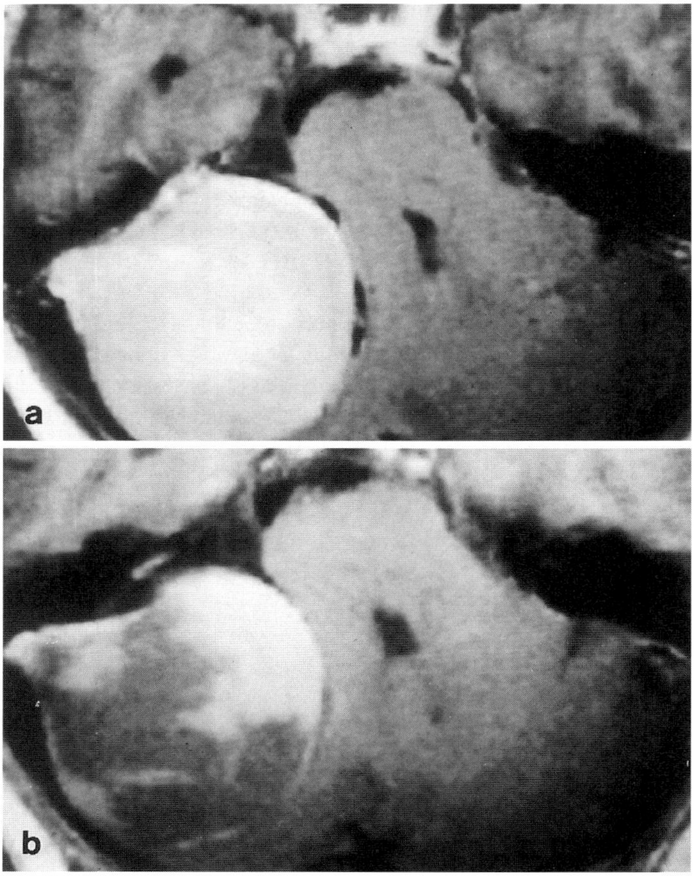

Fig. 2. Contrast-enhanced T1-weighted axial MR image (TR = 500 ms; TE = 20 ms) shows a large tentorial meningioma extending to the cerebellopontine angle (**a**). Follow-up MR obtained on fifth day after embolization with 50–150 mm PVA particles demonstrates an approximately 75% tumor necrosis (**b**)

described previously [9, 10] should be restricted to only a few selected cases. After deflating the balloon, cerebral embolic complications may occur from remaining embolic agent.

The degree of postembolization tumor necrosis could be improved using smaller embolic agent particles (Table 1). This recently described technique has resulted in a significant reduction of intraoperative blood loss, as shown in a larger treated group of meningiomas [10]. Extensive necrosis (Fig. 2), partly with liquefaction of central tumor parts, was confirmed intraoperatively and histologically. Compared to conventional embolization with larger PVA particles a higher incidence of neurologic complications was not encountered.

Much attention has been paid to locating extraintracranial anastomoses during embolization of tumors at the skull base when PVA particles smaller than 150 mm are used. Prior to embolization provocation testing of the central and peripheral nervous system with sodium amytal, it has been recently advocated that sodium methohexital, and lidocaine, respectively, be administered to avoid any inadvertent occlusion of normal brain tissue feeding vessels. Frequent selective contrast material injections should be performed during the embolization procedure, and embolization should be discontinued as soon as the tumor blush disappears. An occlusion of the tumor feeder or flow stasis should not be the goal and comprises unnecessary reflux of embolic agent. Small particles should be used exclusively when the microcatheter is placed close to the tumor nidus and remote from a potentially dangerous anastomosis.

Tumor volume increase, described in meningiomas of the convexity after embolization [10], was observed only in one patient with a skull base lesion. This may be attributed to the protective effect of steroid medication prior to the embolization.

References

1. Djindjian R, Cophignon J, Theron J, Merland JJ, Houdart R (1973) Embolization by superselective arteriography from the femoral route in neuroradiology. Review of 60 cases. Neuroradiology 6:20–26
2. Jungreis CA (1991), Skull-base tumors: ethanol embolization of the cavernous carotid artery. Radiology 181:741–743
3. Manelfe C (1975) Transfemoral catheter embolization of intracranial meningioma. In: Salomon G (ed) Advances in cerebral angiography. Springer, Berlin Heidelberg New York, pp 184–191
4. Mayberg MR, Symon L (1986) Meningiomas of the clivus and apical petrous bone: report of 35 cases. J Neurosurg 65:160–167
5. Richter HP, Schachenmayr W (1983) Preoperative embolization of intracranial meningiomas. Neurosurgery 13:261–268
6. Samii M, Ammirati M, Mahran A et al. (1989) Surgery of petroclival meningiomas: report of 24 cases. Neurosurgery 25:12–17
7. Schumacher M, Gilsbach J, Seeger W, Mennel HD, Voigt K (1979) Techniques and results after embolization of meningiomas. Arch Psychiatr Neurol Sci 227:241–260
8. Sekhar LN, Samii M (1986) Petroclival and medial tentorial meningiomas. In: Scheunemann H, Schürmann K, Helms J (eds) Tumor of skull base: extra- and intracranial surgery of skull base tumors. Walter de Gruyter, Berlin, pp 141–158
9. Theron J, Cosgrove R, Melanson D, Ethier R (1986) Embolization with temporary balloon occlusion of the internal carotid or vertebral arteries. Neuroradiology 28:246–253
10. Wakhloo AK, Jüngling FD, van Velthoven V, Schumacher M, Hennig J, Schwechheimer K (1993) Extended preoperative polyvinyl alcohol microembolization of intracranial meningiomas: assessment of two embolization techniques. AJNR 14:571–582
11. Yasargil MG, Mortara RW, Curcic M (1980) Meningiomas of basal posterior cranial fossa. In: Krayenbühl H (ed) Advances and technical standards in neurosurgery, vol 7. Springer, Vienna, pp 1–115

The Immunological Status of Brain Tumor Patients

W. A. Dauch[1], D. Krex[1], B. Zeithammer[1], and J. Heymanns[2]

Introduction

Nosocomial infections are still a problem in intensive care medicine in general, and in neurosurgical patients with brain lesions in particular [4]. A variety of external factors facilitate germ access into the body, challenging host defense mechanisms which in turn are subject to immunosuppressive influences themselves. Focusing on brain tumor patients, three factors are suspected to cause immunosuppression: the tumor itself, releasing cytokines such as transforming growth factor-β or prostaglandin E [1], the operative procedure and its concomitants [3, 9], and adjuvant corticosteroid treatment [6, 10]. In a prospective observational clinical trial we addressed the question of interaction of these factors and looked for the clinical relevance of immunosuppression regarding nosocomial infections of the lower respiratory tract.

Patients and Methods

A total of 32 adult patients were investigated 2 days before and 2 days after total or subtotal microsurgical resection of an extracerebral benign (meningioma or neurinoma, WHO grade I; $n = 16$) or an intracerebral malignant tumor (astrocytoma, oligodendroglioma, or glioblastoma, WHO grades II–IV; $n = 16$). The influence of the operation was assessed from the comparison of pre- and postoperative findings in patients without corticosteroid pretreatment after stratification for tumor type, using the Mantel-Haenszel or Fisher's test [5]. The influence of dexamethasone (Dx) was assessed comparing the preoperative findings of patients who received the drug preoperatively (for at least 2 days, 8 mg every 4–8 h; $n = 16$) to those who did not ($n = 16$). Since Dx was not given in a random design but according to clinical indications, the two subgroups were not identical in some of their main characteristics (Table 1) and were stratified before statistical analysis. An impression of the influence of the tumor type was derived from the comparison of preoperative findings in patients with benign versus malignant tumors, now stratified for preoperative Dx treatment.

---

[1] Neurochirurgische Klinik, Philipps-Universität, Baldingerstr., 35033 Marburg, Germany.
[2] Abteilung Innere Medizin mit Schwerpunkt Hämatologie, Immunologie und Onkologie, Philipps-Universität, Baldingerstr., 35033 Marburg, Germany.

Advances in Neurosurgery, Vol. 22
B. L. Bauer, M. Brock, M. Klinger (Eds.)

Table 1. Demographic data and diagnosis of patients with and without Dx treatment before preoperative testing.

	With Dx ($n = 16$)	Without Dx ($n = 16$)
Female:male ratio	11:5	8:8
Age:		
< 50 years	3	4
50–65 years	9	7
> 50 years	4	5
Extracerebral tumor (meningioma, neurinoma)	11	5
Intracerebral tumor (astrocytoma, glioblastoma, oligodendroglioma)	5	11

Postoperatively Dx was administered routinely intravenously at 8 mg every 4 h, for at least 3 days. No other cytostatic drugs were given, no antibiotics for prophylaxis, and no irradiation before the operation or within 7 days after it. Blood samples were taken at 8 A.M. (in patients receiving Dx just before they took the drug). A white cell count was performed, differentiating neutrophilic and eosinophilic granulocytes, monocytes, and lymphocytes cytochemically. Lymphocyte subsets were analyzed after density-gradient centrifugation [2], incubation with fluorescein – or phycoerythin-conjugated monoclonal antibodies (Becton-Dickinson, Mountain View CA, USA), and immunofluorescence staining [8], using flow cytometry (FACS Analyser, Becton-Dickinson). Immunoglobulins were quantified by monovalent antisera automatically (Nephelometer, Behring, Marburg, Germany). Simultaneously, cutaneous reaction to seven recall antigens was tested (Multitest Merieux, Lyon, France) and rated as positive when the control area was negative 48 h after the administration, and at least one antigen area showed an induration of more than 2 mm average diameter. Postoperative infection of the lower respiratory tract was diagnosed in patients with leukocytosis (> 1200/μl) and fever for at least 3 days, colonization of the infralaryngeal respiratory tract by bacteria or yeasts, and purulent bronchial secretion. When the signs of infiltration were seen on X-ray films, the infection was diagnosed as pneumonia.

Since data were not normally (gaussian) distributed, median values were used instead of arithmetic means, and nonparametric statistical tests were used. Median values of preoperative findings in patients without Dx pretreatment were set as 100%, and preoperative medians in the Dx group as well as postoperative medians were expressed as a percentage of these baseline data.

Results

In patients without Dx treatment, preoperative test results were usually well within normal limits. A distinct trend towards eosinopenia and elevated IgM levels was

Table 2. Median values of selected immunological parameters in brain tumor patients (percentage of the respective medians of preoperative measurements in patients without Dx pretreatment)

	Before operation with Dx	After operation without Dx	After operation with Dx
Neutrophils	282%	392%	335%
Eosinophils	9%	21%	17%
Monocytes	135%	195%	153%
Lymphocytes	66%	59%	41%[a]
B lymphocytes	83%	86%	86%
T helper cells	32%	38%	18%[a]
T suppressor cells	63%	42%	35%[b]
Natural killer cells	97%	97%	43%[b]
IgG	82%	66%	50%[b]
IgA	64%	70%	46%[b]
IgM	133%	67%	92%

[a] Apparent synergism of operation and Dx.
[b] Possible synergism of operation and Dx.

found, which has been described in brain tumor patients and attributed to malignancy [7]. As Table 2 shows, even after stratification for tumor type Dx-pretreated patients had significantly more neutrophils ($p = 0.008$), fewer eosinophils ($p = 0.039$), and fewer lymphocytes ($p < 0.0001$) in their blood than patients without Dx pretreatment, while monocytes were only insignificantly increased. In the lymphocyte subset analysis, T helper cells were considerably reduced ($p = 0.002$), T suppressor/cytotoxic cells moderately reduced ($p = 0.007$), and neither B lymphocytes nor natural killer cells were altered significantly. Among the immunoglobulins, IgG showed a moderate decrease ($p = 0.008$) while IgA and IgM were not influenced.

When patients without corticosteroid pretreatment were operated on, their immune system incurred similar changes as were seen in Dx-treated patients in the preoperative period. Operation affected the laboratory parameters in Dx-pretreated patients. In total lymphocyte counts and especially in the T helper subset Dx effects and perioperative influences acted synergistically, depressing the median of T helper cell levels from 780 to 140 cells/μl, which is far below the normal range (410–1340 cells/μl). In many other parameters such as neutrophilic and eosinophilic granulocytes, monocytes, B lymphocytes, and IgM, a synergistic interaction of operation and Dx was not detected, indicating something of a "ceiling" (or "floor") effect.

With antigen skin testing, preoperatively and without Dx, almost all patients (13/16) produced at least one positive reaction. Operation alone reduced this number to 4/16, Dx pretreatment alone to 3/16, and after the combination of the two only a single patient of the 16 reacted. Postoperative infection of the lower respiratory tract became apparent in 6 of 32 patients. Five of these had T helper cell levels below 150/μl, while in noninfected patients the majority (20/26) had levels well above this limit. This is a significant difference ($p = 0.011$, Fisher's exact test), indicating an association between severe depression of T helper cells and respiratory tract infection rate after resection of intracranial neoplasms.

The question of tumor type influence on immunological parameters could be addressed in this study only with caution due to the small sample size. After stratification for Dx treatment, we found preoperatively in grades II–IV tumor patients some tendency towards neutrophilia ($p = 0.007$), eosinopenia ($p = 0.020$), and elevated IgM ($p = 0.018$) compared to grade I patients. Of course, these numbers do not indicate whether histological grading itself is responsible for this trend, or the associated features of localization (extra- versus intracerebral) or sex.

Discussion and Conclusions

Immunosuppressive effects of surgical treatment, corticosteroid treatment, and neoplastic disease are well known. We have shown that they are present even in microsurgical operations, in short-term (3–10 days) Dx therapy, and in intracerebral malignancies. When two or all of these factors come together, considerable immunosuppression results. Cellular elements of immunity are much more affected than humoral factors, and the most pronounced synergestic effect was seen, curiously, in T helper cells, which are of paramount importance in specific defense mechanisms. This is why it is not a surprise to observe clinical sequelae: in brain tumor patients, skin reaction to recall antigens is absent, and the nosocomial infection rate is high whenever T helper cell counts drop below a certain level. This level is far below the lower border of the normal range, but it can easily be reached when surgical and corticosteroid treatment are combined.

References

1. Black KL, Chen K, Becker DP et al. (1992) Inflammatory leukocytes associated with increased immunosuppression by glioblastoma. J Neurosurg 77:120–126
2. Böyum A (1968) Separation of leukocytes from blood and bone marrow. Scand J Clin Lab Invest 21, [Suppl 97]:31
3. Cullen BF, van Belle G (1975) Lymphocyte transformation and changes in leukocyte count: effects of anesthesia and operation. Anesthesiology 43:563–569
4. Dauch WA, Landau G, Krex D (1989) Prognostic factors for lower respiratory tract infections after brain-tumor surgery. J Neurosurg 70:862–868
5. DeMaria EJ, Reichman W, Kenney PR et al. (1985) Septic complications of corticosteroid administration after central nervous system trauma. Ann Surg 202:248–252
6. Fauci AS, Dale DC, Balow JE (1976) Glucocorticosteroid therapy: mechanisms of action and clinical considerations. Ann Intern Med 84:304–315
7. Hekim N, Sayin E, Demirkaya E et al. (1981) Serum IgM levels as an index of malignancy in brain tumor patients. Acta Neurochir (Wien) 59:227–230
8. Saunders AM, Chang CH (1986) A new immune monitoring system for the determination of lymphoid cell subsets. Ann NY Acad Sci 468:128–143

9. Seeldrayers PA, Hoyle NR, Thomas DGT (1984) Pre- and post-operative changes in serum immunoglobulin level in neurosurgical patients. Acta Neurochir (Wien) 70:269–274
10. Weston WL, Mandel MJ, Yeckley JA et al. (1973) Mechanism of cortisol inhibition of adaptive transfer of tuberculin sensitivity. J Lab Clin Med 82:366–371

Postoperative Infections After Craniotomy: A Prospective Study with Partial Hair Removal and the Use of Antiseptic Hair Gel and Perioperative Antibiotics

U. Spetzger[1], L. Mayfrank[1], B. Lippitz[1], I. Kreitschmann[1], H. Bertalanffy[1], and J. Gilsbach[1]

Introduction

Surgical wound infections are still serious and sometimes fatal complications in neurosurgery [2, 4, 5, 9, 11, 17, 18, 21, 23]. Several investigations have, however, demonstrated a decrease in the rate of infection using perioperative antibiotic prophylaxis [3, 6, 7, 8, 10, 12, 14, 15, 19, 22]. The conception of modern microneurosurgery that minimization of the operative trauma contributes to improvement in the postoperative outcome as well as psychological and cosmetic aspects leads to a minimization of hair removal [20]. In the context of these improvements this study evaluated the rate of infection by using a standardized method with minimal partial hair removal in the incision line [16], antiseptic hair gel, and perioperative antibiotics in 716 craniotomies.

Materials and Methods

Patients. From February 1991 to November 1992 (21 months) 831 consecutive patients undergoing trepanation at the Department of Neurosurgery, Technical University of Aachen, were investigated. A total of 716 craniotomies in 688 patients were included in the study. The average age of patients was 52 years, with a minimum of 4 months and a maximum of 83 years.

Criteria. The postoperative observation period investigated for surgical wound infection was 6–30 months (mean 19 months). All 716 craniotomies were performed in clean wounds or clean contaminated wounds (paranasal sinuses were opened) [13]. Excluded were shunt operations, traumas, single burr hole trepanations, brain abscesses, and transnasal, transethmoidal approaches.

Treatment. The surgical procedure was standardized. On the evening before surgery the patients were instructed to wash their hair with a polyvidone-iodine shampoo. With the induction of anaesthesia, a single dose of 2 g cefotiam was administered intravenously as perioperative antibiotic prophylaxis. In patients with known hypersensitivity to penicillins or cephalosporines, a single dose of 5 g fosfomycin

[1] Neurochirurgische Klinik, Medizinische Fakultät der RWTH-Aachen, Pauwelsstr. 30, 52057 Aachen, Germany.

Advances in Neurosurgery, Vol. 22
B. L. Bauer, M. Brock, M. Klinger (Eds.)

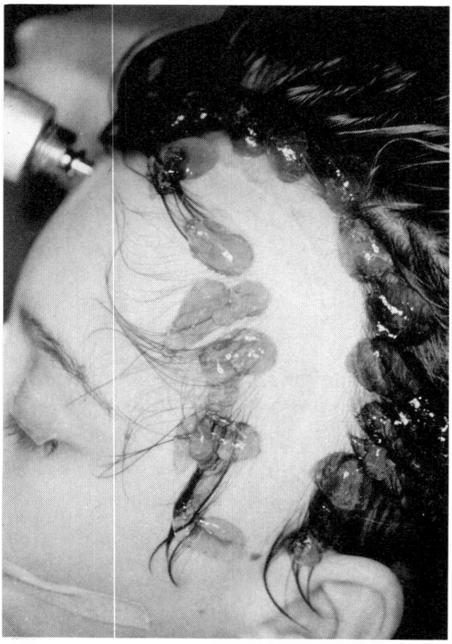

Fig. 1. Partial hair removal along the skin incision and application of the antiseptic hair gel in a 14-year-old boy with a recurrent optic glioma

was given. In accordance with the exact preoperative planning of the approach, the hair was partially removed only 2 cm along the determined incision line, using an electrical clipper and a disposable razor for additional shaving. The head was fixed in a Mayfield clamp, and after positioning of the patient the partially shaved area was cleaned of skin particles and washed with benzine to eliminate the fat on the surface of the hair and the skin. The antiseptic hair gel, which was especially manufactured by us for this purpose, was applied (Fig. 1), and the hair was combed away from the operative field (Fig. 2). The region of the skin incision was cleansed with a polyvidone-iodine solution. The osteoplastic trepanation was performed with a free bone flap, kept in a polyvidone-iodine solution during surgery, and reinserted and fixed with resorbable threads at the end of the operation. The burr holes were refilled with bone dust. The skin was closed with staples. All intradural procedures, except the stereotactic operations, were performed using the operating microscope. In 43 cases (6%) a computer-assisted localizer and intraoperative ultrasound were employed as additional tools to improve the localization and approach to the process.

Infection. A surgical infection during the postoperative follow-up period was defined as a deep wound infection with presence of pus or purulent reaction with microbiological confirmation of bacteria. In these cases surgical wound revision with removal of the bone flap was performed. Brain abscess and a bacterial meningitis were also considered as postoperative deep wound infections and were treated

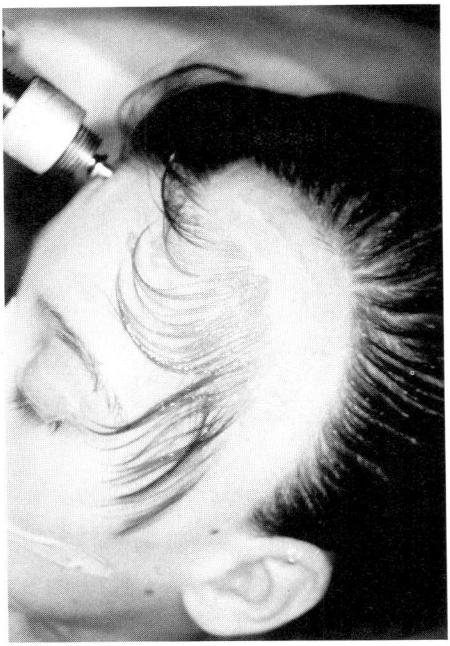

Fig. 2. Combing of the hair away from the operative field, before cleansing the skin with a polyvidone-iodine solution

with puncture and specific antibiotics, respectively. Not included in this evaluation were superficial wound infections without need for further surgical or systemic antimicrobial treatment.

Results

Surgery. The neurosurgical procedures in all 716 craniotomies are shown in Table 1. Histological diagnoses of the supratentorial tumors were 118 (16.5%) menigiomas, 107 (15.0%) gliomas, and 74 (10.3%) metastases and other tumors. Infratentorially located were 36 (5.0%) metastases and 31 (4.3%) other tumors such as hemangioblastomas, meningiomas, and gliomas. The 53 (7.4%) cases with craniotomy in extradural lesions were 18 (2.5%) skull tumors (eosinophilic granulomas, osteogenous metastases), 27 (3.8%) cranioplasties, and 8 (1.1%) infants with skull deformities. Trepanation for aneurysm surgery was performed in 131 (18.3%) cases using pterional, subtemporal, frontal interhemispheric, and various suboccipital approaches. Additionally there were 45 (6.3%) trepanations for intracerebral hematomas and 29 (4.0%) for arteriovenous malformations. Thirty-two (4.5%) craniotomies in cases with neurovascular compression syndromes were performed, including 16 (2.2%) trigeminal, 14 (2.0%) optical, and 2 (0.3%) facial microvascular decompressions. Also 9 (1.2%) cases with extra-/intracranial bypasses

Table 1. Surgical procedures with partial hair removal and use of antiseptic hair gel and perioperative antibiotics in 716 craniotomies

Indication for surgery	*n*	%
Supratentorial tumor	299	41.8
Aneurysm	131	18.3
Infratentorial tumor	67	9.4
Extradural lesion	53	7.4
Stereotaxy	51	7.1
Intracerebral hemorrhage	45	6.3
Vascular decompression	32	4.5
Arteriovenous malformation	29	4.0
STAMCA bypass	9	1.2

were included. The 51 (7.1%) stereotactic procedures were performed in 30 (4.2%) as tumor biopsies and in 21 (2.9%) cases to evacuate intracerebral hematomas.

Infection. The rate of deep wound infection was 1.7% (12/716). Table 2 summarizes the clinical data of these 12 cases. There were 6 patients with single bone flap infections, all treated by surgical revision and removal of the infected bone flap. Except for the cosmetic defect, the problems of prolonged hospitalization and possibly another operation for plastic reconstruction, there were no further drawbacks. Neurological deficits did not occur at any time in these patients. Two patients developed an infection of the bone flap in combination with *Staphylococcus aureus* meningitis. One of them died; the other sustained a severe hemiparesis and aphasia. There was one patient with bone flap infection and brain abscess, with residual seizures and hydrocephalus which required shunting. One of the two patients with bacterial meningitis recovered completely. The second, a 28-year-old woman who had suffered severe subarachnoid hemorrhage (Hunt and Hess grade IV) due to a ruptured basilar artery aneurysm, remained severely disabled. She became paraplegic after developing bacterial meningomyelitis and subsequent spinal abscess because of an infected lumbar cerebrospinal fluid drainage. The onset of surgical wound infection was on an average 55 days postoperatively, with a minimum of 8 days and a maximum of 329 days. Four (33.3%) of the 12 patients had malignant tumors, with consecutive postoperative radiotherapy. The mortality rate due to postoperative deep wound infection was 8.3% (1/12), the rate of permanent disability was 25% (3/12), and 66.7% (8/12) patients recovered completely after adequate treatment of the surgical infection.

Table 2. Postoperative deep wound infections ($n = 12$) in 716 craniotomies

Patient	Sex	Age (years)	Diagnosis	Infection	Onset (day)	Pathogen	Therapy	Outcome
1	F	68	Meningioma	Bone flap	124	*Staphylococcus epidermidis*	Surgery	Complete recovery
2	F	55	Aneurysm	Bone flap	8	None	Surgery	Complete recovery
3	F	28	Aneurysm	Meningitis	15	*Staphylococcus aureus*	Antibiotics	Spinal abscess and paraplegia
4	M	56	Acoustic neurinoma	Bone flap	19	*Streptococcus*	Surgery	Complete recovery
5	M	24	Astrocytoma	Bone flap	10	*Staphylococcus aureus*	Surgery	Complete recovery
6	M	52	Astrocytoma	Bone flap	61	*Staphylococcus epidermidis*	Surgery	Complete recovery
7	M	64	Metastasis	Bone flap and meningitis	36	*Staphylococcus aureus*	Surgery and antibiotics	Sepsis and death
8	M	59	Intracerebral hemorrhage	Bone flap	13	*Staphylococcus aureus*	Surgery and antibiotics	Complete recovery
9	M	42	Cavernoma	Bone flap	329	*Streptococcus*	Surgery	Complete Recovery
10	M	69	Metastasis	Bone flap and meningitis	9	*Staphylococcus aureus*	Surgery and antibiotics	Hemiparesis and aphasia
11	M	70	Meningioma	Bone flap and abscess	21	*Enterococcus*	Surgery and antibiotics	Seizures and hydrocephalus
12	F	2	Leucemia	Meningitis	14	*Staphylococcus epidermidis*	Antibiotics	Complete recovery

Discussion

For the whole spectrum of neurosurgical procedures the reported wound infection rates using perioperative antibiotic prophylaxis range between 0% and 3.1% [3, 8, 9, 13, 15, 16, 19, 22]. Only the investigations of Blomstedt [3], Gaillard [8], and Young [22] focused on major craniotomies, all using complete hair removal preoperatively. Compared to their results the infection rate of 1.7% (12/716) in our study with minimal partial hair removal is favorable. In a recent study Winston [20] has shown a low infection rate of 0.3% (1/313) in cranial surgery without any preoperative hair removal, with the conclusion that shaving is unnecessary [1]. This demonstrates that the surgeon's aversion to hair close to the operative field seems to be unfounded. Certainly these results must be confirmed. A disadvantage of this method [20] is a prolonged surgical closure, because trapping hair in the surgical knots must be avoided. In contrast, our method of partial hair removal along the incision line combines two advantages: easy surgical closure and minor cosmetic deficit.

There has been no controlled study on the rate of infection comparing complete shaving with partial hair removal. Therefore these results are descriptive and represent the outcome of the total surgical procedure, which is affected by and dependent on multiple factors. Our results with an infection rate of 1.7% are comparable to those of Gaillard [8], taking into account the methods used. In the latter investigation with complete preoperative hair removal the infection rate was 3.1% (11/356). There was no case of infection in the 43 patients operated on using a computer-assisted localizer and intraoperative ultrasound despite the additional technical expenditure and prolonged operating time.

Conclusion

We do not believe the rate of postoperative deep wound infection in patients in whom hair is only partially removed to be higher than that in patients in whom hair is completely removed. However, our method incorporates the additional advantage of discharging patients with their hairstyles hardly affected, which is an important part of the patient's body image. We therefore believe that partial hair removal will soon become an accepted method in cranial microneurosurgery with an excellent medical, cosmetic, and psychological outcome and improving the postoperative quality of life.

References

1. Alexander JW, Fischer JE, Boyajian M, Palmquist J, Morris MJ (1983) The influence of hair-removal methods on wound infections. Arch Surg 118:347–352
2. Blomstedt GC (1985) Infections in neurosurgery: a retrospective study of 1143 patients and 1517 operations. Acta Neurochir (Wien) 78:81–90

3. Blomstedt GC, Kyttä J (1988) Results of randomized trial of vancomycin prophylaxis in craniotomy. J Neurosurg 69:216–220
4. Court-Brown CM (1981) Preoperative skin depilation and its effect on postoperative wound infection. J Coll Surg Edinb 26:238–241
5. Cushing H, Eisenhardt L (1938) Meningiomas: their classification, regional behavior, life history and surgical end results. Thomas, Springfield
6. Dempsey R, Rapp RP, Young B, Johnston S, Tibbs P (1988) Prophylactic parenteral antibiotics in clean neurosurgical procedures: a review. J Neurosurg 69:52–57
7. Gaillard T, Gilsbach JM (1991) Intra-operative antibiotic prophylaxis in neurosurgery. A prospective, randomized, controlled study on cefotiam. Acta Neurochir (Wien) 113:103–109
8. Geraghty J, Feely M (1984) Antibiotic prophylaxis in neurosurgery. A randomized controlled trial. J Neurosurg 60:724–726
9. Gilsbach J, Harders A, Mayfrank L, Bertalanffy H (1989) Postoperative mortality in the era of microneurosurgery. In: Frowein RA, Brock M, Klinger M (eds) Advances in neurosurgery, vol 17. Springer, Berlin Heidelberg New York, pp 198–202
10. Haines SJ (1989) Efficacy of antibiotic prophylaxis in clean neurosurgical operations. Neurosurgery 24:401–405
11. Kourtopoulos H, Burman LG (1979) Prophylaxis of neurosurgical infections by improved preoperative disinfection of the scalp. Scand J Infect Dis 11:175–176
12. Malis LI (1979) Prevention of neurosurgical infection by intraoperative antibiotics. Neurosurgery 5:339–343
13. National Academy of Sciences-National Research Council (1964) Postoperative wound infections: the influence of ultraviolet irradiation of the operating room and various other factors. Ann Surg 160 [Suppl]:1–192
14. Savitz MH, Malis LI, Meyers BR (1974) Prophylactic antibiotics in neurosurgery. Surg Neurol 2:95–100
15. Savitz MH, Katz SS (1981) Rationale for prophylactic antibiotics in neurosurgery. Neurosurgery 9:142–144
16. Scherpereel B, Rousseaux P, Bernard MH, Guyot JF (1979) Le non rasage preoperative en neurochirurgie cranienne. Neurochirurgie 24:244–245
17. Tenny JH, Vlahov D, Salcman M, Ducker TB (1985) Wide variation in risk of wound infection following clean neurosurgery. J Neurosurg 62:243–247
18. van Ek B, Bakker FP, van Dulken H, Dijkmans BA (1986) Infections after craniotomy: a retrospective study. J Infect 12:105–109
19. Winkler D, Rehn H, Freckmann N, Nowak G, Herrmann HD (1989) Clinical efficacy of perioperative antimicrobial prophylaxis in neurosurgery – a prospective randomized study involving 159 patients. Chemotherapy 35:304–312
20. Winston KR (1992) Hair and neurosurgery. Neurosurgery 31:320–329
21. Wright RL (1966) Septic complications of intracranial surgery. In: Gurdjian ES (ed.) Cranial and intracranial suppuration. Thomas, Springfield, pp 26–31
22. Young RF, Lawner PM (1987) Perioperative antibiotic prophylaxis for prevention of postoperative neurosurgical infections. A randomized clinical trial. J Neurosurg 66:701–705
23. Zentner J, Gilsbach J, Daschner F (1987) Incidence of wound infection in patients undergoing craniotomy: influence of type of shaving. Acta Neurochir (Wien) 86:79–82

Incidence and Clinical Significance of Postcraniotomy Seizures: Should Prophylactic Anticonvulsants Be Administered? A Review of 910 Operative Cases

H. Wiedemayer[1], G. Becker[1], and D. Stolke[1]

Introduction

Seizures may occur in the course of many neurosurgical diseases. It is the neurosurgeon's responsibility to decide whether or not to start with an anticonvulsant medication. To provide a rational approach to this decision some basic consideration is given to the topics: the incidence of postoperative seizures, risk of seizures in time, danger posed by a seizure, and effectiveness of an anticonvulsant medication. This report presents the data from our own patients concerning these topics and discusses the literature.

Patients and Methods

Data were collected on 910 consecutive patients who underwent a craniotomy in our neurosurgical clinic. Patients with traumatic lesions were excluded. The records were reviewed for age, sex, diagnosis, treatment, complications, history of seizures, and anticonvulsant medication. Generally, patients with a preoperative history of seizures were treated with anticonvulsants, which were continued in the postoperative course. No patient received prophylactic anticonvulsants preoperatively. There were 461 women and 449 men with a mean age of 48 years (range 6 month–83 years). The mean follow-up period was 16 month. The diagnoses are listed in Table 1.

Results

Incidence. A total of 338 patients experienced at least one seizure during the period of observation, for an overall incidence of 37%; thus 572 patients (63%) of the total 910 patients were free of seizures during the whole period of observation. In 204 patients (22%) the epileptic event was generalized tonic-clonic, in 103 (11%) focal, and in 27 (3%) complex partial. Four patients (0.4%) suffered a status epilepticus. Most often the first seizure occurred in the preoperative period: 216 patients (24%). Fifty-six patients (6%) experienced their first seizure in the early postoperative period (from day 0 to day 7 postoperatively), and another 66 patients

---

[1] Universitätsklinikum Essen, Neurochirurgische Klinik und Poliklinik, Hufelandstr. 55, 45122 Essen, Germany.

Advances in Neurosurgery, Vol. 22
B. L. Bauer, M. Brock, M. Klinger (Eds.)

Table 1. Incidence of seizures in patients with no previous history of seizures at the point in time

		Preoperative		Postoperative				Total	
				First week		Later			
	n	*n*	%	*n*	%	*n*	%	*n*	%
Glioma	244	100	41	17	7	20	8	137	56
Aneurysm	179	19	11	6	3	9	5	34	19
Meningioma	141	36	26	13	9	9	6	58	41
Metastasis	114	23	20	8	7	10	9	41	36
Hematoma	68	7	10	4	6	5	7	16	24
Infection	26	11	42	1	4	4	15	16	62
Others	138	20	14	7	5	9	7	36	26
Total	910	216	24	56	6	66	7	338	37

(7%) had their first ictus in the later postoperative course. Of the 338 patients with seizures 114 had more than one epileptic seizure during the period of observation. The seizure recurrence rate is about the same in patients who experienced their first epileptic seizure either in the preoperative or in the later postoperative period (Table 2). In contrast, if the patient experienced his first seizure in the early postoperative period, there was a significantly lower risk of seizure recurrence.

Diagnosis and Location. The incidence of seizures varied considerably depending on the nature and location of the neurosurgical lesion (Table 1). For example, in patients with intracranial infections the overall incidence of seizures was about three times higher than that in patients with aneurysms. Patients with aneurysms of the middle cerebral artery had a significantly higher risk of seizures than those with aneurysms of the posterior circulation (Fig. 1). Patients with gliomas of the frontal lobe had an overall incidence of epilepsy of 69%, in contrast to an incidence of 40% for patients with gliomas of the occipital lobe.

Table 2. Incidence of seizure recurrency in relation to the point in time of the first seizure

	n	Single seizure	Recurrent seizures	
		(*n*)	*n*	%
Preoperative seizures	216	137	79	37
Postoperative seizures				
First week	56	48	8	14
Later	66	39	27	41

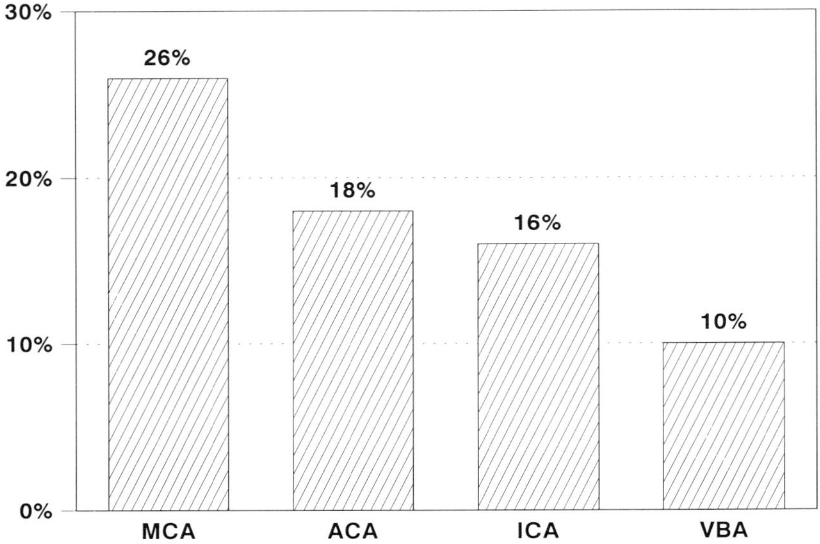

Fig. 1. Incidence of seizures in relation to the location of the aneurysm. *MCA*, Middle cerebral artery; *ACA* anterior communicating artery; *ICA* internal carotid artery; *VBA* vertebrobasilar artery

Early Postoperative Seizures. Of the 910 patients 76 experienced a seizure in the first postoperative week. All 76 were evaluated by cranial computed tomography. In 27 the seizure was considered to be a symptom of a postoperative complication. These complications are listed in Table 3. The epileptic event itself was the cause of a complication in only two; one suffered a skull fracture and another aspiration pneumonia. In the remaining 47 of these 76 patients with an early postoperative seizure the postoperative course was otherwise completely uneventful. Of the 76 patients with an epileptic event in the early postoperative period 56 had no previous history of epilepsy. Of these 56 patients 8 (14%) had recurrent seizures

Table 3. Complications associated with a seizure in the early postoperative period

No complications	47
Seizure associated with	29
Infection	9
Edema	9
Hemorrhage	7
Other	4
Seizure causative for	2
Skull fracture	1
Aspiration Pneumonia	1

during the further period of observation (Table 2). The low incidence of seizure recurrence in this group is in contrast to those patients who suffered their first epileptic seizure in the preoperative or later postoperative period. In these latter patient groups seizure recurrence was observed in 37% and 41%, respectively. A total of 216 patients had suffered at least one seizure in the preoperative period. Of these, 20 experienced an epileptic seizure in the early postoperative period. Despite the fact that these patients were treated with antiepileptic drugs preoperatively, the rate of early postoperative seizures (20 of 216, 9.3%) was roughly the same as in those without preoperative medication (56 of 694, 8.1%).

Risk of Seizures in Time. Figures 2 and 3 demonstrate the risk of seizures in the postoperative period for patients without a previous history of epilepsy. Obviously, there is a high risk of seizures within the first postoperative days, decreasing after day 7 postoperatively (Fig. 2). In the further course the risk of a first epileptic seizure decreased significantly up to the 6th month and slightly up the 12th month postoperatively (Fig. 3). Patients with infections and meningiomas were exposed to a considerably higher risk of a first seizure at 12 months postoperatively than the others. For the total population this risk was about 2%, but for patients with meningiomas 5%, and for those with infections 9% at this point in time.

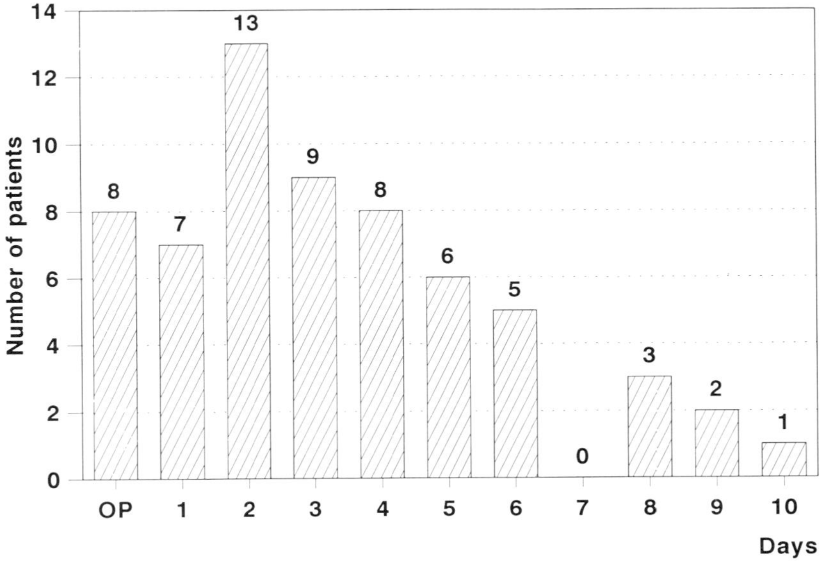

Fig. 2. Incidence of seizures in the early postoperative period in patients with no previous history

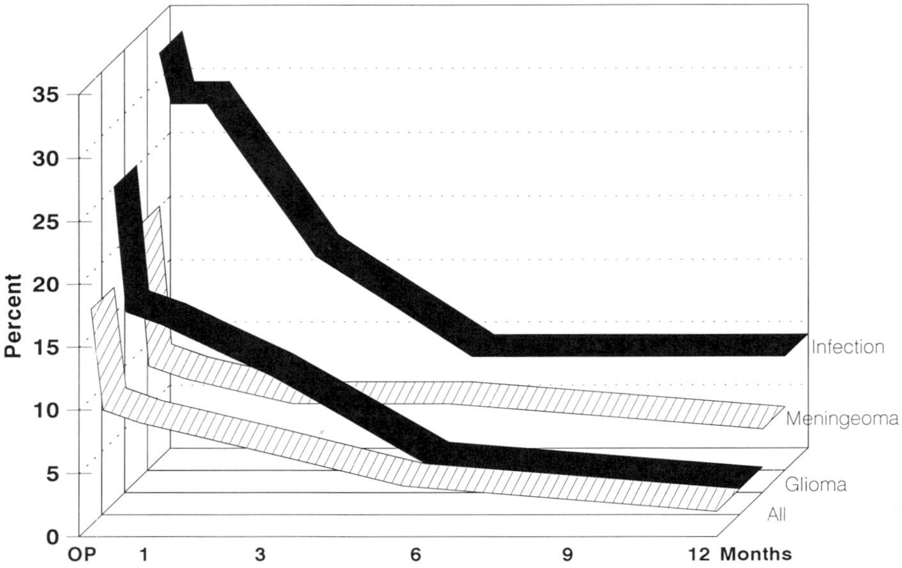

Fig. 3. Percentage risk of seizures in patients with no previous history at the given point in time

Discussion

Incidence. There are several reports that present data on the overall incidence of epileptic seizures in various neurosurgical lesions. As early as in 1940 Penfield and coworkers [13] reported a 45% incidence of epilepsy in patients with intracranial tumors. It is important to know that the frequency of epilepsy varies considerably among the various types of neurosurgical diseases. Infections carry the highest risk of epilepsy. Our own data with an overall incidence of 62% are compatible with those of the literature ranging from 50% to 72% [2, 8, 21]. Gliomas and meningiomas are also associated with a relatively high incidence of seizures [3, 6, 13–15]. The incidence of epileptic events ranges below the average in patients with hematomas and aneurysms. The incidence of 19% in our aneurysm cases is in accord with the figures in the literature, ranging from 15% to 27% [1, 4, 11–19]. However, these general figures are somewhat misleading because the risk of epilepsy is clearly related to the location of the lesion, as demonstrated by the data above.

Postoperative Seizures. The risk of postoperative seizures in patients without a history of previous seizures was 17.6% (122 of 694 patients). This figure is very close to those of Foy and coworkers [4] (146 of 877 patients, 17%) and North and coworkers [9] (17 of 102 patients, 16.7%). Discussing the question of anticonvulsant prophylaxis one must keep these figures in mind. It is only this group of patient with de novo epilepsy postoperatively which may benefit from routine prophylactic anticonvulsants at all. All other patients, roughly 80%, receive the drugs unnecessarily. The risk of postoperative seizures decreases consistently with the passage of time after surgery. The first postoperative week is clearly the period of the highest probability of a first epileptic event. In patients with postoperative de novo epilepsy the first seizure has occurred within the first week in 46%, within 2 months in 60%, within 6 months in 80%, and within 1 year in 89%. These figures are in accord with those of the literature [5]. However, patients with infections and meningiomas continue to be at a higher risk even after 12 months postoperatively, according to the findings of Foy and coworkers [5]. These data are of importance when deciding when an anticonvulsant medication should be discontinued postoperatively. Seizures in the early postoperative period are highly associated with postoperative complications. In about 40% of the patients with early postoperative seizures the seizure must be considered a symptom of some kind of intracranial complication. Consequently it is advisable to perform an immediate cranial computed tomography in each case of an early epileptic seizure to rule out a surgically correctable intracranial lesion. In only two patients (0.2%) of the total 910 patients did the seizure itself cause a complication. From these figures one may conclude that the recurrence risk posed by a single seizure is quite low. For patients who experienced their first seizure in the early postoperative period the risk of seizure recurrence is considerably lower than for those with a first epileptic seizure preoperatively or later postoperatively. One may speculate that mainly reversible postoperative alterations such as cortical damage, edema, hematoma, etc. contribute to this type of seizures. Consequently one may withhold antiepileptic treatment and wait until those postoperative alterations have resolved spontaneously or have been corrected surgically.

Prophylactic Anticonvulsants. Routine prophylactic administration of anticonvulsants in patients who undergo a craniotomy is a matter of controversy. What are the possible benefits from prophylactic anticonvulsants? To answer this question three prospective, randomized studies must be considered. North and coworkers [10] studied 281 craniotomy patients (110 traumatic cases) in a double-blind trial with phenytoin (DPH). They found a significant reduction in seizures from day 7 to day 72 in the treated group (10 of 140 patients in the DPH group versus 22 of 141 patients in the placebo group with seizures). From day 1 to day 6 and from day 73 to day 365 there was no significant reduction in seizures in the treated group. Lee and coworkers [7] conducted a randomized trial of DPH versus placebo in 374 craniotomy patients (210 head injuries). Their focus was directed at seizures in the first postoperative days. The incidence of epileptic seizures was lower in the treated group (0.5% versus 2.2% at day 3), but the difference was not statistically significant. Temkin and coworkers [20] studied 404 patients with severe head injuries in a prospective, randomized trial of DPH versus placebo. A significant reduction in posttraumatic seizures was observed in the first week following the trauma (3.6% versus 14.2% seizures). In the period from day 7 up to 2 years following the trauma the incidence of seizures was not significantly different in both groups (27.5% versus 21.1%). The conclusion from these studies is: at its best anticonvulsant prophylaxis can reduce the incidence of postcraniotomy seizures by half for a limited period of time only, roughly for some days or week. This is true only if sufficient doses are administered and serum levels are controlled frequently, as in the clinical trials. In our opinion it is questionable whether these treatment protocols can be applied to routine clinical use. If not, prophylactic anticonvulsants will be without any benefit. Taking into account that the efficiacy of prophylaxis is questionable, that the number of patients who may benefit from prophylaxis is quite small (80% treated unnecessarily), and that anticovulsant drugs have several untoward effects [12], we conclude that the routine use of anticonvulsants for craniotomy patients is not advisible. The neurosurgeon must decide for each individual patient whether or not to administer anticonvulsants, taking into account several factors: the risk for seizures in the individual case, the possible benefits and side-effects of the drug, the compliance of the patient, and his occupational and social situation.

Conclusions

The decision to administer anticonvulsants is based on specific considerations for each individual patient. Some general guidelines may be followed: (a) A routine prophylactic administration of anticonvulsants for each craniotomy patient is not advisible. (b) Neurosurgical patients with more than one epileptic seizure are treated with anticonvulsants according to the general guidelines of antiepileptic treatment. (c) Single seizures in the early postoperative period are considered to be isolated seizures. There is no need for long-term anticonvulsant medication. In each case immediate cranial computed tomography must rule out a surgically correctable complication. (d) An antiepileptic treatment, once started, should be continued for at least 6 and up to 12 months postoperatively. In meningiomas and infections a longer period of treatment should be considered.

References

1. Cabral RJ, King TT, Scott DF (1976) Epilepsy after two different approaches to the treatment of ruptured intracranial aneurysms. J Neurol Neurosurg Psychiatry 39:1052–1056
2. Calliauw L, De Praetere P, Verbeke L (1984) Postoperative epilepsy in subdural suppurations. Acta Neurochir (Wien) 71:217–223
3. Chan RC, Thompson GB (1984) Morbidity, mortality, and quality of life following surgery for intracranial meningiomas. J Neurosurg 60:52–60
4. Foy PM, Copeland GP, Shaw MDM (1981) The incidence of postoperative seizures. Acta Neurochir (Wien) 55:253–264
5. Foy PM, Copeland GP, Shaw MDM (1981) The natural history of postoperative seizures. Acta Neurochir (Wien) 57:15–21
6. Jan M, Bazeze V, Saudeau D, Autret A, Bertrand P, Gouaze A (1986) Devenir des meningiomes intracraniens chez l'adulte. Etude retrospective d'une serie medico-chirurgicale de 161 meningiomes. Neurochirurgie 32:129–134

7. Lee ST, Lui TN, Chang CN, Cheng WC, Wang DJ, Heimmburger RF, Lin CG (1989) Prophylactic anticonvulsants for prevention of immediate and early postoperative seizures. Surg Neurol 31:361–364
8. Legg NJ, Gupta PC, Scott DF (1973) Epilepsy following cerebral abscess. A clinical and EEG study of 70 patients. Brain 96:259–268
9. North JB, Hanieh A, Challen RG, Penhall RK, Hann CS, Frewin DB (1980) Postoperative epilepsy: a double-blind trial of phenytoin after craniotomy. Lancet I:384–386
10. North JB, Penhall RK, Hanieh A, Frewin DB, Taylor WB (1983) Phenytoin and postoperative epilepsy: a double-blind study. J Neurosurg 58:672–677
11. Öhman J (1990) Hypertension as a risk factor for epilepsy after aneurysmal subarachnoid hemorrhage and surgery. Neurosurgery 27:578–581
12. Olanow CW, Finn AL (1981) Phenytoin: pharmacokinetics and clinical therapeutics. Neurosurgery 8:112–117
13. Penfield W, Erickson TC, Tarlov I (1940) Relation of intracranial tumors and symptomatic epilepsy. Arch Neurol Psychiatry 44:300–315
14. Plate KH, Dauch W, Bel S, Mennel HD (1990) Prognose in Meningeomen. Relevanz morphologischer Untersuchungen und klinischer Risikofaktoren. Zentralbl Neurochir 51:57–68
15. Ramamurthi B, Ravi R, Ramachandran V (1980) Convulsions with meningiomas: incidence and significance. Surg Neurol 14:415–416
16. Richardson AE, Uttley D (1980) Prevention of postoperative epilepsy. Lancet I; 650
17. Rose FC, Sarner M (1965) Epilepsy after ruptured intracranial aneurysm. Br Med J 1:18–21
18. Sbeih I, Tamas LB, O'Laoire SA (1986) Epilepsy after operation for aneurysms. Neurosurgery 19:784–788
19. Sundaram MBM, Chow F (1986) Seizures associated with subarachnoid hemorrhage. Can J Neurol Sci 13:229–231
20. Temkin NR, Dikmen SS, Wilensky AJ, Keihm J, Chabral S, Winn HR (1990) A randomized double-blind study of phenytoin for the prevention of posttraumatic seizures. N Engl J Med 323:497–502
21. Zouhar A, Moravek V (1967) Epileptic seizures and EEG findings in patients after brain abscess operation. Cesk Neurol Neurochir 30:248–254

Minimally Invasive Endoscopic Neurosurgery (MIEN)

Current Endoneurosurgery

B. L. Bauer[1] and D. Hellwig[1]

Introduction

Neuroendoscopy is not new. In 1904 the surgeon L'Espinasse [10] performed the first ventriculoscopy for plexus cauterization in two infants with hydrocephalus. He was followed by Dandy [2], Mixter [15], Putnam [16], and Scarff [17], who performed neuroendoscopic interventions mainly for treatment of hydrocephalus either with choroid plexus coagulation or third ventriculostomy. The main disadvantage at that time was the large diameter of the endoscopes and the lack of useful operating instruments. In 1986 Griffith [4] summarized neuroendoscopic techniques and termed the field endoneurosurgery.

Today technological advances in the development of flexible, steerable endoscopes, rigid endoscopes, and auxillary instruments make it possible to perform complex neuroendoscopic procedures through a minimal operative approach without major tissue traumatization. In analogy to the term minimally invasive surgery, coined by Wickham and Fitzpatrick [18] in 1990, we have defined these procedures as minimally invasive (endoscopic) neurosurgery (MIEN) [1]. MIEN refers to neurosurgical interventions in which, through the use of endoscopes, larger openings of intracranial or intraspinal spaces can be avoided. It provides an exciting prospect to some aspects of neurosurgical practice but does not reach the established standards of safety in current microneurosurgery. The history of MIEN has, on the other hand, taught us much about the gap to be bridged between future requirements and today's reality of endoneurosurgery, not only to patients and their surgeons but also to those concerned with health policy and ethical issues. The neurosurgeon, as technical expert and as the patient's advocate, has a special responsibility. His first responsibility must be to respect the trust placed in him, especially when offering new possibilities in therapy.

The development from macrosurgery to microsurgery is now nearly complete. The next step in MIEN is a current project. The instrumental requirements and the pathology suitable for endoscopic approach in neurosurgical practice must be discussed in depth. MIEN must be evaluated according to the standards of classical microsurgical approaches. It offers obvious benefits to patients and to neurosurgeons, but the present situation is characterized not only by a clearcut list of indications but also by unsolved problems of the desirable level of safety and versa-

[1] Neurochirurgische Klinik, Philipps-Universität Marburg, Baldingerstr. 35033 Marburg, Germany.

Advances in Neurosurgery, Vol. 22
B. L. Bauer, M. Brock, M. Klinger (Eds.)

tility of the instruments available compared with the contemporary state of the art in microsurgery.

At present the stringency of the criteria to establish the indication for endoscopic operations on the brain and the spinal cord is just as unsatisfactory as the safety of the instrumentation and the reliability of hemostasis. Neuroendoscopic operations are not small scale, nor are they operations which should be performed by beginners. MIEN requires clinical experience of the whole of microsurgery as a basis for endoscopic operations. This is the only way in which the patient can be spared from wrong indications for surgery and an poor technique, and the only way of enabling definitive control of complications. The position is obscured by various factors such as the ready accessibility of diagnostic methods – computed tomography (CT) and magnetic resonance imaging (MRI) – and the apparently easy performance of the operation. Critical analysis and monitoring (also of training) is therefore urgently necessary. It is astonishing how many indiscriminate allegations can be found in the literature, and how uncritically many unreliable case reports are reproduced in the literature. At present there is excessive concern to establish the cause in the most convenient way. The general thoughtlessness in accepting the printed word as an established fact and in this way "collecting evidence" as well as the indiscriminate consideration of case reports from older literature disregarding our present knowledge entail major dangers and lead to overrating of the method. It is therefore understandable that many experienced neurosurgeons are critical of any new attempt to introduce endoscopic techniques in neurosurgery.

Instrumentation

Endoscopes. At present there are many different flexible, steerable, or rigid endoscopes (encephaloscopes) available for neuroendoscopic interventions. Their specifications vary, and one must choose according to the planned operative application. It is useless to discuss whether to employ flexible or rigid endoscopes in special indications; the optimal solution is to have both available.

Stabilization and Guiding Devices. Neuroendoscopic interventions require a safe and fixed stabilization and guiding system. For free-hand endoscopy we have developed a special self-retaining arm (the Marburg neuroendoscopy device) which provides the necessary stability to the whole endoscopic system during the operative procedure and frees the endoscopist from the fatiguing holding of the instrument. The endoscopic working depth is regulated with micrometer screws. The metallic guiding system consists of a special bougie set with different diameters and guiding tubes of different lengths. The main advantage of this system is that undesired, uncontrolled movements and maneuvers can be avoided, thereby preventing damage of brain tissue. For endoscopic-stereotactic interventions the Marburg neuroendoscopy device is compatible to the stereotactic frame of Mundinger and Birg.

Supplementary Instruments. Today a variety of microinstruments for neuroendoscopic interventions are available: microforceps for biopsy and dissection of cysts and abscess membranes; grasping forceps to remove cyst material and foreign bodies; balloon catheters for cystostomy or ventriculostomy. Hemostasis can be performed using monopolar RF (Manwaring saline torch [11]), bipolar RF, or laser energy. Ultrathin bare laser fibers are used for coagulation, vaporization, or cutting of tissues. Intraluminal ultrasound can be used in combination with neuroendoscopy for special cases with intracerebral space-occupying lesions.

Videorecording and Display. The neuroendoscopic procedure is transmitted permanently by an ultralight microchip camera system to a video unit. In this way the surgeon has a direct (real-time) pictorial recording and a documentation of the intervention.

Operating Room Set-Up. The complexity of operative technique with video and laser technologies demands a highly specialized neuroendoscopic team. Each member plays an important role in the initiation and completion of a successful neuroendoscopic procedure. The neuroendoscopic team consists of a neurosurgeon, anesthesiologist, instrument nurse, circulating nurse for laser application, and a second nurse for camera and video control.

Documentation. It is necessary to have a form of computer-aided documentation for endoscopic interventions. The main goal of such documentation is, in addition to gathering data from centers worldwide involved in neuroendoscopy, to obtain an overview of the total number of endoscopic interventions performed, the indications, operative techniques, complications, and results.

Indications, Patients Selection, and Results

There are special diagnostic and therapeutic indications for intracranial or intraspinal neuroendoscopic interventions. The availability of miniaturized endoscopes and instruments has expanded the field of indications tremendously.

Intracranial Endoscopy

Hydrocephalus. Mixter [15] performed the first third ventriculostomy in 1923. At that time many technical problems had to be solved, and the development of shunting systems replaced this method in treatment of obstructive hydrocephalus. Jones et al. [8] reintroduced third ventriculostomy. Their selection criteria for the intervention are: (a) patients with aqueductal stenosis or other forms of noncommunicating hydrocephalus; (b) the third ventricle must be of adequate width – at least 7 mm in size; (c) no anatomic contraindications to the procedure such as large massa intermedia or a tiny floor of the third ventricle; (d) previous radiotherapy may represent a contraindication; and (e) third ventriculostomy is not indicated in cases of communicating hydrocephalus. From 1979 to 1990 they operated on 54 patients. There was successful outcome in 33 patients, an improvement of neurological signs in 9, and failure in 12. In recent years we have developed in our Department an endoscopic topographic anatomy of the third ventricle on cadaver brains in situ to gain confidence with the anatomic relationships of this region. To date we have performed eight third ventriculostomies in patients with occlusive hydrocephalus, without peri- or postoperative complications and with a marked improvement of neurological symptoms after the intervention.

Endoscopic Stereotaxy. In 1989 Hellwig, Bauer, and coworkers [5, 6] introduced endoscopic techniques in stereotactic neurosurgery and termed this combination endoscopic stereotaxy. They proposed this new technique especially for interventions in the cerebral midline. The indications for endoscopic stereotaxy are biopsy of undiagnosed solid or cystic processes or abscesses, installation of drainage systems, and laser therapy of small intracranial lesions. The advantages of the combination of endoscopic and stereotactic operative technique are: (a) early recognition of intraoperative hemorrhages which allows immediate hemostasis; (b) intraoperative differentiation between normal and pathological brain tissue, and (c) complete evacuation of cystic intracerebral processes and abscesses under visual control. To date we have performed 146 endoscopic stereotactic biopsies, with an intraoperative morbidity of 2.9%. The operative mortality (day 1–3 after intervention) was 1.4%. Histopathological diagnosis was established in 89% of cases, which is 14% higher than that obtained by conventional stereotactic biopsies in our Department [14].

Cystic Intracerebral Lesions. Cystic intracerebral lesions are a domain for neuroendoscopic interventions. This group of pathological intracerebral cavities include colloid cysts, cystic gliomas, cystic craniopharyngeomas, and other dysembryogenetic tumors such as dermoid, epidermoid, and teratoma. The aim of the neuroendoscopic interventions is the evacuation of the cystic parts of the tumor to decrease elevated intracranial pressure (ICP). In many cases these procedures precede the microsurgical resection of the solid tumor parts of the lesion or the capsule. In colloid cysts or solitary cystic craniopharyngeomas, endoscopic interventions have a high success rate without further management (Fig. 1). A total of 46 cystic lesions have been operated on in our Department in endoscopic, partly in endoscopic-stereotactic technique. In some cases an Omaya reservoir was placed for repeated aspiration of the cyst contents. If the cyst contents are of low viscosity there is no problem aspirating them, whereas in high-density cysts aspiration may fail, and the contents may then have to be removed with microforceps or microscissors. It is not necessary to remove the whole cyst membrane because the possibilty of cyst reformation is extremely low. Usually we vaporize the cyst membrane by laser.

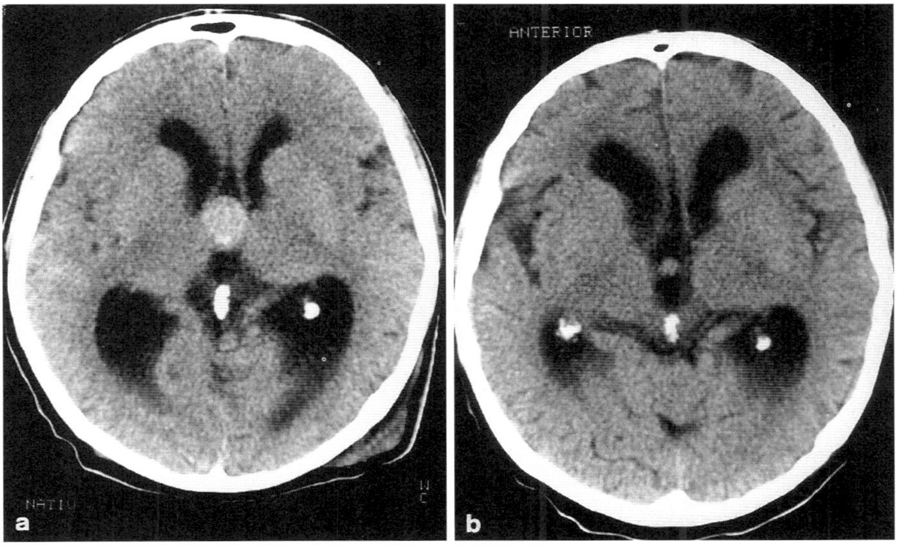

Fig. 1. Cranial CT: colloid cyst of the third ventricle before (**a**) and after (**b**) endoscopic stereotactic evacuation

Intracerebral Hematoma. There is still controversy as to whether massive intracerebral hematomas should be operated on or be treated conservatively. In our opinion, no indication for operation is given in patients with a massive hematoma and increased ICP with impaired consciousness, whereas in patients who are unconscious or have a secondary deterioration of consciousness and in whom herniation is demonstrated there is an emergent indication for surgery. In these cases even if the hemorrhage is not completely evacuated, reduction of the raised ICP leads to an improvement of cerebral blood flow. In our experience, the neurological findings, the size of the hematoma, and the ventricular penetration or hydrocephalus are the determining factors of whether endoscopic intervention is carried out in acute intracerebral hemorrhage. We have operated on 12 patients endoscopically with intracerebral hematoma. Our results allow the following conclusions: (a) the intervention should be performed in the first 48 h after the onset of the bleeding; (b) hematoma volumes of more than 50 ml impair prognosis; (c) more than 50% of the hematoma volume can be removed using this technique; (d) comatose patients do not profit from intervention; and (e) in atypical and unclarified hermorrhages stereotactic biopsy under endoscopic control enables one to clarify the diagnosis (Fig. 2).

Septated Chronic Subdural Hematoma. Successful treatment of nonseptated chronic subdural hematoma (CSH) can be easily achieved by burr-hole trepanation and the insertion of a subdural silicon catheter. Treatment of septated CSH using this

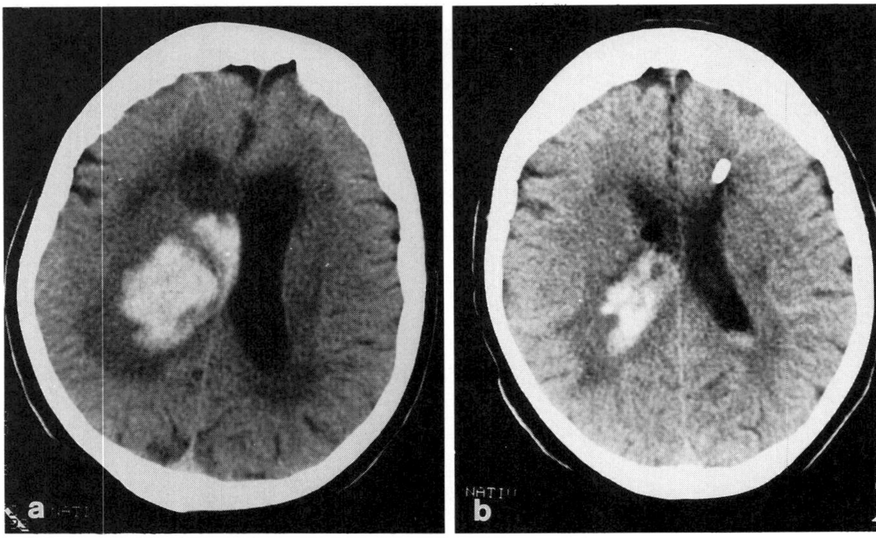

Fig. 2. Cranial CT: hypertensive intracerebral hemorrhage which has ruptured into the ventricular system (**a**) and residual hematoma after neuroendoscopic intervention (**b**)

method may be unsuccessful since the subdivision of the hematoma cavity by neomembranes can limit the complete efflux of hematoma fluid. We have operated on ten patients with septated CSH using endoscopic technique. Seven showed a complete hematoma removal on postoperative CT and three had to be operated on a second time to remove the residual hematoma fluid.

Brain Abscesses. Different strategies in the therapy of brain abscesses have been proposed in recent decades. Abscess puncture and evacuation was first performed by McEwen [13] and improved by Dandy [3]. This procedure was combined with drainage tubes of different consistency. King and Turney [9] were the first to report encephaloscopic intervention in a brain abscess, and we have also used this approach to reduce acute ICP elevation, sample infectious material for microbiological examination, and attempt to cure the lesion by serial puncturing and aspiration. Seven patients with brain abscesses have been treated using endoscopic stereotactic technique. In six patients the abscess were supratentorial, and in one patient the abscess was within the cerebellum. *Staphylococcus* was present in four cases, *Streptococcus* and *Bacteroides* in one case; in one case it was not possible to establish the organism. Postoperatively all patients were treated with the appropriate antibiotics and followed for periods of between 3 and 48 months. The outcome was measured with the Karnofsky Performance Scale. Six patients showed an improvement of 30% or more on this scale. One patient suffered postoperative seizures. One patient died 11 months afte abscess evacuation from sepsis caused by bacterial endocarditis. Postoperative CT and MRI control showed a reduction of the abscess diameter in all patients (Fig. 3).

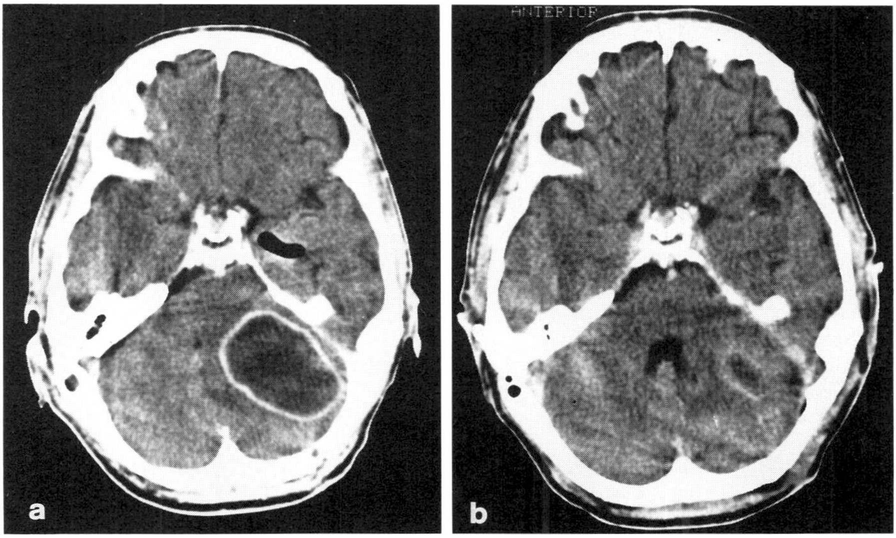

Fig. 3. Cranial CT: left cerebellar abscess (**a**); after endoscopic evacuation only a small abscess cavity remains (**b**)

Intraspinal Endoscopy

Hydromyelia Syringomyelia. Hydromyelia, defined as an increase of fluid in the dilated central canal of the spinal cord, and syringomyelia, the presence of longitudinal cavities in the spinal cord lined by dense gliogenous tissue, are indications for neuroendoscopic techniques. Hüwel et al. [7] have proposed neuroendoscopic interventions in cases of septated syringomyelia. We have performed neuroendoscopic interventions in six patients with septated syringomyelia. In no patient have we seen postoperative worsening of neurological symptoms in the first months after operation; however, there is as yet no long-term follow-up.

Endoscopic Discectomy. Percutaneous endoscopic laser discectomy is increasingly important due to technical advances and the trend to MIEN, with reduced surgical trauma, shorter hospital stay, reduced costs, and early reintegration into work and normal life. This is particularly true with the percutaneous endoscopic treatment of lumbar disc disease as introduced by Mayer and Brock [12] in 1989.

References

1. Bauer BL, Hellwig D (1992) Minimally invasive neurosurgery I. Acta Neurochir (Wien) [Suppl] 54
2. Dandy WE (1922) Cerebral ventriculoscopy. Bull John Hopkins Hospital 33:189

3. Dandy WE (1926) Treatment of chronic abscess of the brain by tapping: preliminary note. JAMA 87:1477
4. Griffith HB (1986) Endoneurosurgery: endoscopic intracranial surgery. In: Symon L (ed) Advances and technical standards in neurosurgery, vol 14. Springer, Berlin Heidelberg New York, pp 2–24
5. Hellwig D, Bauer BL (1991) Endoscopic procedures in stereotactic neurosurgery. Acta Neurochir (Wien) [Suppl] 52:30–32
6. Hellwig D, Bauer BL, List-Hellwig E, Mennel HD (1991) Stereotactic-endoscopic procedures on processes of the cranial midline. Acta Neurochir (Wien) [Suppl] 53:110–114
7. Hüwel NM, Perneczky A, Urban V (1993) Neuroendoscopic diagnostic procedures in operative treatment of syringomyelia. Acta Neurochir (Wien) 123:216
8. Jones RFC, Teo C, Stenning WA, Kwok BCT (1992) Neuroendoscopic third ventriculostomy. In: Manwaring K, Crone KR (eds) Neuroendoscopy, vol 1. Mary Ann Liebert, New York, pp 63–77
9. King JEJ, Turney F (1936) Brain abscess: evolution of the methods of treatment. Ann Surg 103:647
10. L'Espinasse VL (1943) In: Davis (ed) Neurological surgery, 2nd ed. Lea and Febinger, Philadelphia, pp 442
11. Manwaring K (1992) Endoscopic ventricular fenestration. In: Manwaring K, Crone KR (eds) Neuroendoscopy, vol 1. Mary Ann Liebert, New York, pp 79–89
12. Mayer HM, Brock M (1989) Percutaneous lumbar discectomy – the Berlin technique. In: Mayer HM, Brock M (eds) Springer, Berlin Heidelberg New York, pp 107–117
13. McEwen W (1983) Pyogenic infective disease of the brain and spinal cord. Maclehouse and Sons, Glasgow
14. Mennel HD, Rossberg C, Lorenz H, Schneider H, Hellwig D (1989) Reliability of simple cytological methods in brain tumor biopsy diagnosis. Neurochirurgia 32:129–134
15. Mixter WJ (1923) Ventriculoscopy and puncture of the third ventricle. Boston Med Surg J 188:277
16. Putnam T (1934) Treatment of hydrocephalus by endoscopic coagulation of the choroid plexus: description of a new instrument and preliminary report of results. New Engl J Med 22:1373–1376
17. Scarff JE (1952) Nonobstructive hydrocephalus. Treatment by endoscopic cauterization of the choroid plexus. Long term results. J Neurosurg 9:164–176
18. Wickham J, Fitzpatrick J (1990) Minimally invasive surgery. Br J Surg 77:721

Endoscopic Anatomy of the Third Ventricle

T. Riegel[1], D. Hellwig[1], B. L. Bauer[1], and H. D. Mennel[2]

Introduction

Preformed intracranial spaces such as the cerebral ventricles and the subarachnoid cisterns are of particular interest in neuroendoscopy. Since we began our experience in 1989, we have had problems in spacial orientation and identification of endoscopically visible anatomical structures within the ventricular system. As yet there is no endoscopic "cartography" of the ventricular system. For transventricular neurosurgical endoscopic interventions knowledge of the topographic anatomy of the ventricular system is imperative.

Methods and Material

The data for descriptions of the normal endoscopic anatomy in the ventricular system were provided by endoscopic examinations of cadaver brains in situ (Department of Neuropathology, Prof. Dr. H.D. Mennel). Up to now the total number of endoscopic procedures has been 42. Cadavers with intracranial pathologies are excluded from the study.

Technical Equipment. We use flexible and steerable endoscopes with an outer diameter of 3.3–4.0 mm. Most are prototypes developed by Olympus (Tokyo). Supplementary instruments include the ultralight camera system OTV-S2-TV camera, VO-9600 P standard U-matic recorder, and the Trinitron color videomonitor PVM 2043 MD (Sony). For documentation and printouts we use the videoprinter UV-5000 P (Sony). For free-hand ventriculoscopy we have designed an endoscopic guiding system (Fig. 1) for reproduction of endoscopic maneuvers by single lesion of brain substance on the route to the ventricular system.

Approaches to the Ventricular System. For ventricular puncture Kocher's trepanation point [4] 2–3 cm from the midline just anterior to the coronal suture is used. This point is ideal for reaching the foramen of Monro and the third ventricle. Other

[1] Neurochirurgische Klinik, Philipps-Universität Marburg, Baldingerstr., 35033 Marburg, Germany.
[2] Abteilung Neuropathologie, Philipps-Universität Marburg, Baldingerstr., 35033 Marburg, Germany.

Advances in Neurosurgery, Vol. 22
B. L. Bauer, M. Brock, M. Klinger (Eds.)

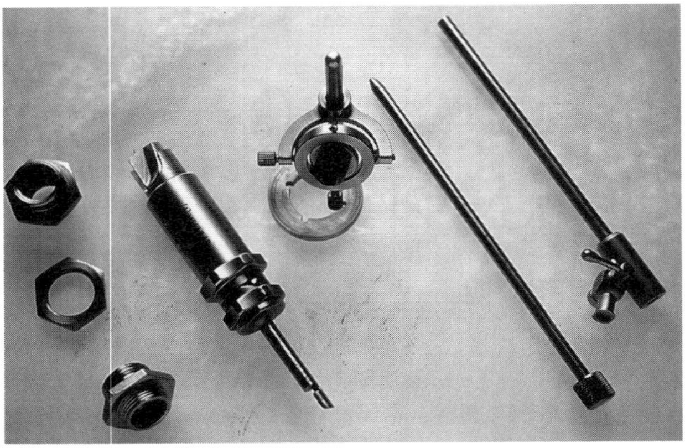

Fig. 1. Our endoscope guiding system with the cardanic joint

well-known approaches through Keen's point (temporal) and Dandy's point (occipital) will be performed in subsequent studies.

Operation Technique. After burr hole trepanation the dura mater is incised. The fixation screw is inserted into the burr hole and connected with a specially developed cardanic joint. The ventricular puncture with the endoscopically guided cannula is performed in neutral position without horizontal or vertical angle adjustment.

Ventriculoscopy. The ultrathin flexible endoscope (diameter 3.3 mm) is introduced, and the guiding tube is pulled back under visual control to the roof of the lateral ventricle and fixed in the cardanic device. The endoscope is connected to the camera system, and the ventriculoscopy is transmitted to the video-unit.

Results

The coronal approach permits endoscopy of the frontal horn including the central part of the lateral ventricle, the foramen of Monro, and the third ventricle. Furthermore it is possible to reach the sylvian aqueduct going further to the fourth ventricle.

Topographic Landmarks

Lateral Ventricle. From the coronal approach one reaches first the central part of the lateral ventricle near the frontal horn. The frontal horn can be distinguished by the lack of choroid plexus. The lateral wall is formed by the caput nucleus caudatus with subependymal veins; medially one finds the septum pellucidum with septal veins. The choroid plexus serves as a landmark for the central part of the

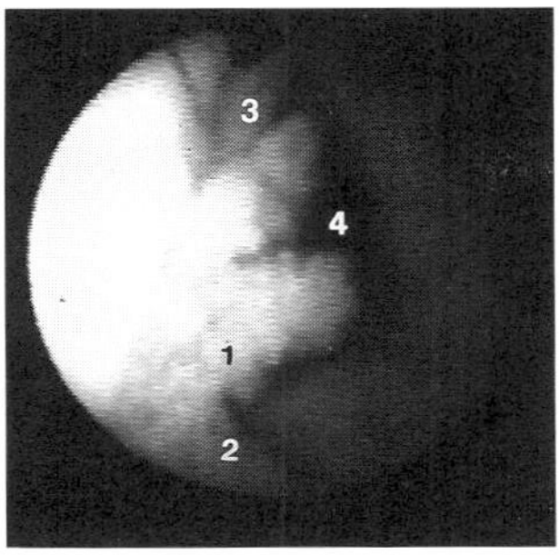

Fig. 2. Typical Y-shaped configuration in the region of the interventricular foramen. *1*, Choroid plexus; *2*, thalamostriate vein; *3*, septal vein; *4* foramen of Monro

foramen of Monro. The plexus is situated at the bottom of the lateral ventricle; the thalamostriate vein is located laterally, and medially one finds the confluence of septal veins. These three structures form a typical Y-shaped configuration [1] which is ideal for orientation (Fig. 2). The foramen of Monro is formed anteriorly by the fornix, and the posterior and lateral border by the anterior tubercle of the thalamus [5]. After angling the flexible endoscope, one locates the central part of the lateral ventricle up to the ventricular trigone. Laterally one finds the corpus nuclei caudati with the thalamostriate vein under the lamina affixa, and the medial border is formed by the fornix and the septum pellucidum.

Third Ventricle. Going through the interventricular foramen, one enters the anterior part of the third ventricle. The mamillary bodies glimmer through the thin ventricular base. This membrane, which is the posterior part of the tuber cinereum, is the location for performing third ventriculostomy [2] (Fig. 3). The optic chiasma and recess and the infundibular recess are visible in the frontal part. Laterally one finds important hypothalamic regions and also parts of the fornix. In the posterior part of the third ventricle the first visible structure may be the interthalamic connection, but this is absent in 25% of cases [3]. Going further under the massa intermedia, one reaches the pineal region. The floor is made up by the posteriorly perforated substance and the uppermost mesencephalic tegmentum. On each side the third ventricle is bounded by the medial surfaces of the thalami [5]. The posterior commissure separates the pineal recess and the habenular commisure from the entrance

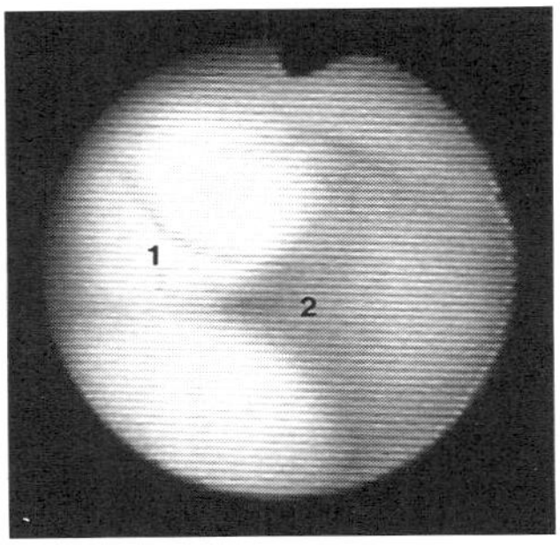

Fig. 3. Location for third ventriculostomy. *1*, Mamillary bodies; *2* premamillary membrane

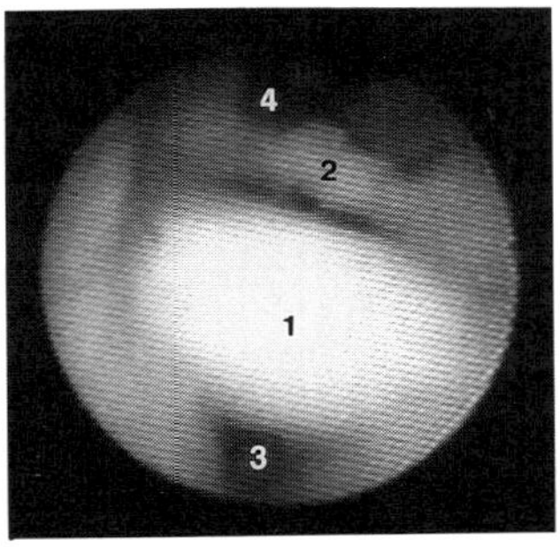

Fig. 4. Posterior wall of the third ventricle. *1*, Posterior commisure; *2*, habenular commisure; *3*, aqueduct; *4*, suprapineal recess

of the aqueduct (Fig. 4) in the small posterior wall. Reaching the suprapineal recess, two longitudinal strips of choroid plexus and branches of the internal cerebral vein project toward the roof of the third ventricle. The roof is formed by the tela choroidea. Below the posterior commisure one finds the entrance of the aqueduct. From there, it is not difficult to penetrate the fourth ventricle. Endoscopic examinations of the fourth ventricle are in preparation.

Topographic Measurements. The endoscopic route from the chosen precoronal trepanation point (outer table of the skull) to the defined ventricular landmarks has been measured in 22 cadavers with a mean age of 68.8 years (10 female and 12 male cadavers). The findings are presented in Table 1.

Discussion

We decided to study cadaver brains in situ with the idea of simulating physiological relationships. The brain is without any fixation, and the ventricular system is still filled with CSF. The vessels are sometimes collapsed, and autolytic processes may impair optic conditions, but this model gives an excellent overview of possibility of endoscopic navigation. The ultrathin flexible endoscope allows one to observe and estimate the neuroanatomical structures with less trauma. The flexibility

Table 1. Topographic measurements ($n = 22$)

Landmark	Median (cm)	Range (cm)
Roof of the lateral ventricle	4.50	3.5–5.3
Foramen of Monro	6.10	4.6–6.9
Mamillary bodies	7.70	7.0–8.4
Optic recess	8.80	7.7–9.7
Infundibular recess	8.50	7.5–9.6
Posterior commissure	8.90	7.8–9.7
Pineal recess	9.50	8.4–10.8
Sylvian aqueduct	9.30	8.2–10.0

provides good maneuverability in the ventricular system, but the optical view with endoscopes shows only the directly visible part and does not allow the control of possible lesions of passed parts. In our material we could see lesions of the interthalamic connection and the region of the interventricular foramen, especially after endoscopy within the aqueduct and fourth ventricle.

The identification and measurement of the anatomical landmarks is helpful for the assessment of dimensions and spatial orientation. To reproduce endoscopic procedures and measurements in one case, we have designed the endoscopic guiding system with the cardanic joint. This gives excellent stability to the guiding cannula and reduces brain traumatization.

References

1. Fukushima T et al. Ventriculofiberscope: a new technique for endoscopic diagnosis and operation. J Neurosurg 38:251–256
2. Jones RFC et al. (1990) Neuroendoscopic third ventriculostomy. Neurosurgery 26:86–92
3. Lang J (1992) Topographic anatomy of preformed intracranial spaces. In: Min-Bauer BL, Hellwig D (eds) Minimally invasive neurosurgery. Acta Neurochir Suppl [Wien] 54:1–10
4. Mapstone TB, Ratcheson RA (1985) Techniques of ventricular puncture. In: Wilkins RH, Rengachary SS (eds) Neurosurgery. McGraw-Hill, New York, pp 151–152
5. Netter FH (1983) Nervous system volume. I Anatomy and physiology. The Ciba collection of medical illustrations, vol 30

Endoscopic Approaches to the Suprasellar Region: Anatomy and Current Clinical Application

K. D. M. Resch[1] and A. Perneczky[1]

Introduction

Endoscopy belongs to the so-called minimally invasive techniques in neurosurgery and today has become a necessary tool in providing the neurosurgeon a new anatomical dimension by revealing the topographic anatomy under endoscopic conditions. In endoscopic neuroanatomy the general roadmaps have been described already [13]. As Yasargil has pointed out, the change of neurosurgery from a macro- to a microtechnique has not been a question merely of the technical tools [16]. There are some fundamental differences between endoscopic topographic anatomy and microsurgical anatomy; one sees everything in a fish-eye perspective with a broad-angle view and perspective. As endoscopy represents the key-hole principle par excellence, the so-called contralateral approaches play an important role in the use of endoscopy in neurosurgery.

The topographic landmarks with endoscopy differ from those of microsurgery not only in the decreased field of overview but also in the often unusual viewing angles of anatomic regions. Neighboring structures disappear from view while progressing to a deeper level, orientation is difficult, and rotation of the picture is easy and does not necessarily represent the true position – all of which may lead to mistakes. Neuroendoscopic strategies and instrumentation have undergone substantial progress in recent years, and the indications for routine use of endoscopy in neurosurgery are growing constantly at many centers in the world [1, 3–7, 10, 12]. This increases the need for a description of the intracranial and spinal anatomy under endoscopic conditions. The suprasellar region offers an excellent example for demonstrating the special endoscopic anatomy and for discussing the endoscopic approaches of the key-hole strategy (Figs. 1–4).

Materials and Methods

Endoscopic explorations were carried out and in 53 specimens the results documented by photographs and analyzed by video. The first three explorations and initial endoscopic training were performed in plastinated specimens, which are preserved using a plastic impregnation technique [8, 14, 15]. The other procedures

[1] Neurochirurgische Universitätsklinik, Langenbeckstr. 1, 55131 Mainz, Germany.

Advances in Neurosurgery, Vol. 22
B. L. Bauer, M. Brock, M. Klinger (Eds.)

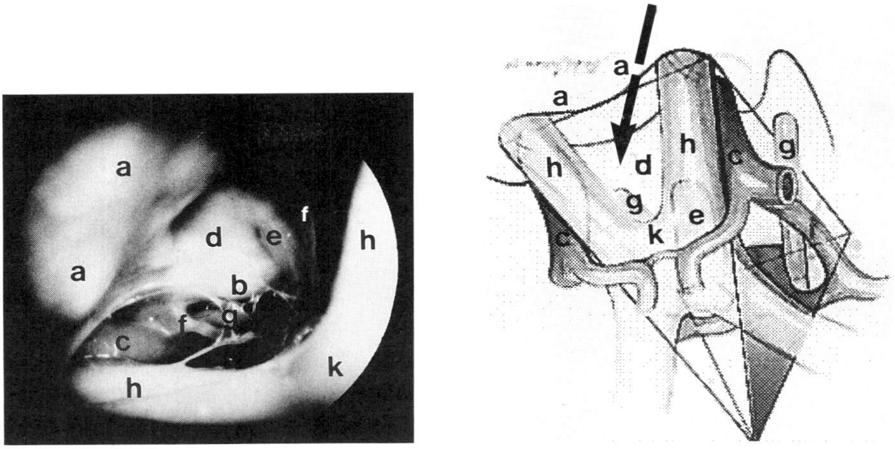

Fig. 1. *a*, Tubercle of sella; *b*, posterior clinoid process; *c*, carotid artery; *d*, diaphragma of sella; *e*, pituitary stalk; *f*, superior hypophyseal artery; *g*, oculomotor nerve; *h*, optic nerve; *k*, optic chiasm

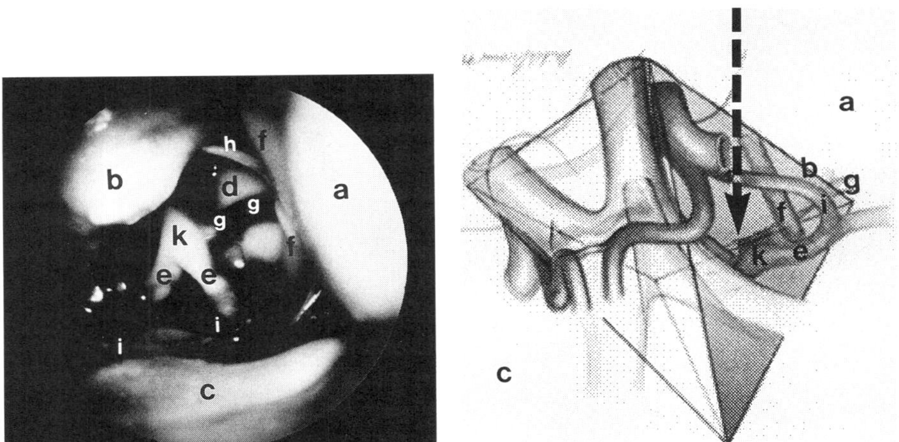

Fig. 2. *a*, Temporal lobe; *b*, posterior clinoid process; *c*, frontal lobe; *d*, pons; *e*, posterior cerebral artery; *f*, oculomotor nerve; *g*, superior cerebellar artery; *h*, arachnoid membrane; *i*, right posterior communicating artery

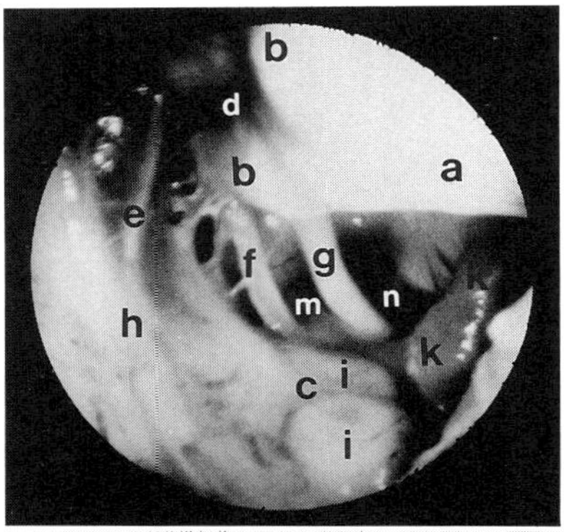

Fig. 3. *a*, Clivus; *b*, posterior clinoid process; *c*, premammillarian area; *d*, diaphragma of sella; *e*, pituitary stalk; *f*, posterior communicating artery left (contralateral); *g*, oculomotor nerve left (contralateral), *h*, tuber cinereum; *i*, corpus mammillare; *k*, basilar artery; *m*, posterior cerebral artery left (contralateral); *n*, superior cerebellar artery left (contralateral)

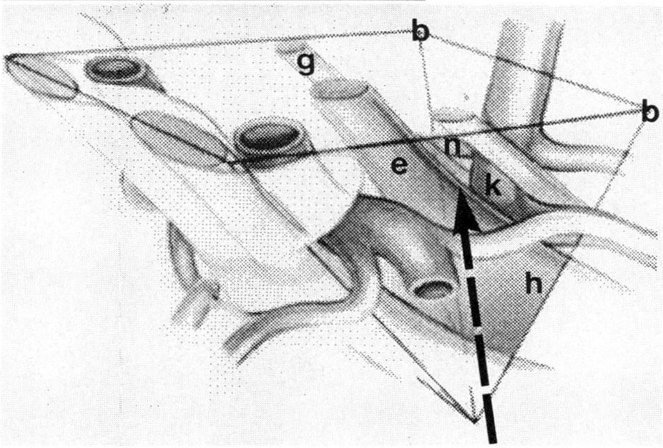

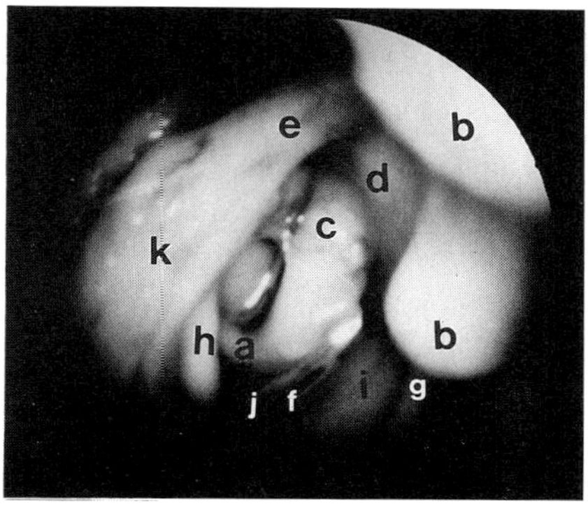

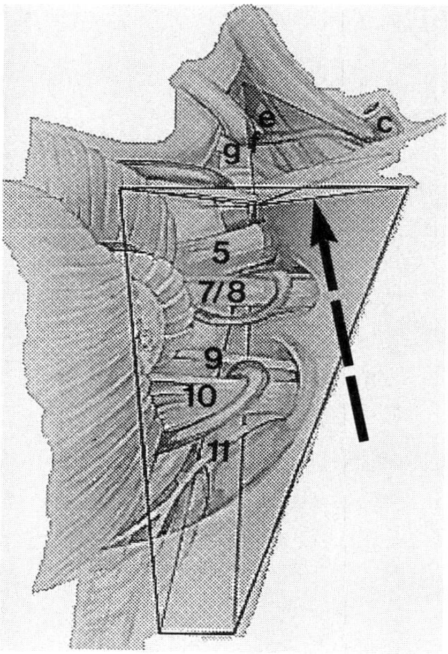

Fig. 4. *a*, Anterior cerebral artery left; *b*, posterior clinoid process; *c*, carotid artery; *d*, diaphragma of sella; *e*, pituitary stalk; *f*, posterior communicating artery left, *g*, oculomotor nerve left; *h*, optic tract; *i*, temporal lobe (uncus) left, *j*, anterior choroid artery left

were performed in fresh cadavers. The technical equipment consisted of: rigid endoscopes of 4 mm 0°, 30°, 70° and 6 mm 5° with canals for irrigation, suction, and instruments; flexible scopes of 3.5, 2.8, 2.0, and 0.8 mm; photo-video system; and microsurgical instrument set. The different approaches that have been used for endoscopic dissection represent the "suprasellar pyramid," which allows the neurosurgeon to enter the region between the structures through preexistent spaces as though through windows [11, 12].

Results

The endoscopic approaches to the suprasellar region are associated with the windows possible between structures. The following endoscopic routes have been used:

Fronto-paramedian Route. Burr hole: 1 cm supraorbital, 1 cm paramedian; target structures:

0° optic

- Anterior communicating artery
- Optic chiasm
- Both optic nerves
- Pituitary stalk
- Basilar tip, pons (anterior aspect)

30°–70° optic

- Hypothalamus
- Optic tract
- Oculomotor nerve

Fronto-laterobasal Route. Burr hole: in the linea temporalis and 5 mm above eyebrow; target structures:

0° optic

- Ipsilateral optic nerve (anterolateral aspect)
- Contralateral optic nerve (posteromedian aspect)
- Ipsilateral internal carotid artery (anterolateral aspect)
- Contralateral internal carotid artery (median aspect)
- Contralateral posterior communicating artery
- Contralateral oculomotor nerve
- Optic chiasm
- Contralateral A1
- Contralateral M1
- Contralateral parahippocampal gyrus

Pterional Route. Burr hole: pterion (sphenofrontal margin); target structures:

0° optic

- Ipsilateral optic nerve
- Ipsilateral olfactory tract
- Contralateral olfactory tract
- Ipsilateral interior carotid artery (lateral aspect)
- Ipsilateral posterior communicating artery
- Anterior choroidal artery
- Ipsilateral A1
- Basilar tip and both oculomotor nerves
- Posterior cerebral and superior cerebellar artery
- Pituitary stalk
- Opposite trigeminal nerve (superior median aspect)
- Opposite facial nerve (anterior superior aspect)
- Opposite internal auditory meatus
- Contralateral trochlear nerve

30°–70° optic

- Retrosellar region
- Upper clivus
- Opposite abducens nerve

Subtemporal Route. Burr hole: 2 cm in front of external auditory meatus, close to temporo-zyomatic process; target structures:

0° optic

- Interior carotid artery ipsilateral
- Posterior communicating artery ipsilateral
- Oculomotor nerve ipsilateral
- Anterior choroid artery ipsilateral
- Ipsilateral trochlear nerve
- Crus cerebri ipsilateral
- Posterior cerebral artery ipsilateral
- Pituitary stalk (lateral aspect)

30°–70° optic

- Tuber cinereum
- Infundibulum
- Mammillary bodies
- Optic chiasm

Retromastoid Infratentorial Route. Burr hole: close behind the occipitomastoid margin (asterion) target structures:

0° optic

- Ipsilateral cerebellopontine angle
- Ipsilateral trigeminal nerve (inferior posterior aspect)
- Contralateral posterior communicating artery
- Contralateral oculomotor nerve (median aspect)
- Contralateral optic tract
- Tuber cinereum and infundibulum (posterior aspect)

30°–70° optic

- Mammillary bodies
- Basilar artery
- Cavum meckelii ipsilateral
- Ipsilateral abducens nerve

The clinical application of endoscopy in the suprasellar region during key-hole surgery makes possible microsurgical dissection behind the structures without retraction. The visual control offered by endoscopy thus allows one to work around the corner during microsurgical procedures. We generally use the endoscope in cases of tumor or aneurysm in the suprasellar region. In tumor cases endoscopy plays an important role in the end phase of resection; it permits control of each corner behind the structures of the "pyramid" and, in cases with retrosellar extension, a view of the clivus without drilling off the dorsum sellae. In cases of large and giant aneurysms one can control the backside of the lesion and view the important structures and perforators covered by the aneurysm sac. Also, the clipping procedure can be viewed by controlling the tip of the clip. Our experience (A.P.) with endoscopically assisted key-hole surgery in the suprasellar region includes 27 tumor cases (meningiomas, craniopharyngeomas, and suprasellar adenomas) and eight vascular cases (six giant aneurysms and two cases with multiple aneurysms).

Discussion

Although neuroendoscopy was used as early as 1910 by Espinasse [1, 3, 7], the development of surgical endoscopy in neurosurgery is behind that in other disciplines [2]. This is due to the enormous precautions necessary for safety when working intracranially and to the very small spaces. Nevertheless, endoscopy is well suited for working in a space such as the suprasellar area because atraumatic approach actually allows entry through a keyhole, and because neuroendoscopy is the logical development from a key-hole microsurgical point of view [11, 12]. The main field of neuroendoscopy is generally the ventricle system [7, 10], but in our Department it is endoscopically assisted key-hole surgery [12]. Neuroendoscopy will not easily become popular, however, if roadmaps for its use are not available [9]. As can be seen in retrospect, microneurosurgery originally encountered the same problems.

Yasargil emphasizes the point that "the problems are not only technical, but start with the anatomical difficulties and concepts" [16].

Conclusion

Before starting clinical endoscopy it is indispensible to study the anatomy in specimens under endoscopic conditions. The suprasellar area is a rather ideal model for endoscopy of a subarachnoidal cistern, presenting anatomic windows through which to enter, where the view is difficult in microsurgery. This is especially the case in the posterior part or the retrosellar part. The need for flexible endoscopes is not as great as was previously thought. Regarding safety and future needs the lens scope presents better optical conditions intracranially and is much easier to guide. The intracranial use of flexible endoscopes appears sensible but is not safe for microsurgery through burr holes. The enormous paralax effect of the endoscope provides a special three-dimensional view of the working space, and acquaintance with this can be developed very quickly by training on cadavers. At the moment there are few endoscopes that genuinely deserve the name neuroendoscope. The endoscope of the future must assure a level of safety comparable to that found in microsurgery through a burr hole. Endoscopy confirms the aphorism of Leonardo da Vince: "To see is to understand".

References

1. Bauer BL, Hellwig D Minimally invasive neurosurgery I. Acta Neurochir Suppl (Wien) 54
2. Buess G (ed) (1990) Endoskopie. Von der Diagnostik bis zur neuen Chirurgie. Deutscher Ärzteverlag, Cologne
3. Caemaert J, Abdullah J, Calliauw L, Carton D, Dhooge C, van Coster R (1992) Endoscopic treatment of suprasellar arachnoid cysts. Acta Neurochir (Wien) 119:68–73
4. Cohen AR (1993) Endoscopic laser third ventriculostomy. N Engl Med 328:552
5. Del Valle Robles R Neuroendoscopy for intraventricular cysticercosis. Minimal invasive techniques in neurosurgery, abstracts, p 44
6. Gaab MR A universal neuroendoscope: development, clinical experience and perspectives. Minimal invasive techniques in neurosurgery, abstracts, p 48
7. Griffith HB (1986) Endoneurosurgery; endoscopic intracranial surgery. Springer, Vienna New York, pp 3–23 (Advances and technical standards in neurosurgery, vol 14).
8. Hagens G von (1985/1986) Heidelberg plastination folder. Anatomisches Institut I, University of Heidelberg
9. Heilmann CB, Cohen AR (1991) Endoscopic ventricular fenestration using a "salin torch". J Neurosurg 74:224–229
10. Manwaring KH, Crone KR (eds) (1992) Neuroendoscopy, vol 1. Liebert, New York
11. Perneczky A (1992) Planning strategies for the suprasellar region. Philosophy of approaches. Neurosurgeons 11:343–348
12. Perneczky A (1993) Neuroendoscopy: update and future. Official Joint Meeting Belgian, German and Dutch Neurosurgical Societies, abstracts, p 65
13. Perneczky A, Tschabitscher M, Resch KDM (1993) Endoscopic anatomy for neurosurgery. Thieme, Stuttgart

14. Resch KDM, Perneczky A (1990) The use of plastinated specimen in planning microsurgical approaches to the skull and brain base. J Int Soc Plastination 4
15. Resch KDM, Perneczky A (1993) Use of plastinated craniums in neuroendoscopy, J Int Soc Plastination vol 6:15–16
16. Yasargil MG (1984) Microneurosurgery, vol 1. Thieme, Stuttgart

Stereotactic-Endoscopic Therapy of Colloid Cysts

P. C. Warnke[1], F. J. Hans[1], V. Jaiswa[2], F. W. Kreth[1], and C. B. Ostertag[1]

Introduction

There exists considerable controversy regarding the optimal therapy of colloid cysts of the foramen of Monro [9, 13]. Whereas some authors propose an aggressive surgical approach as the appropriate and definitive therapy [4, 12], others suggest a less invasive stereotactic approach employing cyst aspiration [1, 10]. The stereotactic approach is undoubtedly associated with significantly lower morbidity and mortality, but it seems that complete aspiration of the cyst content can be achieved only in 50%–80% of cases. In almost 100% of cases open transcallosal or transventricular resection of the cyst results in complete resection of the whole cyst but carries the risk of severe neuropsychological sequelae [6, 7]. Regarding this dilemma we have analyzed our patient material of colloid cysts in terms of the morbidity/mortality of stereotactic cyst aspiration as well as the therapeutic endpoint. Concerning the therapeutic results we used a somewhat different approach; in our opinion a good result in this benign disease with rare recurrence is not characterized by complete ablation of the cyst and optimal appearance on computed tomography (CT) or magnetic resonance imaging but by a patient status without neurological symptoms, without obstruction of the CSF pathways, and with a Karnofsky index of 100. Thus we analyzed our data according to both criteria, complete aspiration and functionally excellent results.

Materials and Methods

Between 1978 and 1992 49 patients with colloid cysts were operated on in our Department. The mean age was 47.2 ± 9.4 years, and there were 24 men and 25 women. Of these, 21 were referred to us already harboring shunts. Most patients presented with a history of fluctuating headaches and/or mental disturbances. Diagnosis of a space-occupying lesion in the plane of the foramen of Monro was established by CT or magnetic resonance imaging. The vast majority of cysts (45 of 49) had a hyperdense appearance on CT. All cysts were well demarcated. Patients were treated by CT-guided stereotactic aspiration using the Riechert system. The stereotactic procedure was carried out under local anesthesia. Target localization was

---

[1] Neurochirurgische Universitätsklinik, Abt. für Stereotaktische Neurochirurgie, Hugstetter Str. 55, 79106 Freiburg, Germany.
[2] 6376, Sedör B, Posket 9, Vasant Kuns, New Dehli 110037, India.

Advances in Neurosurgery, Vol. 22
B. L. Bauer, M. Brock, M. Klinger (Eds.)

performed using a standard CT scanner (Siemens Somatom DR and Siemens HiQ) with the head ring attached to the scanner table.

After exact target localization the patient was transferred to the operating suite, and the stereotaxic guidance system was attached to the base ring. Usually trepanation was performed on the right side in front of the coronal suture. In 15 of the 49 cases aspiration was performed in conjunction with endoscopic visualization of the cyst. In these cases a rigid endoscope (Storz) was used which could be introduced via the stereotactic arc of the Riechert system, thus visualizing the target trajectory. The endoscope (type Hopkins forward viewing with a diameter of 2.6 mm)

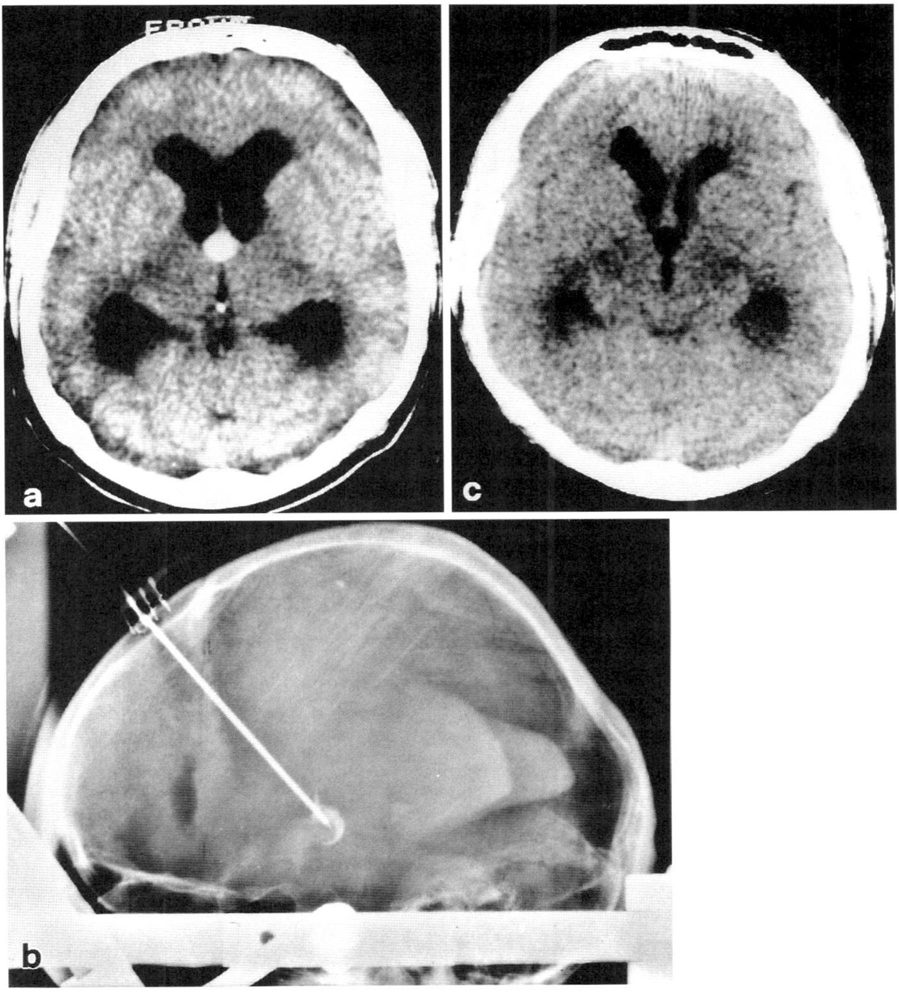

Fig. 1 a–c. Stereotaxic colloid cyst aspiration. **a** CT appearance of colloid cyst before treatment. **b** Stereotactic aspiration and ventriculography. The cyst is made visible by injection of contrast media. **c** Postoperative CT scan showing complete aspiration of the cyst was used to inspect the right frontal horn of the ventricle and to locate the thalamostriate vein and the vessels of the choroid plexus. If no blood vessels were overlying the cyst, a sharp trocar was then used for puncture. If the cyst was not encountered centrally by the chosen trajectory, angles of the stereotactic arc were adjusted so that the cyst was positioned in the center of the viewing field of the endoscope. In all cases the cyst was aspirated under fluroscopic visualization. Intraoperative ventriculography was performed in all cases to document reopening of CSF pathways (Fig. 1). Stereotactic surgery was performed in all cases under local anesthesia. Follow-up was carried out by clinical and CT examination; the mean follow-up period was 5.2 years. Patient charts and follow-up CT scans were analyzed for neurological symptoms, morbidity/mortality, Karnofsky index, completeness of cyst aspiration, and recurrence of cyst.

Results

Of the 49 patients cystes in 40 could be aspirated completely in the first session. No stereotactic aspiration was possible in two patients because of the enormous viscousity of the cystic fluid. The two patients were referred to open microsurgical cyst resection, which was performed successfully in both cases. In six patients only partial aspiration despite heavy irrigation of the cyst with saline was possible (volume reduction > 50% in three cases). In one case, although complete cyst aspiration was possible, there was still obstruction of the CSF pathways, and a shunt implantation was necessary. In three patients a recurrence of the cyst was observed within the first year after stereotactic aspiration. A second aspiration was performed successfully, and so far no recurrence has been detected.

There was no mortality in our group but a transient morbidity consisting of increased headache, blurred vision, and in one case diplopia (6% of cases). Figure 2 illustrates the contribution of the endoscope to the therapeutic outcome. According to our criteria of excellent results (no neurological symptoms, no obstruction of

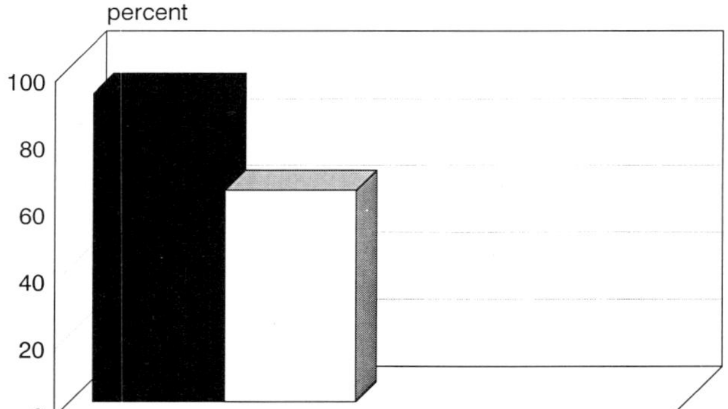

Fig. 2. Percentage of excellent results of stereotaxic colloid cyst aspiration using the endoscope (*filled bar*) versus the use of the fluoroscope only (*open bar*)

CSF pathway, Karnofsky index 100) we achieved an excellent result in 63% of cases using solely the fluroscope for a cyst aspiration. As small cysts tended to be more mobile and were therefore able to swing out of the stereotactic trajectory and also seemed to have a firmer capsula, the endoscope was used in these cases, and under endoscopic guidance we were able to improve our outcome to 92% excellent results. Although this did not reach statistical significance (*t*-test) because of group size inhomogeneity, it strongly indicates that in selected cases with the above characteristics the endoscope can improve the results of stereotactic cyst aspiration considerably.

Discussion

In this largest retrospective series of colloid cysts treated by stereotactic aspiration we have shown in 92% of patients that using fluoroscopic and/or endoscopic guidance of stereotactic aspiration excellent results can be achieved without any mortality and a considerably lower morbidity than has been reported for open microsurgical procedures (Table 1) although cyst aspiration did not always result in complete aspiration of the cyst content, but only in 82%. With the exception of the report by Mathiesen [9] stereotactic aspiration did not lead to a higher number of secondary procedures after primary treatment than did open surgery (Table 1). Compared to the results of open microsurgical resection the rate of complete aspiration is somewhat lower in our group (Table 1); our group ranges favorably among the reported stereotactic therapy results. This may be due to two variables: we used the endoscope in a higher percentage of patients than reported by other

Table 1. Reports in the literature on morbidity, mortality, percentage of complete cyst resolutions, and percentage of secondary procedures required after primary treatment of colloid cysts by surgical removal or stereotactic aspiration

	Morbidity %	Mortality %	Complete resolution %	Second procedure %
Stereotactic aspiration				
Bosch (1978) [1]	0	0	100	–
Mohadjer (1987) [10]	17	0	75	8
Ostertag (1990) [11]	7	0	80	–
Kondziolka (1991) [8]	0	0	50	32
Mathiesen (1993) [9]	31	0	19	81
Warnke, present series	6	0	82	6
Transcallosal/transcortical resection				
Jeeves (1978) [7]	50	0	75	25
Fritsch (1988) [4]	0	0	63	32
Camacho (1989) [2]	27	0	100	–
Symon (1990) [12]	31	0	100	–
Yasargil (1990) [13]	5	5	100	–

authors, [8] and in comparison to the latest report on stereotactic colloid cyst aspiration [9] we used a stereotactic approach with intraoperative fluoroscopic and/or endoscopic control of the cyst aspiration and concomitant ventriculography. This allows an intraoperative variation of the trajectory which is not possible by CT-guided stereotactic approach alone [3]. Thus therapeutic results in the treatment of colloid cysts by stereotactic aspiration are comparable to those can be achieved by open microsurgical resection [1]. Furthermore, these results were achieved with a significantly lower morbidity and mortality than has been reported in surgical series [2, 5].

Conclusions

Stereotactic aspiration of colloid cysts resulted in excellent clinical outcome in more than 90% of the cases in our large series. As these results were achieved without any mortality and with a low transient morbidity a stereotactic approach could be the primary therapeutic strategy for colloid cysts. In addition to the clinical results and the morbidity/mortality rate a contemporary issue in medicine is cost effectiveness; in these terms stereotactic treatment of colloid cysts is far superior to open resection. Microsurgical transventricular or transcallosal resection is still indicated in those cases in which stereotactic aspiration using current imaging technologies and endoscopic guidance fails; however, this is the case in only a small minority of patients.

References

1. Bosch A, Rähn T, Backlund EO (1978) Treatment of colloid cysts of the third ventricle by stereotactic aspiration. Surg Neurol 9:15–18
2. Camacho A, Abernathy CD, Kelly PJ, Laws ER (1989) Colloid cysts: experience with the management of 84 cases since the introduction of computed tomography. Neurosurgery 24(5):693–700
3. Eiras-Ajuria J, Alberdi-Venas J (1991) Traitement endoscopique des lesions intracraniennes. A propos de 8 cas. Neurochirurgie 37(4):278–283
4. Fritsch H (1988) Colloid cysts – a review including 19 own cases. Neurosurg Rev 11(2):159–166
5. Gorrido E, Fahs GR (1990) Cerebral venous and sagittal sinus thrombosis after transcallosal removal of a colloid cyst of the third ventricle: case report. Neurosurgery 26(3):540–542
6. Hodges JR, Carpenter K (1991) Anterograde amnesia with fornix damage following removal of IIIrd ventricle colloid cyst. J Neurol Neurosurg Psychiatry 54(7):633–638
7. Jeeves MA, Simpson DA, Geffen G (1979) Functional consequences of the transcallosal removal of intraventricular tumours. J Neurol Neurosurg Psychiatry 42:134–142
8. Kondziolka D, Lunsford LD (1991) Stereotactic management of colloid cysts: factors predicting success. J Neurosurg 75(1):45–51
9. Mathiesen T, Grane P, Lindquist C, von Hoht H (1993) High recurrence rate following aspiration of colloid cysts in the third ventricle. J Neurosurg 78(5):748–752
10. Mohadjer M, Teshmar E, Mundinger F (1987) CT-stereotaxic drainage of colloid cysts in the foramen of Monro and the third ventricle. J Neurosurg 67:220–223

11. Ostertag CB (1990) Surgical techniques in the management of colloid cysts of the third ventricle. The stereotaxic endoscopic approach. In: Symon L, Calliauw L, Cohadon F et al. (eds) Advances and technical standards in neurosurgery, vol 17. Springer, Vienna New York, pp 143–148
12. Symon C, Pell M (1990) Surgical techniques in the management of colloid cysts of the third ventricle. The transcortical approach. In: Symon L, Calliauw L, Cohadon F et al. (eds) Advances and technical standards in neurosurgery, vol 17. Springer, Vienna New York, pp 122–132
13. Yasargil MG, Sarioglu AG, Adamson TE, Roth P (1990) Surgical techniques in the managment of colloid cysts of the third ventricle. The interhemispheric-transcallosal approach. In: Symon L, Calliauw L, Cohadon F et al. (eds) Advances and technical standards in neurosurgery, vol 17. Springer, Vienna New York, pp 133–142

Minimally Invasive Therapy of Symptomatic Cavum Vergae and Other Midline Cysts: Stereotactic Cystoventriculostomy

J. R. Moringlane[1], E. Donauer[1], and W. I. Steudel[1]

Introduction

Cysts of the cavum septi pellucidi and cavum vergae are believed to be secondary cavities following the closure of the commissural plate [7] or the involution of the prosencephalic commissures in the 4th month of gestation [9–11]. The embryonal portion of the septum pellucidum and also the cavities disappear in the 30th–40th weeks of gestation. In 20% the anterior portion persists as a cavum septi pellucidi and in 2%–3% the posterior cavity as a cavum vergae cyst [6, 8]. Midline cysts are regularly observed in premature and newborn infants [1], but ultrasonography reveals no cyst after the 3rd month of life [5, 8, 9]. In adults such cavities are found in 2%–3% of autopsy series (Fig. 1). Arachnoidal cells, glial fibers with fibrillary astrocytes, are the components of the cyst wall.

Cysts of the cavum vergae and septum pellucidum may communicate with the ventricular space and cause the occlusion of cerebrospinal fluid (CSF) pathways and provoke symptoms and signs of intracranial hypertension or other neurological disorders. The traditional method of treatment described by Dandy [2] consists in creating a communication between the ventricular space and the cyst via a frontal approach. We report on the minimally invasive technique of computed tomography (CT) guided stereotactic internal drainage.

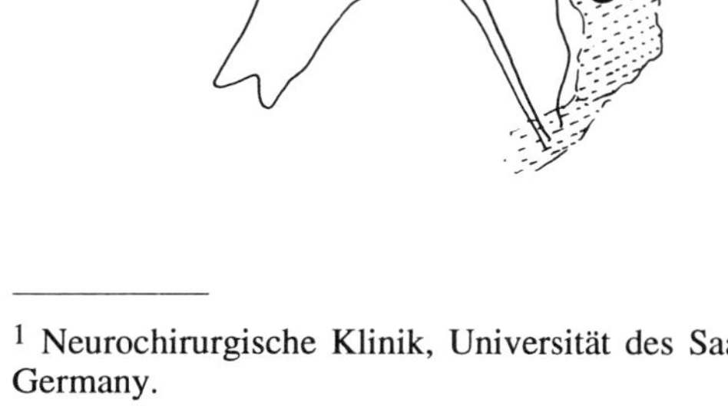

Fig. 1. Topographic anatomy of midline cysts. *1*, Cavum septi pellucidi; *2*, cavum vergae; *3*, cavum veli interpositi

[1] Neurochirurgische Klinik, Universität des Saarlandes, Oscar-Orth-Str., 66421 Homburg, Germany.

Advances in Neurosurgery, Vol. 22
B. L. Bauer, M. Brock, M. Klinger (Eds.)

Materials and Methods

Patients. Eight patients with midline cysts, cavum vergae, or cavum vergae and cavum septi pellucidi were treated at our institution. One 1-year-old boy had a space-occupying cyst combined with agenesia of the corpus callosum. There were three adult women aged 22 (two cases) and 36 years, one man aged 45 years, and four children (one boy and three girls) aged between 6 months and 11 years. Symptoms in adults were headache (one case), visual problems (one case), eye muscle weakness (two cases), paresia of one arm (one case), and hypoesthesia (one case). Symptoms in children were developmental disturbance (three cases), macrocephaly (three cases), seizure (one case), eye muscle weakness (one case), and headache in the case of the 11-year-old girl.

Imaging Studies. The presence of the midline cyst was demonstrated in infants by ultrasound scan and magnetic resonance imaging (MRI). In adults and in the 11-year-old girl MRI and CT had revealed the presence of the cavity. In all cases the lateral ventricles were compressed and displaced laterally. As a result the frontal horns were narrow and the occipital and temporal horns enlarged.

Stereotactic Technique. Stereotactic surgery was performed under general anesthesia in the children and under local anesthesia in the adults. Following fixation of the head ring to the skull of the patient CT was carried out. The coordinates of a target point within the cyst in one of the caudal slices were obtained. Via a 6-mm frontal opening a cannula was introduced through the lateral ventricle into the cyst. The clear aspect of the cyst content and intraoperative laboratory examination of the fluid confirmed the nature of its CSF. By injecting a few drops of contrast medium the topographical anatomy of the ventricular space and of the cyst was visualized (Fig. 2). Additional endoscopic monitoring and video documentation was obtained in two adults. Using the guiding support of the instrument, a catheter with a Rickham reservoir at the proximal end and provided with additional perforations was inserted into the cyst through the lateral ventricle. Intraoperative real-time ultrasound imaging was used in infants with open fontanelle. In these cases postoperative ultrasound was also carried out. All other patients underwent CT and MRI in the postoperative period.

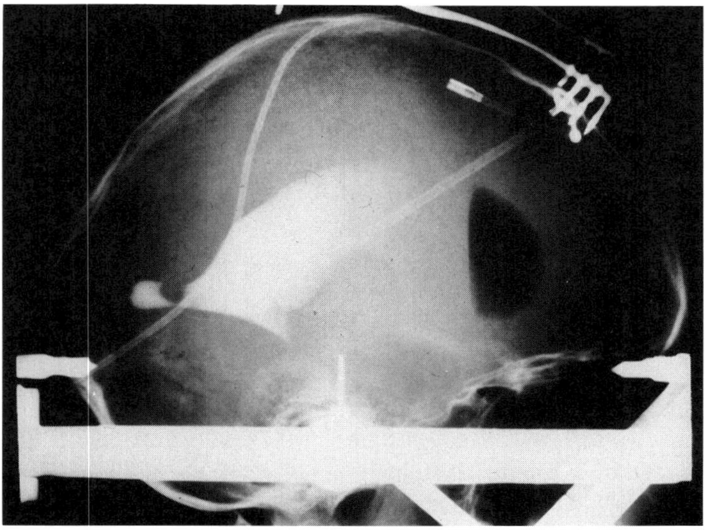

Fig. 2. Intraoperative X-ray contrast medium study showing the lateral ventricle and the caudal border of a cavum vergae cyst

Results

There were no complications due to the surgical procedure. Follow-up time ranged between 1 month and 7 years. In infants head circumference and psychomotoric development returned to normal. In adults headache and other symptoms disappeared. CT and MRI showed gradual normalization of ventricular size after 6 months–1 year and a small remnant of the cavity (Fig. 3).

Discussion and Conclusion

Imaging modalities such as CT, MRI, and ultrasound provide thorough information on cerebral lesions and on their topographical anatomy. Diagnostic procedures may be carried out without discomfort for the patient and without complications. Traditional methods of treatment for space-occupying midline cysts are invasive, time consuming, and not exempt of complications. Imaging-guided, stereotactic, minimally invasive techniques offer the advantages of precise localization and exact definition of midline cysts. A safe pathway may be chosen, and the lack of orientation during free-hand procedures is overcome by the use of a system of coordinates [3] which facilitates the use of guided laser probes and of endoscopy.

Long-term follow-up of stereotactic cystoventriculostomy in infants cannot be reported at the present time. In the cases followed between 2 and 7 years, good re-

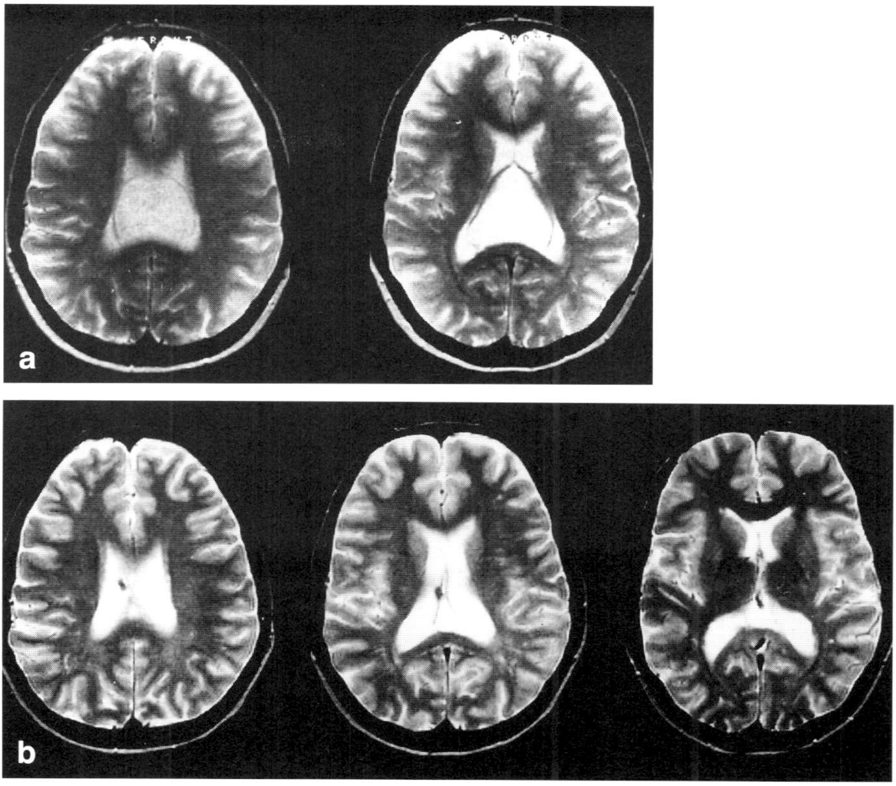

Fig. 3 a, b. Cavum vergae cyst on T2 weighted MRI. **a** Before treatment. The lateral ventricles are displaced by a large triangularly shaped midline cyst. **b** Two years after cystoventriculostomy. The size and the morphology of the ventricles are normal. A minute portion of the cyst (posteriorly) is visible. (From [4])

sults remain stable. Should the communication become obliterated, a second stereotactic procedure could be proposed.

References

1. Bohlayer R, Straßburg HM, Sauer M (1983) Das Cavum septi pellucidi and Cavum Vergae beim Säugling – eine Untersuchung mit der zweidimensionalen Sektor-Echo-Enzephalographie. Klin Padiat 195:92–96
2. Dandy W (1931) Congenital cerebral cysts of the cavum septi pellucidi and the cavum vergae. Diagnosis and treatment. Arch Neurol Psychiatr 25:44–66
3. Donauer E, Moringlane JR, Ostertag CB (1986) Cavum vergae cyst as cause of hydrocephalus, "almost forgotten"? Successful stereotactic treatment. Acta Neurochir (Wien) 83:12–19

4. Donauer E, Moringlane JR, Huber G, Voges M, Ostertag CB, Steudel WI (1993) Behandlungsergebnisse der Zysten der Mittellinie nach minimal invasivem Vorgehen. Klin Neuroradiol 3:85–90
5. Farruga S, Babcock DS (1981) The cavum septi pellucidi: its appearance and incidence with cranial ultrasonography in infancy. Radiology 139:147
6. Larroche J, Baudey J (1961) Cavum septi pellucidi, cavum vergae, cavum veli interpositi: cavites de la ligne mediane. Etude anatomique et pneumoencephalographique dans la periode neonatale. Biol Neonatl 3:193
7. Rakic P, Yakovlev PJ (1968) The development of corpus callosum and cavum septi in man. J Comp Neurol 132:45–72
8. Schwidde PT (1952) Incidence of cavum septi pellucidi and cavum vergae in 1032 human brains. Arch Neurol Psychiatr 67:625–632
9. Shaw CM, Alvord EC (1969) Cavum septi pellucidi and vergae: their normal and pathological states. Brain 92:213–224
10. Sonntag I (1971) Anlagebedingte Gehirnanomalien der Mittellinie. Nervenarzt 42:10
11. Zellweger H (1951) Die cisterna interventicularis und ihre klinische Bedeutung. Helv Paediat Acta 6

Magnetic Resonance Imaging-Guided Interstitial Laser Therapy in Brain Tumors

M. Bettag[1], F. Ulrich[1], and T. Kahn[2]

Introduction

Laser-induced interstitial thermotherapy (LITT) is a minimally invasive technique of local brain tumor destruction. The concept of interstitial hyperthermia was first evaluated in experimental studies by Bown in 1983 [6]. For a safe clinical application it is mandatory to define the extent of thermally mediated laser-induced damage to the tissue. Jolesz and coworkers studied the sensitivity of magnetic resonance imaging (MRI) to visualize laser-induced tissue changes [7]. MRI proved to be well suited for monitoring LITT due to its high soft-tissue contrast and its sensitivity for temperature changes. In this paper we report our experiences with MRI-guided LITT in eight patients with intracranial tumors.

Patients and Methods

Eight patients with intracerebral neoplasms were treated by LITT. There were two women and six men with a mean age of 51 years and age range of 24–74 years. The admission criteria of the patients were as follows: (a) supratentorial localization of the tumor, (b) approximately spherical configuration of the tumor, (c) maximum diameter of the tumor under 35 mm, and (d) histological diagnosis by preceeding stereotactic biopsy. Tumors within the posterior fossa were excluded because neoplasms in this localization could have been treated only in prone position, which is not feasible within the magnet. Tumors with hemorrhage were excluded because with the applied wavelength of 1064 nm blood may lead to carbonization at the tip of the light guide. The tumor diameter was limited to 35 mm or less due to the limited maximum diameter of the laser-induced lesion.

The histology of the tumors treated by LITT was heterogenous. There were three astrocytomas WHO II, one astrocytoma WHO II or III, one astrocytoma WHO III, one astrocytoma WHO IV, and two brain metastases. Localization of the tumors was hemispherical in six cases, with four tumors infiltrating the central motor cortex. There was one tumor in the corpus callosum and one thalamic tumor. The diameter of the tumors varied from 18 to 34 mm, with a mean of 25.1 mm.

---

[1] Neurochirurgische Klinik, Heinrich-Heine-Universität Düsseldorf, Moorenstr. 5, 40225 Düsseldorf, Germany.
[2] Institut für Diagnostische Radiologie, Heinrich-Heine-Universität Düsseldorf, Moorenstr. 5, 40225 Düsseldorf, Germany.

Advances in Neurosurgery, Vol. 22
B. L. Bauer, M. Brock, M. Klinger (Eds.)

The main neurological symptoms on admission were epileptic fits in four cases, progressive hemiparesis in three, and psychological disorders in one.

Prior to laser therapy all patients had serial stereotactic tumor biopsy followed by implantation of an applicator probe according to stereotactic calculations. After this procedure the awake patients were referred to the MRI Department. LITT was performed using a cw 1064 nm ND:YAG laser (Medilas 4060N, Dornier Medizintechnik, Germering) and a special light guide with a circumferential beam characteristic. The laser unit was installed outside the MRI room and connected with the laser fiber. Afterwards, the patients were placed on the MRI table, and the laser fiber was introduced into the center of the tumor via the applicator probe according to calculated stereotactic coordinates. The position of the laser fiber and the applicator probe was controlled by multiplanar reconstructions of a three-dimensional turbo-FLASH sequence. Interstitial laser irradiation was then started. To monitor the laser therapy a T1-weighted FLASH sequence with an acquisition time of 15 s was used. After calculation of the images the sequence was started again and repeated during the course of LITT. The reconstructed images were displayed on a second console, thus allowing a simultaneous acquisition and evaluation of the procedure. The images were analyzed regarding the size and localization of areas with changed signal intensity. According to these data, the duration of LITT could be determined.

In our patients we used a laser power of 4–5 W, with an exposure time of 10–20 min. The laser energy used was 1440–6000 J, with a mean of 3560 J. After finishing the laser irradiation, measurements of the two-dimensional FLASH sequence were continued for 15–20 min. MRI follow-up studies were performed 24 h, 4–6 days, 3–5 weeks, 3–4 months, 6 months, and 1 year after therapy.

Imaging Results

In all patients we were able to identify and localize the position of the light guide and the applicator probe by multiplanar reconstructions of a three-dimensional turbo-FLASH sequence. During LITT typical changes in signal intensity occurred, and a dynamically altering lesion with a zonal architecture was noted. A gradually increasing central zone of high signal intensity next to the light guide was surrounded by an increasing area of reduced signal intensity. The temporal development of these areas varied. The central lesion was seen first 1–5 min after starting laser therapy (mean time 3.1 min). At the end of the procedure, the maximum diameter varied between 5 and 22 mm (mean 12.6 mm). The peripheral low signal intensity zone was noted after 1–5 min (mean 3.0 min), with this area increasing up to 18–30 mm (mean 23.6 mm). T1-weighted images after gadolinium-DTPA showed a spherical enhancing rim at the border of the peripheral zone. The area surrounded by this rim was considered to be the total lesion. There was no significant correlation between lesion size and amount of laser energy used. The laser-induced lesion was 64.5%–130% (mean 101%) of the tumor size. Follow-up studies showed an increase in total lesion size of 4.5%–9.5% (mean 7.2%) within

4–6 days after LITT. After this initial increase the size and signal intensity decreased continuously. The laser-induced lesion appeared more homogenous 18–76 days following LITT, and the zonal architecture was no langer visible. However, the enhancing rim after gadolinium-DTPA remained present in all follow-up studies. In all patients follow-up studies revealed a marked reduction in tumor size. In the patients with an astrocytoma of WHO II there has been no hint of tumor progress until now (follow-up period 4–18 months). However, in the patients with malignant glioma recurrences occured 2 and 12 months after LITT. The patients with brain metastases died due to complications of their primary carcinoma. In one of these two patients no recurrence was detectable; in the older patient a small recurrence starting at the periphery of the laser lesion had developed.

In seven of the eight patients follow-up studies showed a slight to severe increase of perifocal edema on T2-weighted images. There was neither a correlation between grading of the tumor and severity of edema nor between laser energy used and severity of edema. Follow-up studies never showed an increase in perifocal edema directly after LITT. The punctum maximum of edema was 4–7 days after laser therapy and in one case delayed after 27 days. In all patients the laser-induced edema regressed completely within 15–40 days.

Six of the eight patients perioperatively received steroids (hydrocortisone 12–32 mg/day). In four patients steroids were administered for 6–12 weeks. In all of these patients the edema regressed completely. One patient received steroids only for 9 days, and a delayed edema developed 4 weeks after LITT. After a further course of steroids the edema completely regressed within 2 weeks. Two patients received no steroids perioperatively. One patient showed a moderate increase in edema after 4 days that made administration of steroids necessary; the edema then regressed within 2 weeks. In the other patient there was only a slight increase in perifocal edema so that no steroids had to be given; the edema regressed within 25 days.

Clinical Results

In seven of the eight patients neither clinical deterioration nor any pain occurred. After LITT all patients could be referred to the ward; no patient required intensive care. One patient's condition deteriorated during laser therapy. He had an increase in preexisting hemiparesis and partial aphasia. Neurological symptoms improved over the next 4 days. In all patients with an astrocytoma of WHO II we observed clinical improvement in terms of reduction in epileptic fits and improvement in the EEG findings. The patients with high-grade malignant gliomas showed no change in clinical symptoms until recurrence. Both patients with brain metastases died due to complications of their primary carcinoma.

Discussion

The role of LITT in the therapeutic work-up of brain tumors must still be defined. Only a few preliminary reports have been published about the clinical application of LITT in brain tumors [2, 4, 5, 11, 14]. In our series, LITT was of low intraoperative morbidity and no mortality. A marked tumor reduction was obtained in all patients. Although definite conclusions regarding the value of LITT cannot be drawn based on our study, it seems that LITT is of benefit in patients with low-grade gliomas. On the other hand, in malignant gliomas laser therapy can be effective only in combination with other treatment modalities (e.g., radiotherapy, chemotherapy) [12].

MRI is obviously well suited to demonstrate laser-induced tissue changes in real time [1, 7]. The value of MRI in monitoring LITT depends on the ability of MRI to localize the laser fiber exactly, to assess laser-tissue interactions correctly, to predict the final lesion size, and to assess the temporal evolution of the laser-induced lesion.

In our study, we were able to define and localize the position of the laser fiber in all patients using multiplanar reconstructions of a three-dimensional sequence. MRI was reliable in revealing the evolution of a laser-induced lesion. This lesion always had a typical zonal architecture that was in accordance with experimental results [3, 13]. The size of the lesion measured on two-dimensional FLASH scans during therapy readily corresponded to the total lesion size on three-dimensional Turbo-FLASH scans after therapy. Hence, it was possible to predict the total lesion size based on measurements intraoperatively.

In conclusion, our results show great promise in the value of MRI in monitoring LITT. However, the quantification of temperature especially in the periphery of the induced lesion and within the surrounding viable brain must still be studied. There are several approaches to reach this goal. Diffusion-sensitive MRI has been shown to be sensitive to temperature [8, 9]. T1-relaxation measurements with an acquisition time of seconds are another possibility of approaching this goal [10].

References

1. Anzai Y, Lufkin RB, Castro DJ, Farahani K, Jabour BA, Layfield LJ, Udkoff R, Hanafee WN (1991) MR imaging-guided interstitial Nd:YAG laser phototherapy: dosimetry study of acute tissue damage in an in vivo model. JMRI 1:553–559
2. Ascher PW (1990) Interstitial thermotherapy of brain tumours with Nd:YAG laser under real time MRI control. SPIE 1200:242–245
3. Bettag M, Schober R, Sabel M, Ulrich F, Schwarzmaier HJ, Hessel S (1992) Laser-induzierte interstitielle Thermotherapie – experimentelle Untersuchungen am Rattenhirn. Lasermedizin 8:58–62
4. Bettag M, Ulrich F, Fürst G, Langen UJ, Roosen N, Kiwit JCW, Hessel S, Mödder U, Bock WJ (1991) Gadolinium-DPTA-enhanced MRI and positron emission tomography of stereotactic laser-induced interstitial thermal therapy of cerebral gliomas. Neuroradiology 33:37–39

5. Bettag M, Ulrich F, Schober R, Bock WJ (1991) Stereotactic laser therapy in cerebral gliomas. Acta Neurochir (Wien) 52:81–83
6. Bown SG (1983) Phototherapy of tumors. World J Surg 7:700–709
7. Jolesz FA, Bleier AR, Jakab P, Ruenzel PW, Huttl K, Jako GJ (1988) MR imaging of laser-tissue interactions. Radiology 168:249–253
8. LeBihan D, Breton E, Lallemand D, Aubin ML, Vignaud J, Laval-Jeantet M (1988) Separation of diffusion and perfusion in intravoxel incoherent motion MR imaging. Radiology 168:497–505
9. LeBihan D, Delannoy J, Levin RL (1989) Temperature mapping with MR imaging of molecular diffusion: application to hyperthermia. Radiology 171:853–857
10. Nekolla S, Gneiting T, Syha J, Deichmann R, Haase A (1992) T1 maps by k-space reduced snapshot-FLASH MRI. J Comput Assist Tomogr 16:327–332
11. Roux FX, Merienne L, Leriche B, Lucerna S, Turak B, Devaux BC, Chodkiewicz JP (1992) Laser interstitial thermotherapy in stereotactical neurosurgery. Lasers Med Sci 7:121–126
12. Salcman M, Ebert PS (1991) In vitro response of human glioblastoma and canine glioma cells to hyperthermia, radiation, and chemotherapy. Neurosurgery 29:526–531
13. Schober R, Bettag M, Sabel M, Ulrich F, Hessel S (1993) The fine structure of zonal changes in experimental Nd:YAG laser-induced interstitial thermotherapy. Lasers Surg Med 13:234–241
14. Sugiyama K, Sakai T, Fujishima I, Ryu H, Uemura K, Yokoyama T (1990) Stereotactic interstitial laser-hyperthermia using Nd-YAG laser. Stereotact Funct Neurosurg 54/55:501–505

Early Experiences with Percutaneous Nucleus Pulposus Denaturation in Treatment of Lumbar Disc Protrusions: An Alternative Neurosurgical Concept

P. Simons[1], E. Lensker[1], and K. von Wild[1]

Introduction

For the treatment of lumbar disc disease one would favor a minimally invasive method, if possible even without producing peridural scars. Various techniques have been developed, ranging from chemonucleolysis to percutaneous discectomies using forceps by an entry up to 8 mm in diameter. The advantages and disadvantages are well known and have been published elsewhere. In 1986 Ascher introduced a method of decompressing the affected nerve by reducing the volume of the herniation and nucleus using a 1064-nm Nd-YAG Laser [1]. Our prospective study evaluated the results of this treatment as a possible standard neurosurgical procedure, using a modified setting with intradiscal saline irrigation.

Materials and Methods

Between 7 July 1992 and 16 September 1992, 50 patients entered our prospective study, following a pilot study in animal and postmortem models [3]. All patients suffered from a typical sciatica, confirmed by nuclear resonance imaging and resistant to extensive conservative therapy. The patients' ages were between 26 and 65 years; 26 were men and 24 women. We operated on 55 lumbar discs (4 x L3–4; 31 x L4–5; 20 x L5-S1). Patients were operated in the operating room under sterile conditions and using fluoroscopy. After placing a 2.1-mm needle in the center of the disc, by the standard dorsolateral approach, we performed a discometry and a discography to exclude perforation. We then connected the laser fiber with a standard infusion system and a 1.2-mm inner needle. Inner needle and fiber were inserted in the 2.1-mm needle (already positioned), ensuring that the fiber tip extended out only 1–2 mm. Using a Medilas 40/60 Fibertom (MBB Medizintechnik, Munich) 1064-nm Nd-YAG laser, we administered single-shot pulses of 10 W and 1-s duration with continuous pressure saline irrigation. Total energy administered was up to 1200 J per disc. Bedrest was provided on the day of operation, and dismissal was on the second day. The results were scored according to the following criteria: *very good*: no neurological deficit, free of pain, return to work; *good*: minor complaints, no medication needed, return to work; *satisfactory*: under strain more complaints, return to part-time work, needing medication;

[1] Neurosurgical Department, Clemenshospital, Duesbergweg 124, 48153 Münster, Germany.

Advances in Neurosurgery, Vol. 22
B. L. Bauer, M. Brock, M. Klinger (Eds.)

failure: major complaints or microdiscectomy needed, did not return to work. We first evaluated the patients on the dismissal day to obtain information on the immediate decompressing effect of the laser denaturation.

Results

Of the 50 patients, the results in 37 were considered as very good, in 11 as good, in 1 as satisfactory, and in 1 as a failure (reoperated). A follow-up examination was carried out 62–265 days postoperatively (mean 184 days). The same criteria were used. Four patients could not be reached, and thus only 46 were evaluated. Of these, 28 were considered as very good, 3 as good (together 67%), 11 as satisfying, and 4 as failures (3 were reoperated, showing free fragments). We evaluated the subjective findings using the Visual Analogue Scale [4]; the three patients reoperated on were excluded. The postoperative improvement in sciatica was very marked ($p < 0.001$; Fig. 1). Even more important to us was the decompressive effect on the nerve roots. Paresis was reduced to 30% of the preoperative level and hypesthesia and Laseque's sign was reduced to half (Fig. 2).

Complications. At follow-up magnetic resonance imaging showed in one patient, who still had low back pain but no longer sciatica, a lesion of the upper endplate of the fourth and the lower endplate of the third lumbar vertebral body, without any inflammatory signs, after laser denaturation at L3-4 (probably caused by a direct heat lesion). Retrospectively the patient complained of lumbar pain during the operation, which is quite unusual during laser denaturation. Complications due to the puncture or damage to the nerves or retroperitoneal structures did not occur.

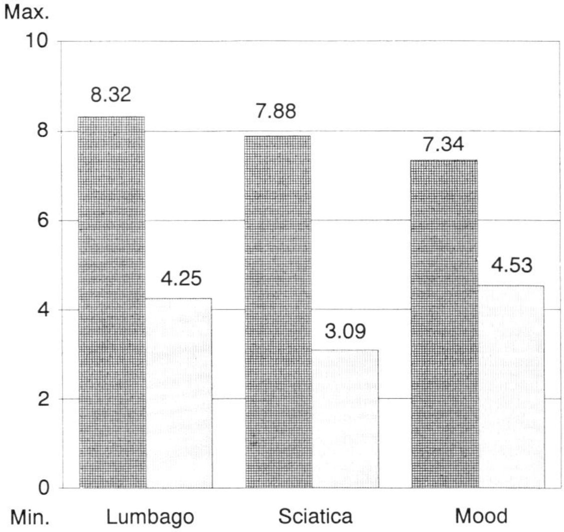

Fig. 1. Results in 43 patients on the Visual Analogue Scale, ranking from 0 = minimal (no low back pain, no sciatica, good mood) to 10 = maximal (severe low back pain, severe sciatica, bad mood), comparing pre- and postoperative findings. *Dark columns*, preoperative; *light columns*, postoperative

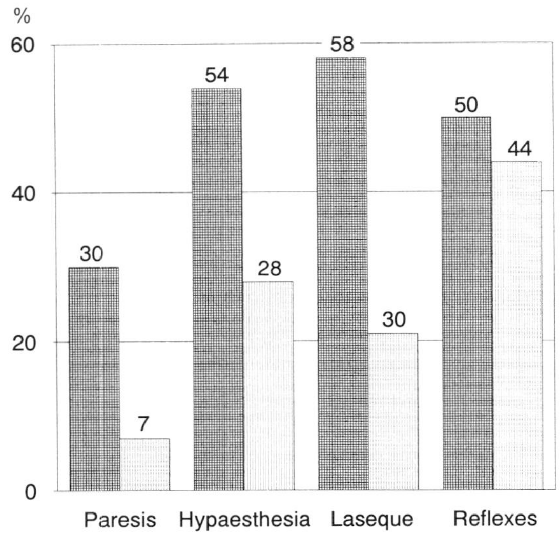

Fig. 2. Percentage of 43 patients showing nerve root compression measured by various neurological symptoms. *Dark columns*, preoperative; *light columns*, postoperative

Discussion

To explain our method one must understand something of laser physics. Laser light administered to tissue is partly reflected and partly passes unchanged, but the effective part is that which is absorbed. The energy of a 1064-nm Nd-YAG laser is only partly (approximately 30%) absorbed in the nearly white nuclear tissue. A typical energy-effect curve can therefore be seen as follows. Administering the laser energy in the nucleus, the nucleus first heats up to 60–70 °C, causing a denaturation of tissue [1, 2]. The radius of this heating is about 4–5 mm around the fiber tip. At the endplates temperatures of approximately 20–30 °C are measured. On the recommendation of J. Hellinger (personal communication) we administered moderate energy per pulse (10 W/s) at 5-s intervals. In this way heat lesion of the endplates can be avoided. With the laser in progress a carbonization of tissue at the laser tip appears at approximately 500 J. Thus more energy is absorbed, and the temperature rises. The tissue immediately adjacent to the tip is even vaporized. To avoid a residual debris of carbonized tissue – causing severe lumbar pain for several days to weeks – and to cool the disc while also letting the laser light flow to the deeper parts we use a pressure saline infusion. In treating the lumbar disc protrusions we attempt to achieve two goals: reduction in intradiscal pressure and retrieval of the herniated mass. We thus reach our first goal – pressure reduction – by vaporization and the second goal – mass reduction – by denaturation.

Our experimental study shows the advantages and risks of this irrigation modification [3]. In a typical laser treatment the fluid returns clear until approximately 500 J; thereafter the fluid turns brown and bubbles out of the needle. Carbonized cells are verified histologically in the collected fluid. In this prospective study on 50 patients there was an excellent immediate decompression effect: 97% rated as very good or good at the day of dismissal. At the follow-up (mean 184 days) 67% were in this group, thus indicating that a mass reduction was achieved with nerve root decompression showing a promising long-term effect. No severe complications occurred. The one patient with the endplate lesion showed the benefit of cooling and the need to stretch the interpulse interval in the case of any low back pain occurring during laser.

Conclusion

Laser denaturation using a 1064-nm Nd-YAG laser in a pressure saline infusion set with pulses of 1 s duration and 10 W, up to a total of 1200 J, seems a simple and effective method to reduce lumbar nerve root compression in a clinical setting. Our 67% very good and good results at follow-up together with the low complication rate justifies the further use of this method to treat selected patients with lumbar disc herniation, thus avoiding peridural scar formation.

References

1. Ascher PW (1991) Laser trends in minimally invasive treatment atherosclerosis, disk herniation. J Clin Laser Med Surg 2:49–57
2. Choy DSJ, Ascher PW, Saddekni S, Alkaitis D, Liebler W, Hughes J, Diwan S, Altman P (1992) Percutaneous laser disc decompression. A new therapeutic modality. Spine 17(8):949–956
3. Lensker E, von Wild K, Simons P, Hobik HP, Lehmann RR Effect of the 1064-nm Nd-YAG Laser on lumbar intervertebral disc tissue: experimental pilot study. Adv Neurosurg 22 (in press)
4. Scott J, Huskisson EC (1979) Accuracy of subjective measurements made with or without previous scores: an important source of error in serial measurements of subjective states. Ann Rheum Dis 38:558–559

Experimental Neurosurgery

Effect of the 1064–nm Nd-YAG Laser on Lumbar Intervertebral Disc Tissue: Experimental Study for Assessing the Operation Concept

E. Lensker[1], P. Simons[1], K. von Wild[1], H. P. Hobik[2], and R. R. Lehmann[3]

Introduction

Increasing importance is being given to minimally invasive, percutaneous methods in the treatment of patients with therapy-resistant lumboischialgiae [8]. Using the dorsolateral approach, various procedures have been developed to decompress the affected nerve root. While chemonucleolysis decomposes the intervertebral disc tissue by a chondrolytic enzyme, other methods reduce the disc volume mechanically by forceps or automated probes. In 1986 Ascher was the first to use laser radiation clinically to decompress intervertebral discs [4]. Good results have been reported although various types of lasers and parameters are in use [1, 4, 9–11]. Nevertheless, there are considerable discrepancies in the conception of this method. Does the mechanism work on thermally achieved volume reduction only or must additive effects also be taken into account? Even the problem of serious complications that may arise has not yet been finally answered [6]. We considered these questions on the basis of our hospital-specific method in an experimental study.

Material and Methods

We use the Nd-YAG laser with a wavelength of 1064 nm at a power level of 10 W. Between each single set of pulses of 1 s we pause for 2–3 s. The laser fiber contacts the tissue as a bare fiber. By means of a modified infusion system NaCl solution is consecutively irrigated.

For this study we used human cadaver intervertebral discs provided by the Forensic Medicine Institute, Münster. These had been taken out 36 h after death, most recent on the day of treatment, or after refrigeration at 4 °C on the next day. Disqualification criteria were an age of younger than 18 years or older than 70 years, pathological alterations in the lumbal part of the spine, or traumatically caused lesions.

The electron microscopic investigations were performed with swine discs due to their availability for the laser procedure 3 h postmortem, and these were fixed in

[1] Abt. Neurochirurgie, Clemenshospital, Duesbergweg 124, 48153 Münster, Germany.
[2] Institut für Pathologie, Clemenshospital, Duesbergweg 124, 48153 Münster, Germany.
[3] Institut für Anatomie, Westfälischen Wilhelms-Universität Münster, Vesaliusweg 2–4, 48149 Münster, Germany.

Advances in Neurosurgery, Vol. 22
B. L. Bauer, M. Brock, M. Klinger (Eds.)

3% glutaraldehyde immediately thereafter. To compensate for their smaller volume the total energy supply was reduced from the clinical dose of 1200 J to only 600 J.

Radiation Distribution

To evaluate the spread of radiation in the tissue, a lumbar intervertebral disc was dissected on one side from its endplate while the adjacent vertebral body of the contralateral side was fixed on a specially prepared board. This gave us the possi-

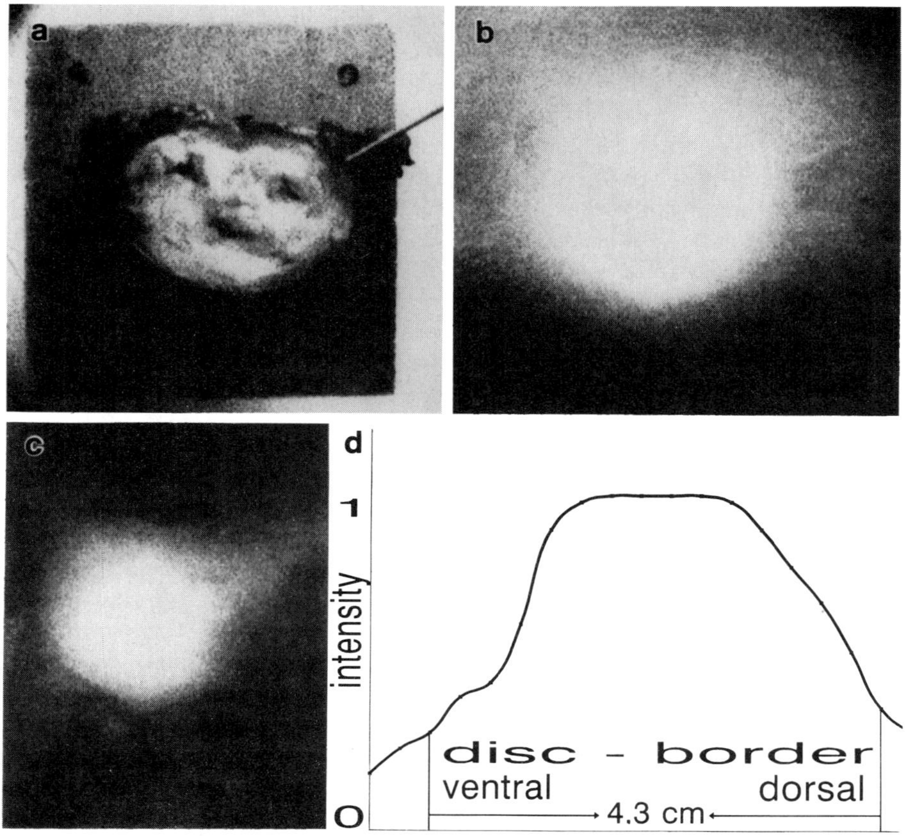

Fig. 1. a Native infrared top view of a dissected intervertebral disc mounted on our fixation board. The laser fiber is centered in the nucleus pulposus with the cannula coming from the upper right. **b** Radiation distribution at the beginning of the laser period. Penetrating laser light reaches the whole disc without detectable intensity decrease in the periphery. **c** Radiation distribution after administration of half the clinical dose (600 J) **d** Scanning graph of picture **c** illustrating the decrease in spread in the dorsoventral direction. The plateau of maximal intensity descends nonlinearly to the disc border

bility to direct the laser fiber into the middle of the disc by means of a pilot cannula. Using a camera (type N 2606, Hamamatsu) equipped with a C 2400-03 detector suitable for the near infrared light of our laser, we investigated the radiation spread in the tissue without taking into account any thermal effects.

Results. At the beginning of the laser procedure, the whole disc flashes without giving evidence of a significant decrease in intensity in the peripheral parts. After administering half the clinical dose the radiation is more concentrated in the center of the disc although the scattered laser light still reaches the outer zone (Fig. 1).

Mass Effect

Isolated segments of the lumbar part of the spine were weighed before and after radiation by means of digital scales permitting an accuracy of 0.001 g. Under clinical standard conditions the laser energy level was varied, from 10 to 15 to 20 W.

Results. Mass reduction correlated with the amount of energy administered but generally ranges at about 2 g. Doubling of the clinical level resulted in an increase of only 0.26 g, from 1.84 to 2.1 g.

Thermal Effect

Using an automated water bath, unilateral dissected discs were warmed to exactly 34 °C. This temperature represents the turning point of our thermographic film. After positioning the cannula tip in the center of the nucleus pulposus, the film was attached to the prepared tissue and the laser activated. The period of laser pulses varied from 1 to 2 s and those of the intermittent pauses from 2 to 5 s. We then observed a colored contour, delineating the outer border of the laser-heated scope (Fig. 2).

Results. (a) The intervertebral disc operates as a thermal accumulator because of additive effects. (b) The velocity of thermal saturation and the maximal expansion of the heated area depend strongly on the laser output. (c) Heated irrigation or tissue fluid can flow through degenerative fissures into the periphery of the annulus fibrosus.

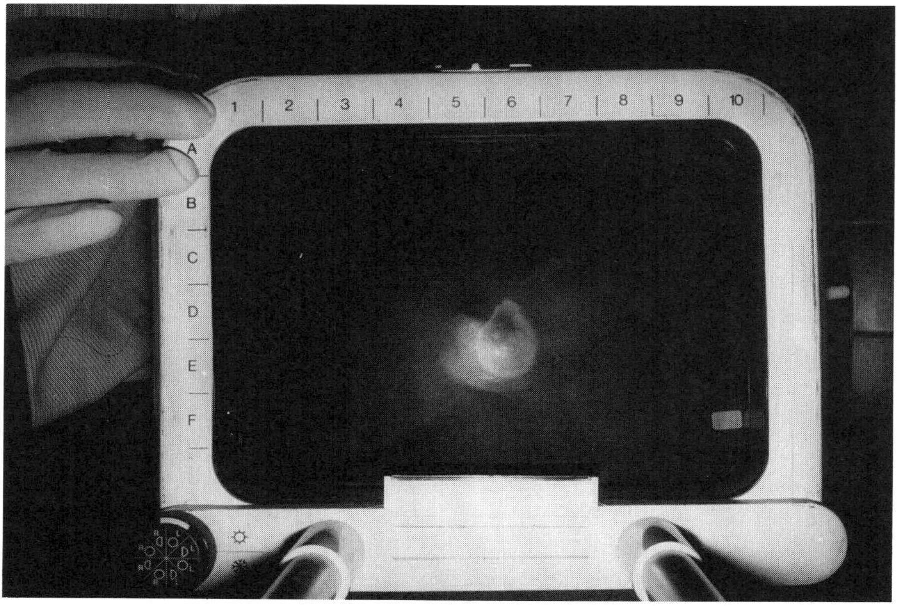

Fig. 2. Thermographic picture showing the irregular shape of heating due to degenerative changes within the annulus fibrosus

Tissue Reactions

Histologic specimens were made from human discs subjected to laser light by staining with hematoxylin-eosin and azan. Not only general laser-induced tissue alterations should be examined but also the irrigation effect compared with nonirrigated specimens. Electron microscopic examination of the swine discs took place with a magnification of 1150–15500 and was used to determine the radiation penetration depth morphologically. Cellular and intercellular alterations of the nucleus pulposus and the annulus fibrosus were compared with congruent native tissue at distances of 3–15 mm from the fiber tip.

Results. Slide preparation of the nonirrigated disc shows a superficial carbonization zone with an adjacent vacuolated area (Fig. 3). In still deeper parts necrotic tissue can be identified. On the other hand, carbonized products are removed to a large extent when irrigating subsequently. Only sporadic carbonized particles can be discovered histologically. A nonlaminated necrosis with structural tissue disorder is dominant. The electron microscopic picture of a typical vital cell of the nucleus pulposus shows large intracytoplasmic vacuoles containing proteoglycans [5]. The oval nucleus is encircled by typical filaments (Fig. 4). A comparable cell from the tissue subjected to laser light shrinks to a dysmorphous structure of approximately the size of the vital nucleus. The annulus fibrosus consists mainly of

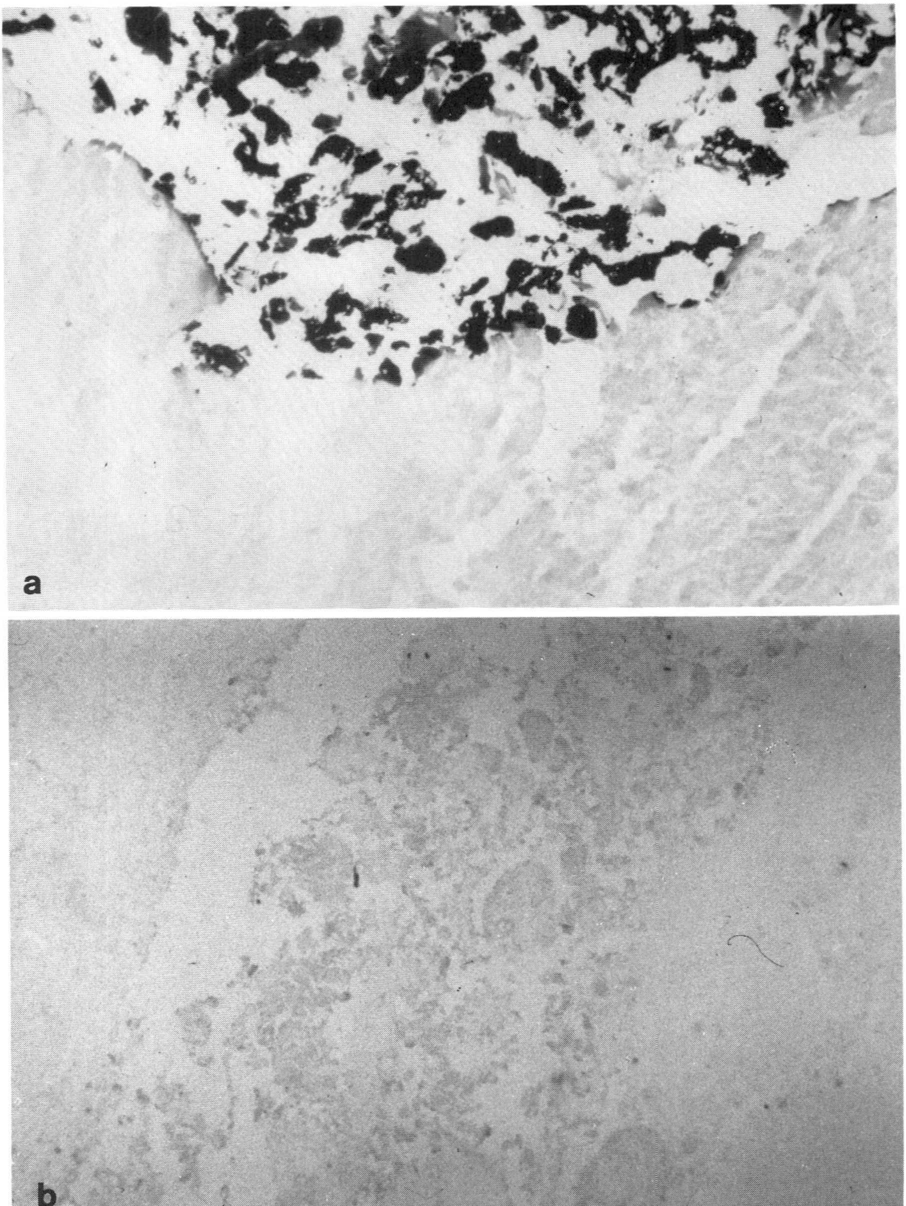

Fig. 3. a Hematoxylin and eosin stained histological specimen of the lasered disc without consecutive irrigation. Carbonized particles can be detected as a nearly continuous layer on the surface of the tissue. The adjacent vacuolated zone is generated thermally due to gas formation during vaporization. **b** The irrigated specimen by contrast shows an irregular necrosis with only sporadic dispersed carbonized products

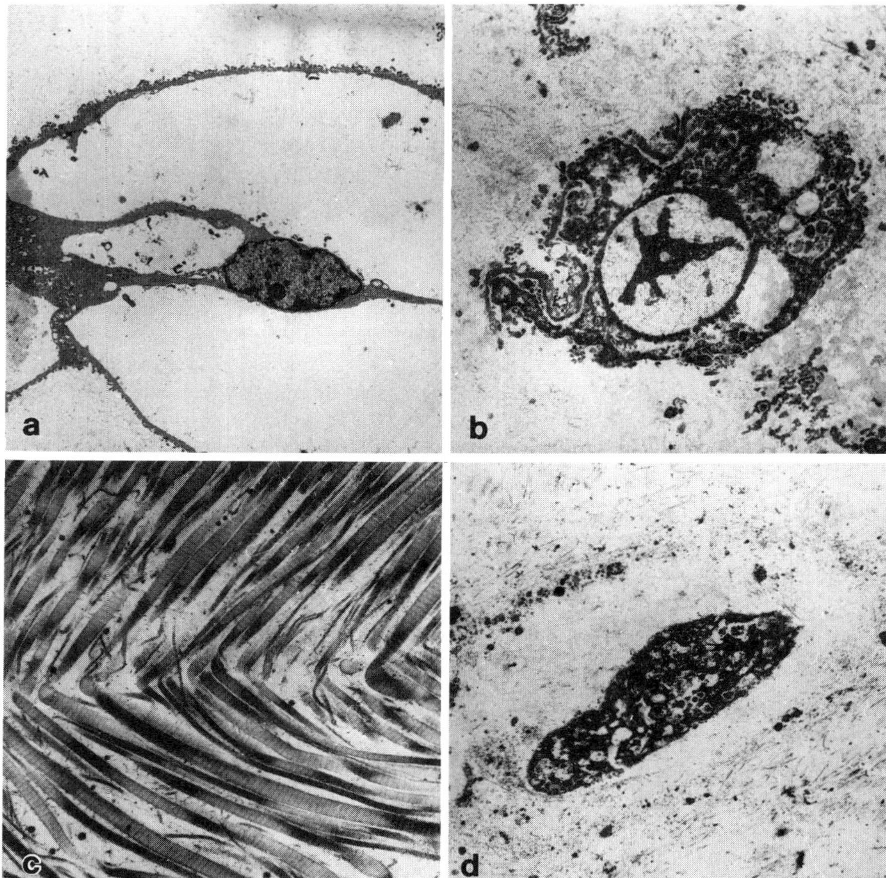

Fig. 4. a Electron micrograph of native nucleus pulposus. Picture of a vital cell with large intracytoplasmatic vacuoles containing recently synthesized proteoglycans. The active cell nucleus is structured into eu- and heterochromatin and surrounded by typical filaments. x 1150. **b** Electron micrograph of lasered pulposus. Equivalently radiated cell to demonstrate irreversible cell death. The avital organelles have shrunk and are of mostly unidentifiable origin. x 2650. **c** Electron micrograph of native annulus fibrosus. Typical collagen fibers in the outer annulus fibrosus with fish-bone profile. This cross-cross arrangement ensures the resistance of torsional and flexional deformity and prevents rupture. x 2650. **d** Electron micrograph of lasered annulus fibrosus. The radiated cell of a congruent zone with **c** is irreparably damaged. The surrounding collagen fibers are affected and due to insufficient cross-connections out of function. x 2650

transversely cross-linked collagenous fibers with the characteristic fish-bone profile. Even the cells of the outer annulus, at a distance of more than 15 mm to the fiber tip, are crumpled and necrotic. The intercellular collagenous fibers are damaged and disintegrated.

Discussion

Nd-YAG laser radiation penetrates deep into the tissue. Vorwerk and colleagues investigated the optical properties of degenerated intervertebral disc tissue at a wavelength of 1064 nm [14]. In accordance with our results, they found relatively high remission (30.3%) and scattering (38,7%) in addition to low absorption (31%) coefficients. This confirms that the effect of the laser is not only local but reaches the complete disc. The radiation spread changes with the formation of carbonization products on the superficial tissue. The decrease in scattering is a consequence of higher absorption on darkly burned material [14].

A reproducible mass reduction can be achieved by means of laser [3]. Brinckmann and collegues reported the change of some mechanical parameters from discectomy [23]. Disc height and intradiscal pressure decrease whereas radial disc bulge increases proportionally to the excised tissue. Regarding our clinical removal of 2 g they assessed a reduction in height of 1.6 mm, in pressure of 33%, and a further bulge of 0.4 mm. Due to gas formation during the laser procedure we must consider an initial rise in intradiscal pressure [4]. It is clinically significant that disc space narrowing reduces the contact force on a nerve root from a root protrusion [13]. This may explain the patient's immediate pain relief.

The real extension of tissue damage by laser can be ascertained only by electron microscopic examinations. Compared with the light microscope alterations can be detected twice as deep [7]. We established that the volume reduction due to laser light is achieved only with a profound necrosis of the intervertebral disc. The extent to which the penetrating radiation or only the heating is responsible for this cannot be finally answered today.

According to Siebert there is no temperature rise over 50 °C at a distance of more than 4 mm to the fiber tip [12]. Our studies support the view that surrounding neurovascular structures do not seem to undergo thermal damage, but with higher outputs the outer annulus fibrosus lies in the scope of warming. Preoperative discography is reasonable for the detection of preexistent annulus defects with the risk of warm leaks.

Consecutive irrigation during the laser procedure entails some risks [11]. The irrigation fluid not only conducts the resulting heat into the extracorporeal but probably also in the peripheral regions of the disc. The removal of carbonization products increases the radiation penetration even further.

Conclusion

1. The surgeon performing the laser decompression must be aware of the physical nature of laser radiation as complications due to uncontrolled distant absorptions may arise.
2. Modifications in the perioperative management such as irrigation or suction may optimize the method.

3. Regular follow-up examinations of the patient are necessary to diagnose possible sequelae as the exchange of necrotic material from the bradytrophic tissue takes a long time to occur.

References

1. Berlien H-P, Müller G (1989) Angewandte Lasermedizin. Lehr und Handbuch für Praxis und Klinik. Ecomed, Landsberg
2. Brinckmann P, Grottenboer H (1991) Change of disc height, radial disc bulge, and intradiscal pressure from discectomy. An in vitro investigation on human lumbar discs. Spine 16(6):641–646
3. Choy DSJ, Altman PA, Case RB, Trokel SL (1991) Laser radiation at various wavelength for decompression of intervertebral disk. Experimental observations on human autopsy specimens. Clin Orthop 267(6):245–250
4. Choy DSJ, Ascher PW, Saddekni S, Alkaitis D, Liebler W, Hughes J, Diwan S, Altman P (1992) Percutaneous laser disc decompression. A new therapeutic modality. Spine 17(8):949–956
5. Humzah MD, Soames RW (1988) Human intervertebral disc: structure and function. Anat Rec 220:337–356
6. Kambin P (1991) Laser nuclear ablation. In: Kambin P (ed) Arthroscopic microdiscectomy. Minimal intervention in spinal surgery. Urban and Schwarzenberg, Munich, pp 133–136
7. Lehmann RR, Willital GH (1990) Morphological alterations following laser resection of abdominal tumors in children. Lasermedizin 0:25–35
8. Mayer HM, Brock M (1988) Behandlung des lumbalen Bandscheibenvorfalls. Die perkutane Diskektomie. Dtsch Arztebl 85(13):853–858
9. Mayer HM, Brock M, Berlien H-P, Weber B (1992) Percutaneous endoscopic laser discectomy (PELD). A new surgical technique for nonsequestrated lumbar discs. Acta Neurochir Suppl (Wien) 54:53–58
10. Philandrianos G, Rose C, Siebert WE (1991) Behandlung des Bandscheibenvorfalls mit dem Laser. In: Siebert WE, Wirth CJ (eds) Laser in der Orthopädie. Einsatzmöglichkeiten der Lasertechnik bei operativen und diagnostischen Verfahren am Bewegungsapparat. Thieme, Stuttgart, New York
11. Siebert WE, Bise K, Breitner S, Fritsch K, Wirth CJ (1988) Die Nucleus-pulposus-Vaporisation – eine neue Technik zur Behandlung des Bandscheibenvorfalls? Orthop Prax 24(12):732–735
12. Siebert W (1993) Percutaneous laser disc decompression: the European experience. Spine State Art Rev 7(1):103–133
13. Spencer DL, Miller JAA, Bertolini JE (1984) The effect of intervertebral disc space narrowing on the contact force between the nerve root and a simulated disc protrusion. Spine 9(4):422–426
14. Vorwerk D, Husemann T, Blazek V, Zolotas G, Günther RW (1989) Laserablation des Nucleus pulposus: optische Eigenschaften von degeneriertem Bandscheibengewebe im Wellenlängenbereich von 200 bis 2200 nm. Fortschr Rontgenstr 151(6):725–728
15. Yonezawa T, Tanaka S, Watanabe H, Onomura T, Atsumi K (1989) Percutaneous intradiscal laser discectomy. In: Mayer HM, Brock M (eds) Percutaneous lumbar discectomy. Springer, Berlin Heidelberg New York, pp 197–204

Cytotoxic Glial Swelling by Arachidonic Acid

F. Staub[1], A. Winkler[1], J. Peters[1], O. Kempski[2], and A. Baethmann[1]

Introduction

Arachidonic acid (AA, 20:4) is a major constituent of membrane phospholipids in brain tissue. Normally, the free fatty acid is present only in a small amount, but it accumulates under adverse conditions, such as ischemia or brain injury [1, 9]. The release of free fatty acid involves activation of phospholipases and breakdown of membrane phospholipids. AA in particular is considered to mediate pathological processes. The polyunsaturated compound is a precursor of prostaglandins, leukotrienes, and oxygen-derived free radicals [11]. In cerebral ischemia concentrations of free AA of up to 0.5 m*M*/kg have been found in brain tissue [9].

Noxious properties of AA have been observed in many investigations. For instance, it has been demonstrated that lipid peroxidation or disturbances of respiration in mitochondria are induced by the fatty acid [2, 6]. Moreover, AA has a significant role in brain edema. The fatty acid has been found to induce swelling of cerebral tissue slices in vitro and to increase permeability of the blood-brain barrier in vivo [3, 10]. Since AA may also be involved in cytotoxic brain edema formation, we have currently investigated the glial cell volume response during administration of the fatty acid. Additional experiments were performed to analyze whether respective effects can be inhibited by blocking of the cyclo- and lipoxygenase pathway or, by inhibition of free radical formation or lipid peroxidation. To assess the specificity of AA (20:4) comparative experiments were made using linoleic acid (18:2) or stearic acid (18:0). The study was carried out in vitro under control of relevant parameters to examine the significance of a single pathophysiological factor in isolation [8]. For this purpose suspension of C6 glioma cells or of astrocytes from primary culture were incubated under continuous recording of pH, pO_2, and temperature with assessment of the cell volume by flow cytometry.

Materials and Methods

C6 glioma cells were cultivated as monolayers in petri dishes using Dulbecco's modified minimal essential medium with the addition of 25 m*M* bicarbonate. The

[1] Institut für Chirurgische Forschung, Klinikum Großhadern, Ludwig-Maximillians-Universität, Marchioninistr. 15, 81366 München, Germany.
[2] Institut für Neurochirurgische Pathophysiologie, Johannes-Gutenberg-Universität, Langenbeckstr. 1, 55131 Mainz, Germany.

Advances in Neurosurgery, Vol. 22
B. L. Bauer, M. Brock, M. Klinger (Eds.)

medium was supplemented with 10% fetal calf serum, 100 IU/ml penicillin G, and 50 µg/ml streptomycin. The cells were grown in a humidified atmosphere of 5% CO_2 and room air at 37 °C. Glial cells for primary culture were prepared from 3-day-old rats according to a modified method of Frangakis and Kimelberg [5]. The culture conditions were identical to those described above. The cells were harvested for the experiment with 0.05% trypson/0.02% EDTA in phosphate-buffered saline and washed twice thereafter. After resuspension in serum-free medium the glial cells were transferred to a plexiglas incubation chamber with electrodes for control of pH, temperature, and pO_2. Details of the method have been published elsewhere [8].

The volume of the glial cells was determined by flow cytometry using an advanced Coulter system with hydrodynamic focusing [7]. The experiments with administration of AA were performed after a 45-min control period used for measurements of normal cell volume and medium osmolality. Subsequently, AA (20:4) was added to the suspension in a dose range of 0.01–1.0 m*M* (final concentration). Cell volume and viability were measured for 90 min during incubation with AA. Comparative studies using linoleic (18:2) or stearic acid (18:0) were made at concentrations of 0.1 m*M*. Further experiments with AA at this concentration were conducted with inhibition of the cyclo- and lipoxygenase pathway by BW755C (0.2 m*M*), with scavenging of superoxide radicals by superoxide dismutase (SOD, 300 U/ml), or during blocking of lipid peroxidation by the aminosteroid U-74389F (0.1 m*M*). Inhibitors were administered to the suspension 15 min prior to addition of AA. In further experiments cell swelling by 0.1 m*M* AA was studied in Na^+-free medium, where Na^+ ions were replaced for this purpose by choline, and bicarbonate by 10 m*M* HEPES.

Results

Administration of AA to the suspension caused an immediate dose-dependent swelling of C6 glioma cells. AA concentrations as low as 0.01 m*M* led to an increase in cell volume to 103.0% ± 1.0% of control within 10 min ($p < 0.01$). A volume increase to 110.0% ± 1.5% (Table 1) or 118.8% ± 1.5% of control was obtained, when the cells were administered with AA at 0.1 or 1.0 m*M*, respectively ($p < 0.001$). After initial and rapid swelling the increased cell volume was largely constant for the remaining observation period (Table 1). Swelling of C6 glioma cells by AA was confirmed in experiments using astrocytes from primary culture. Addition of AA at a dose level of 0.05 or 0.1 m*M* led to a swelling of astrocytes ($p < 0.01$) which was comparable to that of C6 glioma cells. To assess the specificity of the AA-induced glial swelling, cell swelling inducing properties of 0.1 m*M* linoleic (18:2) or 0.1 m*M* stearic acid (18:0) were tested (Table 1). While stearic acid was not found to induce volume changes in the glioma cells, cell volume was significantly increased by linoleic acid ($p < 0.01$). Nevertheless, the volume increase to linoleic acid was only about 50% of that found when AA was administered at the same concentration ($p < 0.05$; Table 1). Additional experiments were performed to analyze mechanisms of the AA-induced glial swelling. Inhibition of the metabolization of AA by cyclo- and lipoxygenase using the dual pathway inhibitor BW755C did not affect glial swelling from AA (Table 1). Administration of SOD to scavenge superoxide radicals did not influence the initial volume response but reduced glial swelling by AA significantly at 60 min after addition of the fatty acid ($p < 0.01$). Preincubation with the aminosteroid U-74389F, however, prevented cell swelling from AA completely ($p < 0.01$). Similar results were obtained when the experiments were conducted with choline for replacement of Na^+ ions in the suspension medium and HEPES as buffer compound instead of bicarbonate (Table 1).

Discussion

The present results demonstrate the powerful potential of AA to induce glial swelling. Exposure of glial cells to the fatty acid led to a dose-dependent cell volume increase at concentrations which have been observed in brain tissue in vivo under pathophysiological conditions, such as focal injury or ischemia [1, 9].

Not only AA but also its metabolites, such as prostaglandins or leukotrienes, can be considered to have mediator functions in the brain under respective circumstances [11]. The present results on inhibition of the cyclo- and lipoxygenase pathway by BW755C suggest, however, that AA itself is the swelling-inducing agent and not these metabolites. On the other hand, since administration of the aminosteroid U-74389F almost completely inhibited cell swelling from AA, lipid peroxidation must be taken into consideration as a major factor in AA-induced cell swelling. Lipid peroxidation commences when oxygen-derived free radicals accumulate in the presence of free fatty acids [2, 4]. It is conceivable that superoxide radicals generated by the conversion of AA interact with AA as substrate, thereby initiating the formation of lipid and lipid peroxide radicals. The marginal success of SOD in reducing glial swelling from AA suggests that superoxide radicals formed in the intracellular compartment are not available for the enzyme since SOD as a large, hydrophilic molecule is unlikely to penetrate the plasma membrane. Accumulation of lipid and lipid peroxide radicals, however, may result in a chain reaction, acting mainly on fatty acids of cell membranes and consequently leading to damage of the double-lipid layer [2]. The results indicate further that the swelling-inducing properties of free fatty acids are related to their number of nonsaturated chemical bonds. Accordingly, the production of superoxide and lipid radicals from free fatty acids by glial cells appears to be directly correlated with the number of nonsaturated bonds. This is supported, albeit indirectly, by findings that formation of reactive radical species is minimal from saturated fatty acids as precursors [4]. Finally, glial swelling from AA was more or less completely prevented when the experiments were conducted in a Na^+-free suspension medium, making obvious the significance of the cellular uptake of Na^+, and thereby water as ultimate mechanism of the AA-induced cell volume increase.

Table 1. Volume response of C6 glioma cells to administration of AA (0.1 m*M*) to the suspension medium (cell volume in percentage of cell size in the last 15 min of the control period; mean ± SEM of four to seven experiments per group)

	Control			Incubation with free fatty acids					
	– 15 min	– 10 min	– 5 min	1 min	5 min	10 min	30 min	60 min	90 min
AA (0.1 m*M*)	100.40	99.93	99.67	104.45	110.04	112.17	111.00	109.58	106.85
	0.26	0.17	0.25	1.16	1.49	1.90	2.23	2.20	1.72
LA (0.1 m*M*)	100.36	99.63	100.01	103.05	106.53	105.88*	105.66	108.22	105.53
	0.61	0.35	0.75	0.71	0.82	0.76	0.82	1.38	1.41
SA (0.1 m*M*)	100.63	99.07	100.30	100.07**	100.45**	99.42**	99.36**	99.46**	100.25**
	0.37	0.64	0.28	0.54	0.96	0.26	1.44	2.13	2.23
AA (0.1 mM) +BW755C	99.88	99.90	100.23	103.84	109.60	111.18	112.36	107.57	106.91
	0.29	0.20	0.33	1.77	1.58	2.04	2.32	2.58	3.86
AA (0.1 m*M*) + SOD	99.84	100.25	99.91	104.59	108.28	109.42	106.79	103.19**	103.05
	0.09	0.44	0.43	2.03	1.98	1.17	0.82	1.03	0.80
AA (0.1 m*M*) + U-74289F	100.27	99.40	100.33	99.41**	100.10**	98.93**	99.47**	100.97**	101.39**
	0.33	0.49	0.35	0.70	1.29	1.35	1.37	1.11	1.53
AA (0.1 m*M*) Na^+-free medium	98.63	101.25	100.12	100.87**	101.65**	103.77**	100.01**	102.00**	103.46
	0.75	0.40	0.44	0.46	0.41	0.86	1.82	1.99	2.51

* $p < 0.05$ versus AA (0.1 m*M*); ** $p < 0.01$ versus AA (0.1 m*M*).
AA, Arachidonic acid; LA, linoleic acid; SA, stearic acid.

Conclusion

Taken together, the present data demonstrate the powerful properties of AA to induce cytotoxic swelling in glial cells obtained from an established cell line and from primary culture. The findings confirm that release and accumulation of the fatty acid in the brain under pathological conditions such as ischemia or trauma play an important role in glial swelling. The present data on quantitative dose-response relationships of glial swelling by AA provide a basis for specific methods of treatment, such as employment of aminosteroids to inhibit lipid peroxidation.

Acknowledgments. The excellent technical and secretarial assistance of Ingrid Kölbl, Helga Kleylein, and Monika Stucky is gratefully acknowledged. We appreciate the generous gifts of BW755C by Dr. Cooke, Wellcome Research Laboratories, Beckenham, Kent, UK, and of U-74389F by Dr. McCall, Upjohn Laboratories, Kalamazoo, MI, USA.

References

1. Baethmann A, Maier-Hauff K, Schürer L, Lange M, Guggenbichler C, Vogt W, Jacob K, Kempski O (1989) Release of glutamate and of free fatty acids in vasogenic brain edema. J Neurosurg 70:578–591
2. Braughler JM, Hall ED (1989) Central nervous system trauma and stroke. I. Biochemical considerations for oxygen radical formation and lipid peroxidation. Free Radic Biol Med 6:289–301
3. Chan PH, Fishman RA (1978) Brain edema: induction in cortical slices by polyunsaturated fatty acids. Science 201:358–360
4. Chan PH, Chen SF, Yu ACH (1988) Induction of intracellular superoxide radical formation by arachidonic acid and by polyunsaturated fatty acids in primary astrocytic culture. J Neurochem 50:1185–1193
5. Frangakis MV, Kimelberg HK (1984) Dissociation of neonatal rat brain by dispase for preparation of primary astrocyte cultures. Neurochem Res 9:1689–1698
6. Hillered L, Chan PH (1988) Role of arachidonic acid and other free fatty acids in mitochondrial dysfunction in brain ischemia. J Neurosci Res 20:451–456
7. Kachel V, Glossner E, Kordwig G, Ruhenstroth-Bauer G (1977) Fluvo-Metricell, a combined cell volume and cell fluorescence analyzer. J Histochem Cytochem 25:804–812
8. Kempski O, Chaussy L, Groß U, Zimmer M, Baethmann A (1983) Volume regulation and metabolism of suspended C6 glioma cells: an in vitro model to study cytotoxic brain edema. Brain Res 279:217–228
9. Kinouchi H, Imaizumi S, Yoshimoto T, Motomiya M (1990) Phenytoin affects metabolism of free fatty acids and nucleotides in rat cerebral ischemia. Stroke 21:1326–1332
10. Unterberg A, Wahl M, Hammersen F, Baethmann A (1987) Permeability and vasomotor response of cerebral vessels during exposure to arachidonic acid. Acta Neuropathol (Berl) 73:209–219
11. Wolfe LS (1982) Eicosanoids: prostaglandins, thromboxanes, leukotrienes, and other derivatives of carbon-20 unsaturated fatty acids. J Neurochem 38:1–14

Posttraumatic Brain Edema: Effects of the Novel Cl^- Transport Blocker Torasemide and the Inositol Triphosphate Analogue PP56

M. Stoffel[1], S. Berger[1], F. Staub[1], J. Eriskat[1], and A. Baethmann[1]

Introduction

Brain edema leading to intracranial hypertension is of major concern in cerebral disorders, such as head injury, stroke and brain tumors. Although cerebral tissue water content can be lowered by hypertonic solutions, for example, by mannitol, hypertonic saline, and glycerol, the treatment does not prevent further formation of edema. Methods of treatment may be more beneficial which also ameliorate breakdown of the blood-brain barrier and extravasation of edema fluid. This might be accomplished by inhibition of the formation or release, respectively, of mediator compounds which enhance development and persistence of brain edema.

The present experiments were conducted to study the therapeutic efficacy of two novel pharmacological agents on vasogenic brain edema in rats subjected to an acute cerebral lesion. Torasemide is a newly developed loop diuretic. It is an inhibitor of the $Na^+/K^+/Cl^-$ cotransporter and of Cl^- channels in kidney epithelial cells [15]. Therapeutic effects of torasemide were observed in intracranial hypertension from water intoxication in vivo as well as in cytotoxic glial swelling from acidosis in vitro [10, 14]. PP56 (D-myo-inositol-1,2,6-triphosphate) is an isomer of the intracellular second messenger IP_3. The compound, however, is probably not a competitive antagonist of IP_3 as it does not affect release of Ca^{2+} in cells [5]. Antiedematous properties of PP56 were found in peripheral organs in experimental inflammation or burns [6]. Further, PP56 antagonizes vasoconstriction of neuropeptide Y (NPY), a potent constrictor of rat or human cerebral arteries [4]. PP56 was studied here with regard to reduction in vasogenic brain edema from an acute cerebral lesion. For this purpose the cryolesion model was substantially refined in rats with improved reproducibility of the insult by employment of a computer-controlled stepper motor during induction of the lesion.

Materials and Methods

Preparation. Fifty-four male Sprague-Dawley rats of 250–350 g b.w. were anesthesized by ether followed by intraperitoneal chloral hydrate. The animals spontaneously breathed room air supplied with additional oxygen. A catheter was introduced into the tail artery for monitoring of blood pressure and to obtain blood

[1] Institut für Chirurgische Forschung, Klinikum Großhadern, Marchioninistr. 15, 81366 München, Germany.

Advances in Neurosurgery, Vol. 22
B. L. Bauer, M. Brock, M. Klinger (Eds.)

samples for determination of blood gases and hematocrit. Another catheter in the right jugular vein served for infusions of fluid and drugs. Body temperature was maintained at 38.5 °C by a servocontrolled heating pad. The animals's head was fixed in a stereotactic holder for preparation of a circular trephination (diameter 6 mm) of the left temporal skull leaving the dura mater intact. A metal probe (diameter 4.5 mm) was attached to a stereotactic device powered by a computer-controlled stepper motor. The probe cooled to –68 °C by a dry ice/acetone mixture was placed onto the exposed brain surface for 15 s.

Protocol. Administration of treatment started prior to induction of the lesion in both groups; treatment was given by a blinded investigator. Untreated animals with trauma (n = 12) were continuously infused with 0.5 ml saline/h. Animals with PP56 (Perstorp Pharma, Lund, Sweden) received either 40 mg/kg b.w. (low dose; $n = 10$) or 120 mg/kg b.w. (high dose; $n = 10$) dissolved in physiological saline (0.5 ml/h) which was continuously administered intravenously from 1 h prior to until 24 h after lesion. Animals with torasemide (Boehringer Mannheim, Germany) received either 1 mg/kg b.w. (low dose; $n = 10$) or 10 mg/kg b.w. (high dose; $n = 10$) at 30 min prior and 6 h after trauma. At 24 h after trauma the aminals were reanesthetized and killed by exsanguination. The cerebrum was rapidly removed and separated in the median plane. The hemispheres were placed into an air-tight glass vial for gravimetrical determination of fresh weight of the tissue. Water content of blood plasma or the brain specimen was obtained by the dry/wet weight method (drying at 110 °C for 24 h). Na^+ and K^+ contents of dried tissue specimen were determined by flame spectrophotometry. Hemispheric brain swelling was determined as increase in weight of the traumatized hemisphere over that of the contralateral hemisphere. Data are given as mean ± SEM. Unpaired data were analyzed by the Kruskal-Wallis test, paired data by the Friedman-Quade test. A level of $p < 0.05$ was considered significant.

Results

Systemic Parameters. No differences in systemic blood pressure were found among the various groups during the control period. Following treatment, however, a dose-dependent increase in mean arterial pressure was found ($p < 0.05$) in animals receiving torasemide within 90 min after first administration of the drug (Fig. 1) whereas PP56 had no effect. PP56 and torasemide at either high or low dose were without other effects, for example, on blood gases, hemoglobin, and hematocrit. Body weight was found to decrease by 8% within 24 h after trauma in all groups (Table 1).

Cerebral Water and Electrolytes. In animals with focal lesion the water content of the traumatized hemisphere was increased by approximately 1% compared to the contralateral hemisphere ($p < 0.001$). In untreated controls the water content of the

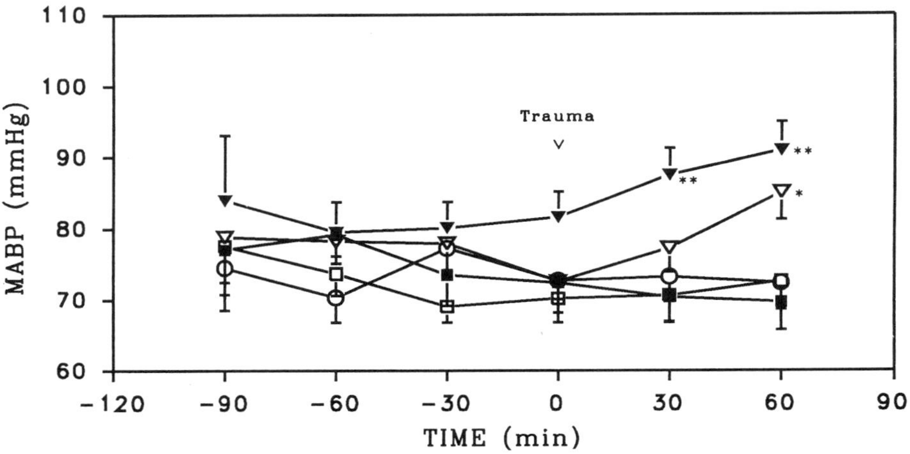

Fig. 1. Course of arterial blood pressure in untreated controls with a cryogenic lesion and following various treatments. $^{*}p < 0.05$ versus control; $^{**}p < 0.01$ versus control. Mean ± SEM. ○, Control, ∇, torasemide low dose, ▼ torasemide high dose; ❑, PP56 low dose; ■, PP56 high dose

Table 1. Blood pressure, hemocrit, arterial blood pH, and body weight subjected to a focal cold lesion of the brain under low-dose (LD) and high dose (HD) torasemide (Tora) and PP56

Group	Mean arterial pressure (mmHg)	Hemocrit (%)	pH –lg[H+]	Body weight (g)
Prior to Trauma				
Control	77.2 ± 3.5	43.6 ± 0.9	7.33 ± 0.01	312 ± 11
Tora LD	77.9 ± 3.7	43.5 ± 1.0	7.35 ± 0.01	328 ± 11
Tora HD	80.1 ± 3.7	42.3 ± 0.6	7.34 ± 0.01	312 ± 9
PP56 LD	67.0 ± 3.1	43.8 ± 0.9	7.31 ± 0.02	335 ± 14
PP56 HD	73.5 ± 4.3	43.3 ± 0.8	7.32 ± 0.01	309 ± 16
60 min after trauma				
Control	72.4 ± 3.3	44.4 ± 0.9	7.34 ± 0.01	–
Tora LD	85.1 ± 3.8*	42.8 ± 1.0	7.37 ± 0.01	–
Tora HD	90.9 ± 4.0**	43.6 ± 0.5	7.37 ± 0.01	–
PP56 LD	67.0 ± 3.7	46.7 ± 0.9	7.36 ± 0.01	–
PP56 HD	69.7 ± 3.9	42.9 ± 1.0	7.33 ± 0.01	–
24 h after trauma				
Control	–	43.1 ± 1.3	–	289 ± 11
Tora LD	–	42.2 ± 0.9	–	302 ± 10
Tora HD	–	42.4 ± 1.2	–	282 ± 10
PP56 LD	–	42.9 ± 0.7	–	310 ± 13
PP56 HD	–	42.9 ± 1.0	–	280 ± 15

$^{*}p < 0.05$ versus control; $^{**}p < 0.01$ versus control.

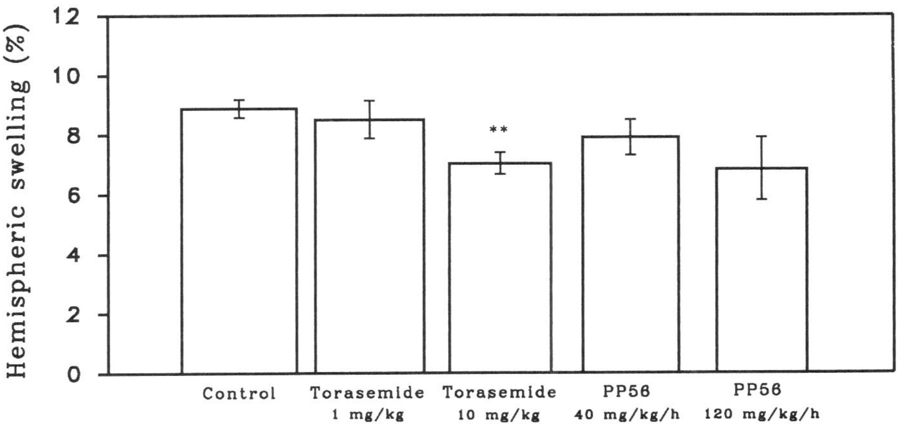

Fig. 2. Swelling of traumatized hemispheres, given as percentage increase in weight over that of the contralateral hemisphere, in untreated controls with trauma and animals with torasemide or PP56 at high- or low-dose treatment. $^{**}p < 0.01$ versus control. Mean ± SEM

injured (left) hemisphere was 81.25% ± 0.14% g/100 g f.w., while 79.93% ± 0.08% g/100 g f.w. were found in the control hemisphere. Low-dose PP56 had no effect on the cerebral water content of either hemispheres. High-dose PP56 had a tendency to lower the water content of the exposed and nonexposed hemispheres, however, without attaining statistical significance. Low-dose torasemide had no influence on the formation of brain edema in the traumatized hemisphere. On the other hand, high-dose torasemide was found to reduce the water content of the traumatized hemisphere to 80.82% ± 0.13% g/100 g f.w. ($p = 0.09$ versus control). The tissue electrolytes were in accordance with extravasation of a plasmalike edema fluid from disruption of the blood-brain barrier. Hence, the Na^+ content was increased whereas K^+ was decreased in the traumatized hemisphere of experimental animals with and without treatment.

Hemispheric Brain Swelling. In untreated controls the freezing lesion led to an increase in weight of 8.89% ± 0.29% over that of the contralateral hemisphere. Hemispheric swelling was somewhat attenuated by PP56, resulting in an increase in weight of 7.9% ± 0.60% ($p = 0.0646$) in the low-dose group, and of 6.85% ± 1.05% ($p = 0.3932$) in the high-dose group. High-dose torasemide afforded significant inhibition of hemispheric swelling from the lesion to 7.04% ± 0.36% ($p < 0.005$), whereas low-dose treatment had no effect. Hemispheric swelling amounted in the latter group to 8.51% ± 0.63% (Fig. 2).

Discussion

Torasemide. Loop diuretics, such as furosemide, which is related to the currently studied agent, have been found to reduce the cerebral water content, computed tomography hypodensity of injured cerebral regions, and intracranial pressure in animals with a focal brain lesion [3]. Loop diuretics may prolong bulk movement of fluid across the blood-brain barrier into blood [13], which is therapeutically utilized to enhance dehydration by hyperosmotic solutions [12]. Similarities between furosemide and torasemide notwithstanding, it must be noted that torasemide is more lipophilic than furosemide, allowing entrance into the brain through the intact blood-brain barrier [34]. Specific mechanisms of torasemide may relate with inhibition of the $Na^+/K^+/Cl^-$ cotransporter and Cl^-/HCO_3^- antiporter at the blood-brain barrier and other interfaces in brain tissue, resulting among others in antagonization of CSF production [8].

PP56. Aside from inhibition of edema formation in peripheral tissue, PP56 has properties which may be relevant for the brain. It is an antagonist of NPY, a polypeptide which is widely distributed in central nervous tissue [2]. NPY is a potent vasoconstrictor of cerebral arteries. Its systemic administration has been found to lower cerebral blood flow in rats and rabbits [4]. Abel et al. [1] consider NPY to have a role in vasospasm from subarachnoid hemorrhage. This, however, is not supported by the studies of Pluta et al. [11] on relationships between plasma and CSF levels of NPY and appearance of delayed vasospasm from subarachnoid hemorrhage. On the other hand, significant release of NPY has been demonstrated in experimental head injury in rats [9]. Observations that PP56 blocks NPY vasoconstriction in vitro and in vivo [7] might be noteworthy in this context. It is, nevertheless, difficult to reconcile with inhibition of vasogenic brain edema, since edema formation is markedly influenced by the regional tissue perfusion. Inhibitory effects of NPY on tissue perfusion, however, may be counteracted by enhancement of necrosis formation from severe blood flow disturbances. It is conceivable then that enhancement of brain tissue necrosis by the release of NPY facilitates edema formation. The limited efficacy of PP56 on vasogenic brain edema might thus be explained by these antagonistic, admittedly hypothetical mechanisms, namely, inhibition of the blood flow reduction resulting from release of NPY and, thereby, of necrosis formation. Further information is certainly required on the function of NPY in secondary brain damage, such as vasogenic brain edema from ischemia and trauma.

Conclusion

Taken together, the present findings on novel methods of brain edema treatment using an experimental screening procedure not only are promising as far as enhancement of treatment specificity is concerned but also pertinent as to information on mechanisms underlying edema formation. While the effects of PP56 did not yet attain statistical significance, the results on torasemide confirm that Cl^- channels and activation of $Na^+/K^+/Cl^-$ cotransport mechanisms play a pathophysiological role, for example, by enhancement of blood-brain barrier permeability to small solutes. Although pretreatment with torasemide was found to attenuate vasogenic edema formation at 24 h after trauma, it is not known yet whether the agent is also effective if administered postinsult. Respective investigations are presently being carried out in this laboratory.

References

1. Abel PW, Han C, Now BD, McDonald JK (1988) Neuropeptide Y: vasoconstrictor effects and possible role in cerebral vasospasm after experimental subarachnoid hemorrhage. Brain Res 463:250–258
2. Adrian TE, Allen JM, Bloom SR, Ghatewi MA, Rossor MN, Roberts GW, Croe TJ, Tatemoto K, Polak JM (1983) Neuropeptide Y distribution in the human brain. Nature 306:584–586
3. Albright AL, Latchaw RE, Robinson AG (1984) Intracranial and systemic effects of osmotic and oncotic therapy in experimental cerebral edema. J Neurosurg 60:481–489
4. Allen JM, Todd N, Crockard HA, Schon F, Yeats JC, Bloom SR (1984) Presence of neuropeptide Y in human circle of Willis and its possible role in cerebral vasospasm. Lancet 2:550–552
5. Authi KS, Gustafsson T, Crawford N (1989) The effects of inositol-1,2,6-triphosphate (PP56) on the calcium sequestration properties of human platelets. Thromb Haemost 62:250–256
6. Claxson A, Morris C, Blake D, Sirén M, Halliwell B, Gustafsson T, Löfkvist B, Bergelin I (1990) The anti-inflammatory effects of D-myo-inositol-1,2,6-triphosphate (PP56) on animal models of inflammation. Agents Actions 29:68–70
7. Edvinsson L, Adamsson M, Jansen I (1990) Neuropeptide Y antagonistic properties of D-myo-inositol-1,2,6-trisphosphate in guinea pig basilar arteries. Neuropeptides 17:99–105
8. Javaheri S (1991) Role of NaCl cotransport in cerebrospinal fluid production: effect of loop diuretics. J Appl Physiol 71:795–800
9. McIntosh TK, Ferriero D (1992) Changes in neuropeptide Y after experimental traumatic brain injury in the rat. J Cereb Blood Flow Metab 12:697–702
10 Plangger C (1992) Effect of torasemide on intracranial pressure, mean systemic arterial pressure and cerebral perfusion pressure in experimental brain edema of the rat. Acta Neurol Scand 86:252–255
11. Pluta RM, Deka-Staarosta A, Zauner A, Morgan JK, Muraszko KM, Oldfield EH (1992) Neuropeptide Y in the primate model of subarachnoid hermorrhage. J Neurosorg 77:417–423
12. Roberts PA, Pollay M, Engles C, Pendleton B, Reynolds E, Stevens FA (1978) Effects on intracranial pressure of furosemide combined with varying doses and admininstration rates of mannitol. J Neurosurg 66:440–446
13. Schettini A, Stahurski B, Young HF (1982) Osmotic and oncotic loop diuresis in brain surgery. J Neurosurg 56:679–684
14. Staub F, Peters J, Kempski O, Schneider GH, Schürer L, Baethmann A (1993) Swelling of glial cells in lactacidosis and by glutamate: significance of Cl^--transport. Brain Res 610:69–74
15. Wittner M, Di Stefano A, Schlatter E, Delarge J, Greger R (1986) Torasemide inhibits NaCl reabsorption in the thick ascending limb of the loop of Henle. Pflugers Arch 407:611–614

Cell Migration of Neural and Neoplastic Cells Transplanted into the Adult Rat Brain

R. Bjerkvig[1,2], K. Marienhagen[2], P.-H. Pedersen[2], A. J. A. Terzis[3], and H. Arnold[3]

Introduction

During embryonic development a complex interplay takes place between the primitive neural ectoderm and surrounding mesodermal tissues. This process is characterized by generation of neuroblasts from the early neuroepithelium which first migrate and then differentiate into mature neural cells in the various regions of the central nervous system (CNS). Extensive cell migration, as observed for fetal cells during development, is a property which is also observed in malignant brain tumor cells in vivo [2–4, 9, 13, 22]. Glioma cells, for instance, show a tendency to migrate along fiber tracts of the white matter and along blood vessels [2, 9], and it is at present unclear whether this migration is enhanced by specific biological properties of the tumor cells or by specific anatomical structures in the brain itself. Of particular interest is the fact that also fetal brain cells, upon transplantation into the adult brain, show a tendency for extensive migration within the CNS [11, 12, 18]. In addition, it has been shown that tumor cells can possess specific fetal phenotypic properties [14, 19] which may be acquired during the process of transformation and differentiation. In the present study we therefore compared the migratory patterns of fetal brain cells and glioma cells transplanted into the adult CNS. To visualize the transplanted cells within the brain they were stained with the carbocyanine dye 1,1'-dioctadecyl-3,3,3',3'-tetramethylindocarbocyanine perchlorate (DiI), which is nontoxic and integrates within the plasma membrane of individual living cells [15–17]. Upon cell division the dye is evenly distributed among the daughter cells.

Materials and Methods

Animals. BS-IX rats [10] of both sexes with weights between 250 and 350 g were kept on a standard pellet diet, given tap water ad libitum, and caged in pairs at constant temperature and humidity on a 12-h light and dark schedule.

Cells. (a) Fetal rat brain cells were obtained from 18-day-old fetuses of inbred BD-IX rats. The brains were removed aseptically, cleaned of meningial coverings, and

---

[1] Institute of Anatomy and Cell Biology, University of Bergen, Norway.
[2] Gade Institute, Department of Pathology, University of Bergen, Norway.
[3] Department of Neurosurgery, University of Lübeck, Germany.

Advances in Neurosurgery, Vol. 22
B. L. Bauer, M. Brock, M. Klinger (Eds.)

placed into sterile petri dishes containing phosphate-buffered saline (PBS) free of calcium and magnesium. The brain tissue was then minced, washed in PBS and dissociated by serial trypsination (0.025% trypsin, Whittaker Bioproducts, Walkerville, MD), and the resulting single cell suspension was counted electronically using a Coulter counter (Coulter Electronics, Luton Beds, UK). It has been shown that the viability of the fetal cells after this procedure is more than 90% as defined by the trypan blue exclusion test [7]. (b) The permanent human glioma cell line GaMG was used [1]. The cells were grown in Dulbecco's modification of Eagle's medium (DMEM; Gibco Life Technologies, Paisley, UK) supplemented with 10% heat-inactivated newborn bovine serum, four times the prescribed concentration of nonessential amino acids, 2% L-glutamine, penicillin (100 UI/ml), and streptomycin (100 mg/ml). They were kept in a standard tissue culture incubator at 37 °C with 100% relative humidity, 95% air, and 5% CO_2. When the monolayer was at confluence, the cells were trypsinized, and the resulting single cell suspension was washed in PBS and counted.

Staining of Cells with the Carbocyanine Dye DiI. To distinguish implanted cells from the host tissue the carbocyanine dye DiI was used as a tracer. The DiI consists of two conjugated rings with a hydrocarbon chain attached to each ring. The two ring structures are linked by three methine groups. An isopropyl group is localized in each ring structure (Fig. 1). This dye is incorporated into lipid bilayers of the living cells and has a maximum absorption at 546 nm and a maximum emission at 563 nm [15–17). We dissolved 2.5 mg DiI in 100% ethalol by sonication. The resulting solution was passed through a 0.5-mm filter and diluted with DMEM to a final concentration of 0.075 mg/ml. The cell suspensions were incubated in DMEM-dye solution for 1.5 h at 37 °C in a rotary mixer. Excessive dye was removed by washing the cells twice in DMEM.

Intracranial Implantation. The rats were anesthetized with a mixture of fentanyl (Hypnorm; Janssen Pharmaceutica, Beerse, Belgium) and midazolam (Dormicum, Roche, Basel, Switzerland) at a concentration of 0.5 mg/100 g body weight each. Half of the dose was given intramuscularly and the other half subcutaneously.

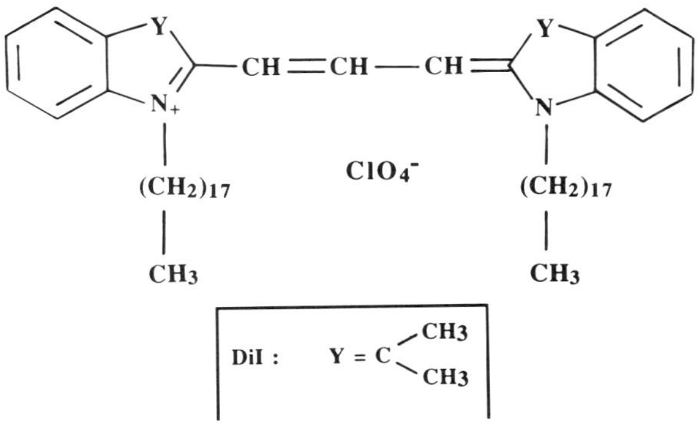

Fig. 1. Chemical structure of the carbocyanine dye DiI

After local anaesthesia with lidocaine (Xylocain 5 mg/ml, Astra Södertalje, Sweden) a skin incision was made. The skull was trephinated using a dental drill of 2.5 mm in diameter. The burrhole was localized 1 mm posterior to the coronal suture and 2 mm lateral to the sagittal suture. The dura mater was cross-incised, and 1 x 10^5 cells in 30 ml saline were injected into the brain at a depth of 2.5 mm by a sterile Hamilton syringe, with a cone-tipped 0.7-mm needle threaded with a Perspex stopper device. Thereafter the skin was closed with nonabsorbable suture. The animals were allowed to recover under a warming lamp before returning to their cages.

Tissue Collection. The rats were killed by CO_2 inhalation 1 h or 7 days after implantation. The brains were removed, washed in PBS, and embedded in Tissue-Tek (Miles Laboratories, Naperville, IL). The tissue was then carefully frozen in isopentane and cooled with liquid N_2. Serial coronal sections of the brains were then performed with 300 μm between the sections collected. The sections were mounted on poly-L-lysine coated glass slides and prepared for fluorescence microscopy.

Control Experiments In Vivo

Implantation of Fluorescent Microspheres Simultaneously with Fetal Rat Brain Cells. We dissolved 1 x 10^5 fluorescent polystyrene microspheres (6.49 ± 0.49 mm in diameter; Polyscience, Warrington, PA) in 30 ml saline. Either in combination with DiI-stained fetal rat brain cells or alone these were injected into the right hemisphere of adult rats, in the same anatomical location as that used for the cell implants. This was done to differentiate between active cell migration and passive displacement of transplanted cells. The distribution of microspheres was studied 1 h or 7 days after implantation.

Capability of Fetal Rat Brain Cells to Phagocytose Microspheres. To determine whether the fetal rat brain cells were able to phagocytose the fluorescent microspheres, 6 x 10^6 cells were incubated together with an equal number of fluorescent microspheres for 24 h in 25 cm^2 tissue culture flasks base-coated with 5 ml 0.75% Dulbecco's noble agar–DMEM solution. The volume of the overlay suspension was 5 ml. The cell-microsphere suspension was then washed in PBS, and the proportion of cells which had internalized microspheres was determined by flow cytometry. With this technique the cells could be identifed by combined flow cytometric measurements of wide- and narrow-angle light scatter. Free microspheres and debris were discriminated from the cells, and the cells were gated to a cytogram for combined measurements of FITC-fluorescence and narrow-angle light scatter [5, 6].

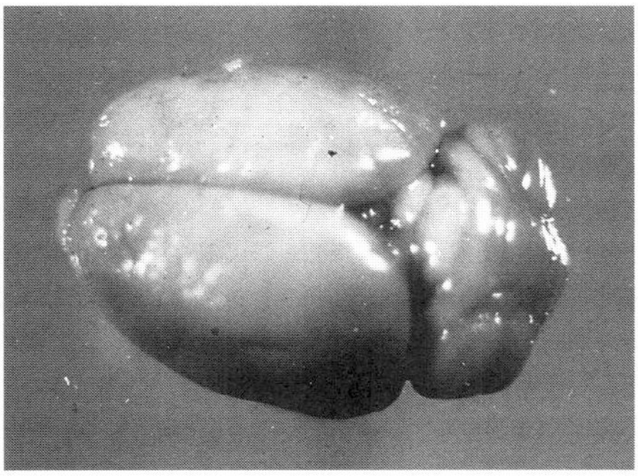

Fig. 2. Macroscopic appearance of the rat brain 1 h after implantation. A pink area around the implantation site is seen. x 3

Results

Macroscopic and microscopic observations of the rat brains 1 h after implantation revealed a pink area around the implantation site, with fluorescent cells localized in the subarachnoidal space (Figs. 2, 3 B). At this time the fetal brain cells and the tumor cells showed the same distribution in the brain (data not shown). Sections observed 7 days after implantation showed both fetal and tumor cells localized in the corpus callosum (Fig. 3 A). In addition, fluorescent cells were observed in the subarachnoidal area over the entire hemisphere (Fig. 3 B). The fetal cells as well as the glioma cells were also observed in the perivascular space around major blood vessels, even in the basal area of the brain (Fig. 3 C). When fluorescent microspheres were implanted alone or together with fetal cells, they were also observed in the subarachnoidal area and in the perivascular space around major blood vessels.

Fetal brain cells may phagocytose microspheres injected together with them. Therefore fetal brain cells were incubated together with fluorescent microspheres in vitro to determine the percentage of phagocytosing cells by flow cytometry. By combining forward-angle light scatter with green fluorescence measurements it was shown that only a small portion ($< 7\%$) of the fetal cells were capable of phagocytosis (Fig. 4)

Discussion

The present study compared the migratory patterns of fetal brain cells and human glioma cells transplanted into the adult brain. To visualize the transplanted cells within the brain the carbocyanine dye DiI was used, which is nontoxic at the concentrations used. The dye is incorporated in the lipid bilayer plasma membrane of individual cells and upon cell division and evenly distributed among the daughter cells [15–17]. These observations confirm the results obtained in earlier transplantation experiments of both fetal and human glioma cells in the CNS. It has been shown, for instance, that grafted specimens may survive, differentiate, and migrate

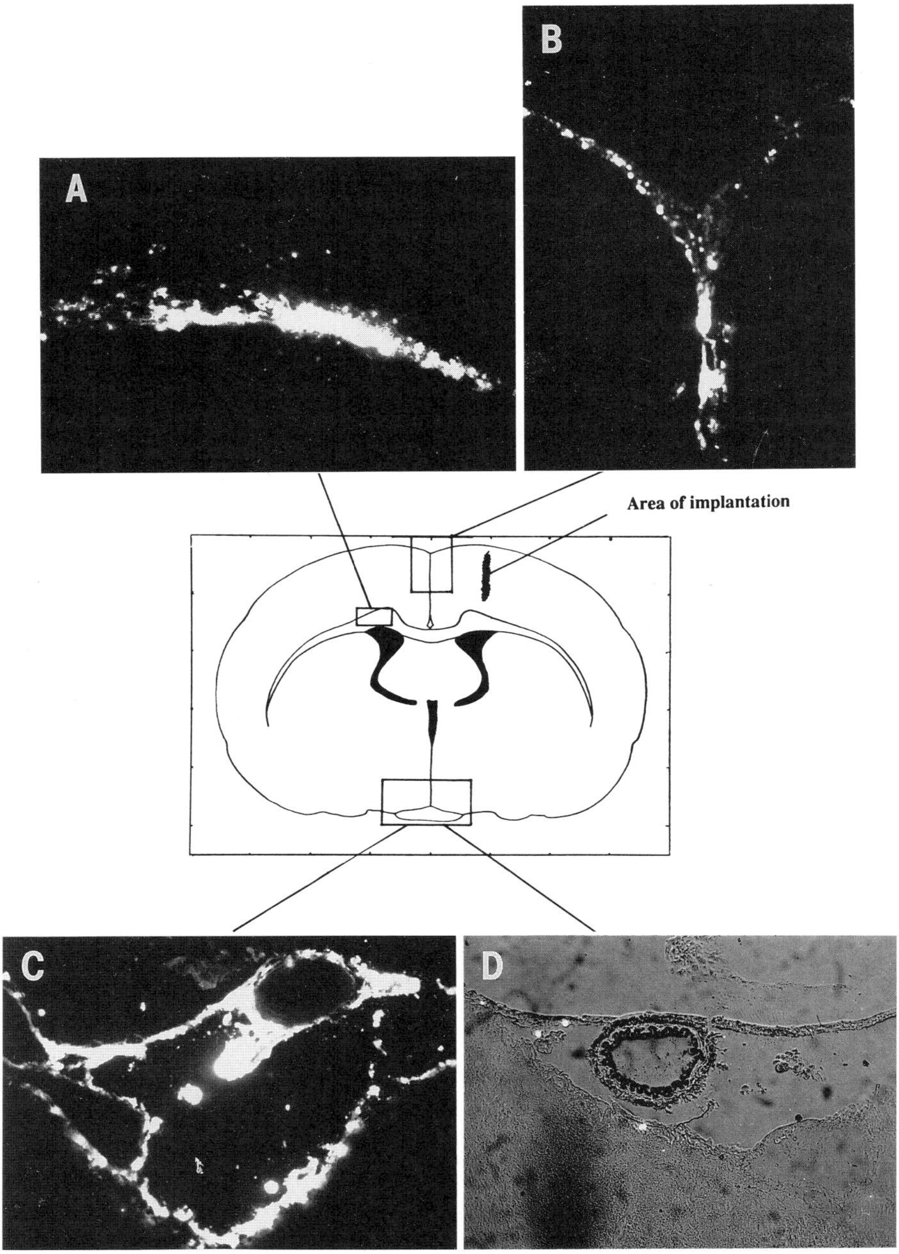

Fig. 3. **A** Fetal cells observed in the subarachnoidal area of the rat brain. **B** Fetal cells migrating over the corpus callosum. **C** Fetal cells localized in the perivascular area at the base of the brain. **D** Fluorescent microspheres observed in the same area. x 35

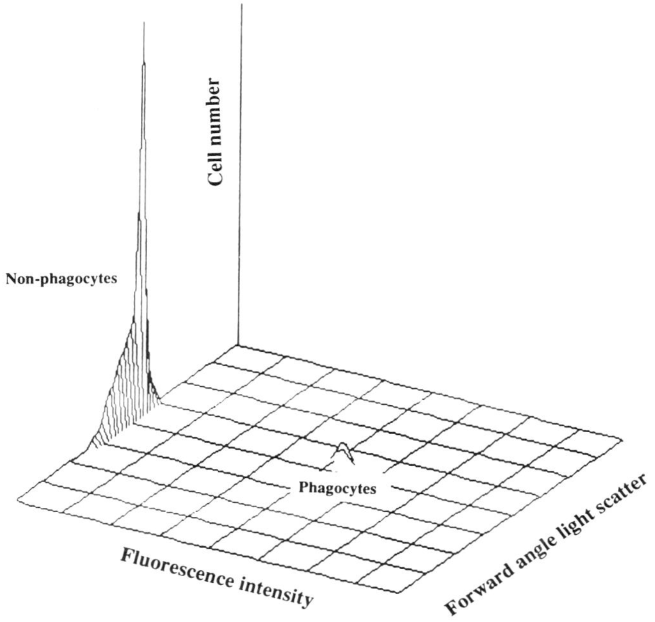

Fig. 4. Combined forward-angle light scatter and green fluorescence measurements showing only a small portion of cells having phagocytosed microspheres

within the adult brain [8, 12, 13]. We have shown that transplanted fetal brain cells may be found at a considerable distance from the implantation site in the rat brain [12, 20]. As also shown in the present study, both fetal cells and glioma cells have a tendency to spread along myelinated fiber tracts, for instance, in the corpus callosum [2, 20, 21]. Both cell types may also spread in the subarachnoid space and along blood vessels. Thus the two cell populations follow the same patterns of migration as have earlier been observed in neuropathological studies of human gliomas [9, 18]. The fact that inert microspheres may also spread within the CNS suggests that cell migration may in part be due to extracellular and cerebrospinal fluid movement within and around the brain, respectively.

Conclusion

Fetal brain cells and malignant glioma cells follow similar migratory paths in the brain. This pattern corresponds well with the invasive characteristics frequently observed in patients with malignant gliomas. The cell migration has a passive "seeding" component since inert microspheres may also spread into certain areas of the CNS.

Acknowledgments. This study was supported by the Norwegian Cancer Society, by the Department of Neurosurgery, University of Lübeck, and by Familien Blix Research Fund.

References

1. Akslen LA, Andersen K-J, Bjerkvig R (1988) Characteristics of human and rat glioma cells grown in a defined medium. Anticancer Res 8:797–804
2. Bernstein JJ, Goldberg WJ, Laws ER (1989) Human malignant astrocytoma xenografts migrate in rat brain: a model for central nervous system. Cancer Research J Neurosci Res 22:134–143
3. Berry M, Eayrs JT (1963) Histogenesis of the cerebral cortex. Nature 197:984–985
4. Berry M, Rogers AW, Eayrs JT (1964) Pattern of cell migration during cortical histogenesis. Nature 203:591–593
5. Bjerknes R, BassŸe CF (1984) Phagocyte C3-mediated attachment and internalization: flow cytometric studies using a fluorescence quenching technique. Blut 49:315–323
6. Bjerknes R, Bjerkvig R, Laerum OD (1987) Phagocytic capacity of normal and malignant rat glial cells in culture. J Natl Cancer Inst 78:279–288
7. Bjerkvig R, Steinsvåg SK, Lærum OD (1986) Reaggregation of fetal rat brain cells in a stationary culture system. I. methodology and cell identification. In Vitro Cell Dev Biol 22:180–192
8. Bjørklund A, Bickford D, Dahl D, Elfman L, Hoffer B, Olsen L (1985) Morphological and functional properties of intracranial cerebellar grafts. In: Bjørklund A, Stenevi U (eds) Neural grafting in the mamalian CNS. Elsevier Science, Amsterdam
9. Burger PC, Dubois PJ, Schold SC, Smith KR, Odom GL, Crafts DC, Giangaspero F (1983) Computerized tomographic and pathologic studies of the untreated, quiescent, and recurrent glioblastoma multiforme. J Neurosurg 58:159–169
10. Druckrey H (1971) Genotypes and phenotypes of ten inbred strains of BD-rats. Arzneimittelforschung 21:1274–1278
11. Emmett CJ, Lawrence JM, Seeley PJ (1988) Visualization of migration of transplanted astrocytes using polystyrene microspheres. Brain Res 447:223–233
12. Goldberg WJ (1987) Transplant derived astrocytes migrate into host lumbar and cervical spinal cord after implantation of E14 fetal cerebral cortex into adult thoracic spinal cord. J Neurosci Res 17:391–403
13. Goldberg WJ, Bernstein JJ (1988) Fetal cortical astrocytes migrate from cortical homografts throughout the host brain and over the glia limitans. J Neurosci Res 20:38–45
14. Haggie JA, Sellwood RA, Howell A, Brich JM, Schor SL (1987) Fibroblasts from relatives of patients with hereditary breast cancer show fetal-like behaviour in vitro. Lancet 1:1455–1457
15. Honig MG, Hume RI (1986) Fluorescent carbocyanine dyes allow living neurons of identified origin to be studied in long-term cultures. J Cell Biol 103:171–187
16. Honig MG, Hume RI (1989) Carbocyanine dyes. Novel markers for labelling neurons. Trends Neurosci 12:336–338
17. Honig MG, Hume RI (1989) DiI and DiO: Versatile fluorescent dyes for neuronal labelling and pathway tracing. Trends Neurosci 12:333–341
18. Kelly PJ, Daumas-Duport C, Kispert DB, Kall BA, Sceithauer BW, Illig JJ (1987) Imaging-based stereotaxic serial biopsies in untreated intracranial glial neoplasms. J Neurosurg 66:865–874
19. Kindler-Rohrborn A, Arens O, Liepelt U, Rajewsky MF (1985) Expression of monoclonal antibody-defined cell surface antigens during rat brain development. Differentiation 30:53–60

20. Marienhagen K, Pedersen P-H, Terzis AJ, Laerum OD, Arnold H, Bjerkvig R (1993) Interactions between fetal rat brain cells and mature brain tissue in vivo and in vitro. J Neuropathol Appl Neurobiol (submitted)
21. Pedersen P-H, Marienhagen K, Mørk S, Bjerkvig R (1993) The migratory pattern of fetal rat brain cells and human glioma cells in the adult rat brain. Cancer Res (submitted)
22. Sidman RL, Rakic P (1973) Neuronal migration, with special reference to developing human brain, a review. Brain Res 62:1–35

Monocyte- and Lymphocyte-Mediated Cytotoxicity After Gene Transfer and Expression of Human Interleukin-2 in a Human Glioblastoma Cell Line

G. Schackert[1], A. Buttler[1], A. Mehrabi[2], H. K. Schackert[2], C. Herfarth[2], and S. Kunze[1]

Introduction

Failing defense mechanisms against malignant tumors are thought to be caused by low immunogenicity of tumor cells and defective T helper cell functions. The concept of associate recognition by Lake and Mitchison [5] posits the necessity of at least two antigens being expressed to achieve a sufficient immune response against the cellular target. In vivo experiments show that expression of a viral antigen together with the putative tumor-associated antigen(s) not only triggers a strong immune response against itself but also remarkably improves immune response mechanisms against the tumor-associated antigen [6]. Local cytokine expression by tumor cells, on the other hand, bypasses a defective T helper function [2] and elicits an effective immune response against tumor cells in animal models [2, 3].

In our previous contribution we discussed the advantage of interferon (IFN)-γ and tumor necrosis factor (TNF)-α mediated monocyte activation and cytytoxicity against human glioblastoma cell lines T739 and T829 and the brain metastasis of a bronchial carcinoma compared to the direct cytotoxic action of both biological response modifiers [7].

In the present investigation we sought to improve the mode of action of biological molecules which mediate the activation of immune effector cells. The aim was to increase local concentration of human interleukin-2 (hIL-2) without having the disadvantages of systemic high levels and resulting severe side effects of the cytokine. In an in vitro model we investigated the possible benefits of local expression of hIL-2 after transfer of the gene into the human glioblastoma cell line T1115 versus systemic administration of hIL-2 in the cytotoxic activation of monocytes and lymphokine-activated killer (LAK) cells.

[1] Department of Neurosurgery, University of Heidelberg, Im Neuenheimer Feld 400, 69120 Heidelberg, Germany.
[2] Department of Surgery, University of Heidelberg, Im Neuenheimer Feld 110, 69120 Heidelberg, Germany.

Advances in Neurosurgery, Vol. 22
B. L. Bauer, M. Brock, M. Klinger (Eds.)

Materials and Methods

hIL-2 Construct

hIL-2 cDNA contained in the 542-basepair *Hin*dIII-*Eco*RI DNA fragment of the pBEH IL-2 vector (kindly provided by Harald S. Conradt, Gesellschaft für Biomedizinische Forschung, Braunschweig, Germany) was cloned into the pUHD 10-1 plasmid [1], resulting in uPHD 10-1 IL-2, where the hIL-2 gene was driven by a CMV promoter/enhancer.

Tumor Cell Line T1115

The human glioblastoma cell line T1115 had been established from a recurrent glioblastoma and was kindly provided by Hans Fischer, German Cancer Research Center, Heidelberg. The tumor cell line was maintained as monolayer culture on plastic in Eagle's basal medium (BME) supplemented with 10% fetal calf serum (FCS), sodium bicarbonate, essential amino acids, L-glutamine, vitamins, HEPES, and penicillin/streptomycin (Biochrom, Berlin, Germany). Cell cultures were incubated in 5% CO_2/95% air at 37 °C. All cultures were free of mycoplasma.

Tumor Cell Line Klon 2

Calcium precipitation was used to cotransfer T1115 cells with pUHD 10-1 IL-2 and pSV2neo [8]. After G418 selection Klon 2 produced 5800 pg hIL-2/100 000 cells per 24 h (hIL-2 ELISA; Biermann, Bad Nauheim, 76 pg = 1 U hIL-2).

Isolation and Culture of Human Peripheral Blood Monocytes and LAK Cells

Mononuclear cells were isolated from peripheral blood of healthy donors by Ficoll (specific gravity d = 1077 g/ml) separation. After allowing the monocytes to adhere for 2 h at 37 °C the nonadherent cells were removed by washing the plates three times with warm (37 °C) RPMI 1640 medium. A monocyte-enriched population adhering to plastic was separated from LAK cells as determined by morphology, hemacolor differential blood analysis, and peroxidase staining. Both cell populations were suspended in RPMI 1640 supplemented with 5% human AB serum and adjusted to a final concentration of 10^6 monocytes or LAK cells. Monocytes or LAK cells 2 x 10^5 were added to each well of 96-well flat-bottomed Microtest III plate (Falcon, Becton-Dickinson, Heidelberg, Germany). All experiments were performed as triplicates. The effector/target ratio was 20:1 in all experiments except the cocultivation experiment (effector/target ratio of 10:1).

In Vitro Activation of Human Effector Cells and Cytotoxicity Assay

Purified monocytes or LAK cells were incubated at 37 °C with hIL-2, TNF-α (1000 U/ml), or IFN-γ (1000 U/ml; all Boehringer Mannheim, Germany) 24 h before addition of radiolabeled target cells (experiment 1) or were coincubated with radiolabeled target cells without preincubation for 3 days. When preincubated with hIL-2, TNF-α (1000 U/ml), or IFN-γ (1000 U/ml), the monocytes were thoroughly washed after 24 h three times with medium, and the radiolabeled target cells were added for 3 days. Blocking of IL-2 activity was facilitated by adding anti-IL-2 receptor CD25, human or anti-IL-2 antibody (both Boehringer Mannheim) to the assay for 3 days. All reagents were free of endotoxin, as measured by Limulus amebocyte assay (Pyroquant, Walldorf, Germany; sensitivity < 0.12 ng/ml).

Target cells in their exponential growth phase were incubated in supplemented BME containing 0.5 μCi/ml [^{3}H]methyl-thymidine (TdR, Amersham, Braunschweig, Germany; specific activity 25 Ci/μmol). After 24 h the cell monolayers were rinsed twice to remove nonbound [^{3}H]TdR. The cells were then incubated for another 2 h in BME, washed twice, stored on ice to extract soluble DNA precursors, and washed again. The cells were harvested by short-term trypsination (0.05% trypsin/0.2% EDTA, Biochrom, Berlin, Germany), washed three times, resuspended in endotoxin-free RPMI 1640 medium (Gibco, Eggenstein, Germany), measured by Limulus amebocyte assay, supplemented with FCS, genamycin, nonessential amino acids, $NaHCO_3$, HEPES, vitamins, L-glutamine, and plated into 96-well plates containing the activated monocytes or LAK cells to obtain an initial effector-to-target ratio of 20:1 or 10:1. Triplicates of radiolabeled cells plated alone served as control. All reagents were free of endotoxin, as measured by Limulus amebocyte assay.

Seventy-two hours after the addition of target cells the cultures were washed three times with PBS, and the adherent viable cells were lysed with 0.2 ml 0.1 *N* NaOH. Samples (100 ml) were added to 2-ml scintillation fluid (Aquasafe 300, Zinsser Analytic, Frankfurt, Germany), and the radioactivity of the lysate was monitored in a Wallac 1410 liquid scintillation counter. The cytotoxic activity of the monocytes or LAK cells was calculated as follows: % cytotoxicity = 100 x ([cpm with control effector cells] – [cpm with activated effector cells])/[cpm with control effector cells]. All data resulted from triplicate measurements and are shown as mean and standard deviation.

Results

Activation of LAK cells and monocytes can be achieved by 24-h preincubation with 100 U/ml IL-2 or TNF-α (1000 U/ml) in combination with IFN-γ (1000 U/ml) and results in cytotoxicity against T1115 ranging from 55% to 65% (Fig. 1). Increasing concentrations of IL-2 in a 3-day incubation assay with effector and target cells facilitate increasing cytotoxicity against T1115 from 24% (5 U IL-2/ml) to 71% (100U IL-2/ml; Fig. 1).

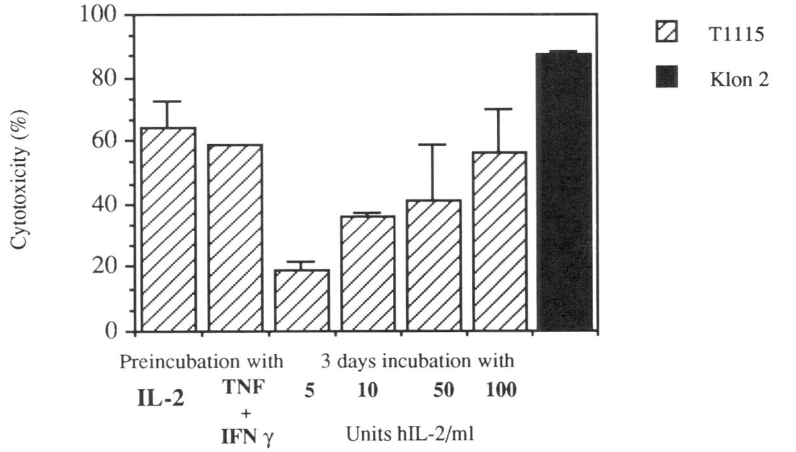

Fig. 1. Monocyte cytotoxicity triggered by endogenous hIL-2 (Klon 2) and by exogenous hIL-2, TNF-α, and IFN-γ

In comparison, cocultivation of Klon 2 with nonstimulated LAK cells results in 86% cytotoxicity in the same assay (Fig. 1) and similar results in a monocyte cytotoxicity assay (data not shown). Klon 2 produces 25.4 U IL-2/ml medium per 24 h in both assays. Addition of anti-IL-2 receptor antibody or anti-IL-2 antibody both result in a significant blocking of cytotoxicity of monocytes which had been coincubated for 3 days with 10 U IL-2/ml. No blocking of monocyte cytotoxicity could be achieved when IL-2 was produced endogenously by Klon 2 (Fig. 2).

Cocultivation experiments of 10 000 T1115 cells with 10 000 Klon 2 cells and nonstimulated monocytes resulted in 57% cytotoxicity against Klon 2 and 53%

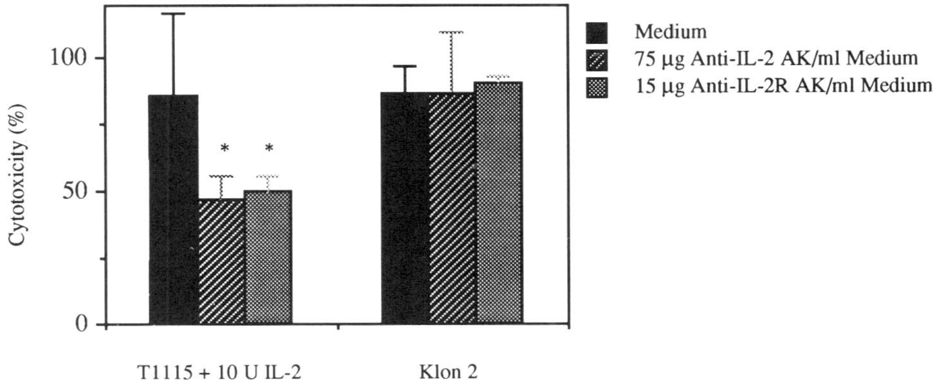

Fig. 2. Effect of anti-IL-2 and anti-IL-2 receptor antibody on monocyte-mediated cytotoxicity. * $p < 0.01$ (t test)

cytotoxicity against T1115. Cytotoxicity against Klon 2 alone was 54%. Similar results were obtained in the LAK assay (data not shown).

Conclusions

Cytotoxic activation of monocytes and LAK cells by IL-2 has been described elsewhere [4]. We demonstrated that endogenous production of hIL-2 by tumor cells (Klon 2) results in a strong cytotoxicity of cocultivated effector cells (monocytes and LAK cells) against Klon 2 tumor cells. Klon 2 cells produced 25.8 U IL-2/ml medium per 24 h in our cytotoxicity assay. The amount of exogenous IL-2 added to the assay was 100 U/ml medium. Since almost equal amounts of IL-2 was blocked only by anti-IL-2 receptor antibody or anti-IL-2 antibodies in an assay in which IL-2 had been given exogenously, we suggest that blocking failed due to high local concentrations of IL-2 around Klon 2 cells which serve as endogenous source for IL-2. Our experiments further suggest that IL-2 produced by Klon 2 may stimulate surrounding effector cells and therefore mediate cytotoxicity very effectively to cocultured T1115 cells which do not produce IL-2. Our findings are in accord with data from animal experiments which show that local production of cytokines by tumor cells activates immune response mechanisms [2, 3]. We conclude that local production is at least as effective as systemic administration of IL-2 in stimulating monocytes and LAK cells against brain tumor cells, and that local production of cytokines may avoid severe systemic side effects of IL-2.

References

1. Deuschle U, Pepperkok R, Wang FB, Giordano TJ, McAllister WT, Ansorge W, Bujard H (1989) Regulated expression of foreign genes in mammalian cells under the control of coliphage T3 RNA polymerase and lac repressor. Proc Natl Acad Sci USA 86:5400–5404
2. Fearon ER, Pardoll DM, Itaya T, Gloumbek P, Levitsky HI, Simons JW, Karasuyama H, Vogelstein B, Frost P (1990) Interleukin-2 production by tumor cells bypasses T helper function in the generation of an antitumor response. Cell 60:397–403
3. Golumbek PT, Lazenby AJ, Levitsky HI et al. (1991) Treatment of established renal cancer by tumor cells engineered to secrete interleukin-4. Science 254:713–716
4. Higashi N, Nishimura Y, Higuchi M, Osawa T (1991) Human monocytes in a long-term culture with interleukin-2 show high tumoricidal activity against various tumor cells. J Immunother 10:247–255
5. Lake P, Mitchison NA (1976) Associate control of the immune response to cell surface antigens. Immunol Commun 5:795–805
6. Schackert HK, Itaya T, Schackert G, Fearon E, Vogelstein B, Frost P (1989) Systemic immunity against a murine colon tumor (CT-26) produced by immunization with syngeneic cells expressing a transfected viral gene product. Int J Cancer 43:823–827
7. Schackert G, Kirsch M, Fischer H, Schackert HK, Kunze S (1993) Comparative study of moncyte mediated cytotoxicity and biological response modifier mediated cytotoxicity against malignant brain tumor cells in vitro. In: Lorenz R, Klinger M, Brock M (eds) Advances in neurosurgery, vol 21. Springer, Berlin Heidelberg New York, pp 312–320

8. Southern PJ, Berg P (1982) Transformation of mammalian cells to antibiotic resistance with a bacterial gene under conrol of the SV40 early region promoter. J Mol Appl Genet 1:327–341

Tissue pO_2 of Normal and Pathological Human Brain Cortex

J. Dings[1], J. Meixensberger[1], H. Kuhnigk[2], and K. Roosen[1]

Introduction

Experimental and clinical investigations have provided substantial insight into hemodynamic changes and alterations in cerebral metabolism following brain damage [4, 7, 10, 11, 13, 14]. However, many questions are still to be answered. As the cerebral metabolism depends mainly on aerobic glycolysis, determination of tissue pO_2 may provide further insight into metabolic status or changes and into cerebral hemodynamics. We therefore monitored brain cortex pO_2 to clarify whether there are differences in tissue pO_2 between normal and pathological human brain cortex, and whether tissue pO_2 is influenced by changes in arterial pO_2 and pCO_2.

Patients and Methods

A total of 43 patients (24 women, 19 men; mean age 48.8 years, range 22–78) with various types of intracranial tumors or vascular malformations were studied. Preoperatively the amount of edema seen on computed tomography and/or magnetic resonance imaging was determined as none, minimal, moderate, or much. The extent of brain swelling after opening the dura mater was classified as none, little, or much. The intraoperative aspect of the cortex was determined as either normal or pathological. According to this classification, normal patients (control) were distinguished from those with pathological findings. Table 1 lists the patients investigated giving age, sex, diagnosis, location, amount of edema, and extent of brain swelling. The pathological group was split into two subgroups: one with moderate or much edema and one with much brain swelling. No patient showed a concomitant cardiovascular or hematological disease.

The brain tissue pO_2 measurements were performed after craniotomy and opening the dura mater. Narcotic conditions were standardized, using fentanyl, dormicum, pancuronium, and sometimes isoflurane for sedation, and analgesia and relaxation. The mean oxygen volume content of the inhaled O_2/N_2 gas mixture was 39%. Except for intubation no barbiturates were used. The sensor used was a

[1] Neurochirurgische Klinik und Poliklinik, Universität Würzburg, Josef-Schneider-Str. 11, 97080 Würzburg, Germany.
[2] Anaesthesiologisches Institut, Universitätskliniken Würzburg, Josef-Schneider-Str. 2, 97080 Würzburg, Germany.

Advances in Neurosurgery, Vol. 22
B. L. Bauer, M. Brock, M. Klinger (Eds.)

Table 1. Characteristics of control and pathological groups

Patient no.	Age (years)	Sex	Diagnosis	Location	Edema[a]	Swelling[b]
1	48	F	Meningioma	Frontal	0	0
2	25	M	Ependymoma	Parietal	0	0
3	23	F	Ependymoma	Temporal	0	0
4	65	F	Meningioma	Parietal	0	0
5	52	F	Meningioma	Frontal	0	0
6	55	F	Meningioma	Frontal	0	0
7	22	F	Cavernoma	Temporal	0	0
8	44	F	Meninigioma	Sella	0	0
9	35	F	Aneurysm	ICA	0	0
10	49	M	Cavernoma	Temporal	0	0
11	48	F	Aneurysm	Multiple	0	0
12	48	F	Aneurysm	Multiple	0	0
13	28	M	Oligoastro-cytoma (WHO III)	Frontal	1	0
14	28	M	Cavernoma	Temporal	0	0
15	43	F	Aneurysm	ACoA	0	0
16	60	F	Meningioma	Sella	0	0
17	54	M	Aneurysm	ACoA	0	0
18	72	F	Cavernoma	Temporal	0	0
19	39	F	Aneurysm	ACoA	0	0
20	46	F	Hypophysis Adenoma	Sella	0	0
21	27	M	Oligodendro-glioma	Temporal	1	0
22	22	M	Aneurysm	MCA	0	0
23	45	M	Metastasis	Frontal	3	2
24	41	M	Meningioma	Frontal	3	0
25	78	M	Metastasis	Frontal	3	1
26	61	M	Metastasis	Temporal	2	0
27	60	M	Glioblastoma	Occipital	2	2
28	45	M	Metastasis	Parietal	1	2
29	62	F	Glioblastoma	Temporal-occipital	3	2
30	57	M	Glioblastoma	Temporal	3	1
31	61	F	Glioblastoma	Temporal-parietal	3	2
32	64	F	Meningioma	Temporal	3	2
33	63	F	Meningioma	Frontal	0	2
34	57	M	Aneurysm	ACoA	0	0
35	62	F	Aneurysm	MCA	0	0
36	63	F	Glioblastoma	Temporal-parietal	2	0
37	44	F	Glioblastoma	Parietal	2	0
38	41	M	Astrocytoma (WHO III)	Frontal	2	0
39	58	F	Glioblastoma	Frontal	2	0
40	38	M	Glioblastoma	Frontal	1	0
41	42	M	Aneurysm	ACoA	0	0
42	65	M	Metastasis	Temporal	2	0
43	58	F	Glioblastoma	Temporal	1	0

ACoA, Anterior communicating artery; ICA, internal carotid artery; MCA, middle cerebral artery.
[a] Scale: 0 = none, 1 = minimal, 2 = moderate, 3 = much.
[b] Scale: 0 = none, 1 = little, 2 = much.

surface sensor coupled to a licox oxygen pressure measuring device (G.M.S. Kiel-Mielkendorf, Germany); the sensor consists of eight platinum cathodes and one silver anode. The oxygen freely diffusing through the sensor membrane and electrolyte solution was reduced at the cathode to hydroxyl ions, changing the polarization current. Current changes were proportional to pO_2. The reaction time was less than 20 s. The measured pO_2 value was the mean of eight individual values of the eight cathodes. The temperature coefficient of the sensor sensitivity was 2.4%–2.5% per degree centigrade. Since a temperature probe was integrated in the sensor, the pO_2 values were corrected automatically when the temperature changed. The sensor has a diameter of 15 mm and height of 11 mm, the measuring surface area has a diameter of 5 mm, and the weight is 2.9 g. Before starting a measurement, a two-point calibration (one at an oxygen pressure of 0 mmHg and one at normal air oxygen pressure) was performed, taking about 45 min.

A placement of the sensor over pial vessels, blood, or cerebrospinal fluid was avoided. The noninvestigated cortex was moistened with saline and covered with wet neurosurgical swabs. First, basal tissue pO_2 was measured, whenever possible, in different areas. The oxygen fraction of the inspired gas was then increased from a mean of 39% to 100% (hyperoxia). At the end $paCO_2$ was decreased by changing ventilating parameters. At the end of each test, when a plateau in tissue pO_2 had been reached, initial ventilating parameters were reestablished. Before, during, and after the test arterial blood gas was analyzed for determination of pH, base excess (BE), paO_2, and $paCO_2$. Mean arterial blood pressure, rectal temperature, and end-expiratory CO_2 were also recorded. Tissue pO_2 and tissue temperature were recorded every 5 s by a connected notebook. Depending on the time required to obtain stable values of tissue pO_2, either both or only one of the tests was performed after determining basic tissue pO_2.

Results

Table 2 gives basic values for the control and pathological groups. The control group ($n = 22$) showed a basic tissue pO_2 or 44.95 ± 14.01 mmHg; the difference

Table 2. Results in control and pathological groups

	Control group ($n = 22$)	Pathological group ($n = 21$)
Tissue pO_2 (mmHg)	44.95 ± 14.01	38.14 ± 26.18
Tissue temperature (°C)	33.77 ± 1.11	32.77 ± 1.86
paO_2 (mmHg)	161.41 ± 29.68	146.81 ± 36.58
$paCO_2$ (mmHg)	31.23 ± 3.32	30.11 ± 2.65
pH	7.50 ± 0.04	7.52 ± 0.04
Base excess	3.14 ± 1.95	4.47 ± 2.71
Mean arterial pressure (mmHg)	89.27 ± 10.58	91.14 ± 9.77
Rectal temperature (°C)	35.93 ± 0.75	36.02 ± 0.98
Endexpiratory CO_2 (mmHg)	3.87 ± 0.64	3.83 ± 0.48

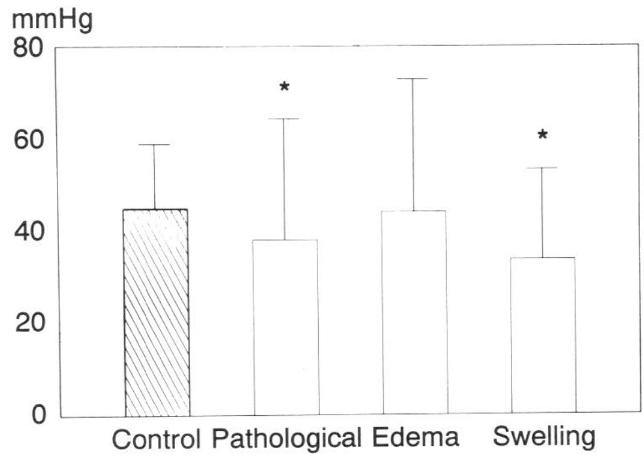

Fig. 1. Tissue pO_2 in the control and pathological groups as well as in the edema subgroup and the subgroup with much brain swelling. Mean ± SD mmHg. * $p < 0.05$

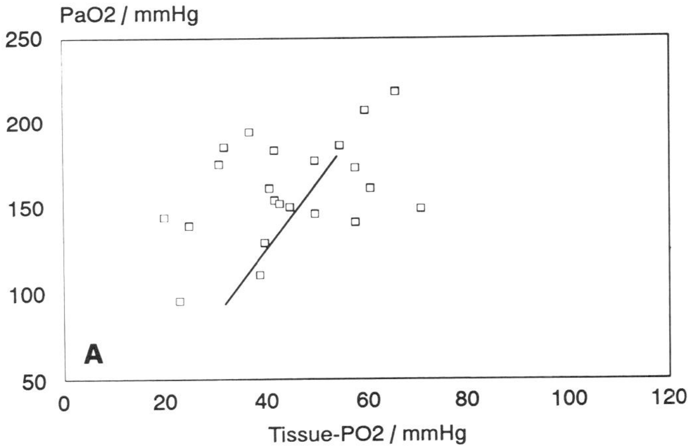

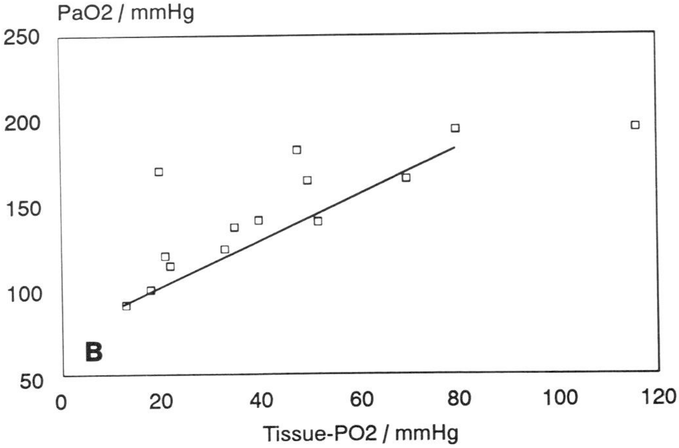

Fig. 2 A, B. Correlation between tissue pO_2 and paO_2. control group ($n = 22$): $r = 0.4247$, $p = 0.0246$ edema subgroup ($n = 14$): $r = 0.7901$, $p = 0.0004$

to the pathological group ($n = 21$) was statistically significant (38.14 ± 26.18 mmHg, $p < 0.05$). Tissue pO_2 values in the control and pathological groups were 20–71 and 13–116 mmHg, respectively. The difference in tissue temperature, pH, and BE between the control and pathological groups was also statistically significant ($p < 0.05$). Figure 1 presents tissue pO_2 values of all four groups. The subgroup with much brain swelling ($n = 7$) revealed the lowest tissue pO_2 values (33.71 ± 19.62 mmHg, $p < 0.05$). In the edema subgroup ($n = 14$) mean tissue pO_2 was 44.14 ± 28.71 mmHg. The correlation between tissue pO_2 and paO_2 in the control group was weak ($r = 0.4247$, $p = 0.0246$) and was increased in the pathological group ($r = 0.7028$, $p = 0.0002$), being highest in the edema subgroup ($r = 0.7901$, $p = 0.0004$; Fig. 2).

On hyperoxia (inhaled oxygen fraction to 100% increased) the change in tissue pO_2 in the control group was 159.7% and in that in the pathological group 290.4% ($p < 0.05$; Fig. 3). There was no significant difference in absolute tissue pO_2 values between the control and pathological groups (101.61 ± 43.69 versus 112.69 ± 71.91 mmHg), nor in absolute paO_2 values (443.93 ± 69.35 versus 410.77 ± 83.40 mmHg). No correlation between tissue pO_2 and paO_2 was seen in the control group ($n = 15$, $r = 0.0354$, $p = 0.04502$) or in the pathological group ($n = 13$, $r = 0.454$, $p = 0.0596$). In the edema subgroup, however, a clear correlation was found ($n = 10$, $r = 0.7021$, $p = 0.0118$). After changing $paCO_2$ from a mean of 31 to one of 25 mmHg, the mean decrease in the control group was 13.75% ± 12.88%. At a mean $paCO_2$ change from 31 to 26 mmHg the pathological group showed only a 6.94% ± 9.48% decrease. Neither the change in percentage tissue pO_2 nor that in absolute $paCO_2$ was statistically significant different between the two groups. As shown in Fig. 4, tissue pO_2 did not change on hyperventilation in two (18%) of the patients in the control group; in the pathological group no reaction in tissue pO_2 was seen in 50% of the patients. The lowest values

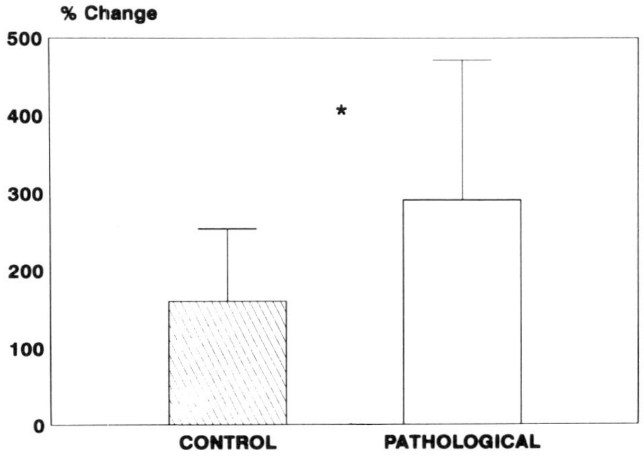

Fig. 3. Percentage change in tissue pO_2 after 100% oxygen (hyperoxia). Mean ± SD. * $p < 0.05$

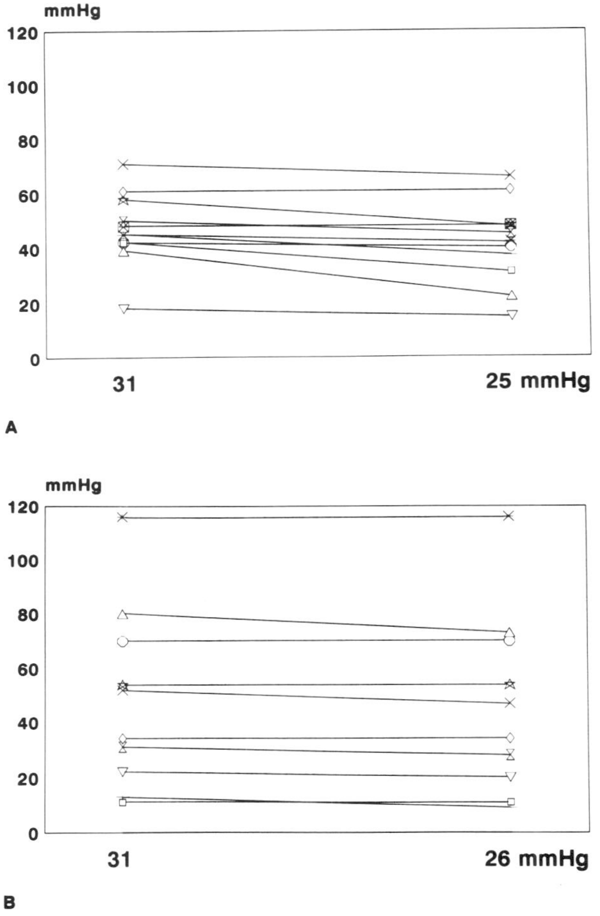

Fig. 4 A, B. Tissue pO_2 before and after decreasing $paCO_2$. Control group (n = 11): decrease from 31 to 25 mmHg. Pathological group (n = 10): decrease from 31 to 26 mmHg. Absolute values

of tissue pO_2 after hyperventilation were found in the pathological group (9 mmHg).

Discussion

Many investigations of brain tissue pO_2 and its regulatory mechanisms have been performed [1–3, 5, 6, 8, 9, 12, 15], but only few reports of in vivo measurements of human brain tissue pO_2 have been published [1–3, 8]. Adams and Severinghaus [1] measured a mean tissue pO_2 of 13 mmHg in 23 patients. When considering the capillary compression and the tissue damage probably induced by the needle electrode which they used (1 mm diameter), not only the low values in general but also the lack of reaction to hyperventilation in 7 of 12 patients could be explained. These findings are in correspondence with our measurements of lowest values in compressed cortex and the lack of reaction to hyperventilation in 50% of patients in the pathological group. Assad et al. [2] studied brain tissue pO_2 in different brain tumors and in the adjacent edematous and compressed cortex. In normal cortex they obtained ($n = 3$) average values of 33–36 mmHg at a paO_2 of 150–170 and a $paCO_2$ of 30 mmHg. The difference to the values that we obtained in normal cortex (44.95 mmHg) may be explained by anesthesia, (non)compensated tissue temperature, or placement of the probe over pial vessels. They also found lowest values in compressed cortex and a wider range of values in edematous cortex. Kayama et al. [8] found a mean tissue pO_2 of 59.8 ± 6.5 mmHg at a paO_2 of 112.7 ± 5.2 mmHg in brain tissue surrounding various kinds of (metastatic) brain tumors. Again, the difference with regard to our results in the pathological group may be caused by the above factors. In six patients Eintrei and Lund [3] obtained a mean tissue pO_2 of 24 mmHg at a paO_2 of 122.25 ± 25.5 mmHg. Few data on human brain tissue pO_2 during hyperoxia and hyperventilation are available [1, 3]. Eintrei and Lund [3] reported an increase as well as a decrease in tissue pO_2 on hyperoxia (100% oxygen). With increasing paO_2 the range of the values became clearly wider. In animal experiments [6, 9, 12] various reactions to hyperoxia have been seen: an increase, no change, or a decrease of tissue pO_2.

These results have led to the postulation of a regulating mechanism for local pO_2. In the present series, the findings of a clear correlation between tissue pO_2 and paO_2 in edematous cortex and the persistence of this correlation on hyperoxia give strong support to this postulation. On hyperventilation the most pronounced changes were seen in the control group (13.75% decrease in tissue pO_2). In this group, however, there were some patients with no reaction, indicating an impaired CO_2 reactivity. Finally, hyperventilation was capable of decreasing tissue oxygen pressure to very low levels in the pathological group, indicating that some patients are at risk from ischemia during hyperventilation.

References

1. Adams JE, Severinghaus JW (1962) Oxygen tension of human cerebral grey and white matter. The effect of forced hyperventilation. J Neurosurg 19:959–963
2. Assad F, Schultheiss R, Leniger-Follert E, Wüllenweber R (1984) Measurement of local oxygen partial pressure (PO2) of the brain cortex in cases of brain tumors. Adv Neurosurg 12:263–266
3. Eintrei C, Lund D (1986) Effects of increases in the inspired oxygen fraction on brain surface oxygen pressure fields in pig and man. Acta Anaesthesiol Scand 30:194–198
4. Enevoldsen EM (1986) CBF in head injury. Acta Neurochir Suppl (Wien) 36:133–136
5. Grote J, Zimmer K, Schubert R (1985) Tissue oxygenation in normal and edematous brain cortex during arterial hypocapnia. Adv Exp Med Biol 180:179–184

6. Ingvar DH, Lübbers DW, Siesjö B (1960) Measurement of oxygen tension on the surface of the cerebral cortex of the cat during hyperoxia and hypoxia. Acta Physiol Scand 48:373–381
7. Jaggi JL, Obrist WD, Gennarelli TA, Langfitt TW (1990) Relationship of early cerebral blood flow and metabolism to outcome in acute head injury. J Neurosurg 72:176–182
8. Kayama T, Yoshimoto T, Fujimoto S, Sakurai Y (1991) Intratumoral oxygen pressure in malignant brain tumor. J Neurosurg 74:55–59
9. Leniger-Follert E, Lübbers DW, Wrabetz W (1975) Regulation of local tissue PO2 of the brain cortex at different arterial O2 pressures. Pflugers Arch 359:81–95
10. Meixensberger J, Brawanski A, Dannhauser-Leistner J, Holzschuh M, Ullrich W (1992) Is there a risk to induce ischemia by hyperventilation therapy? Springer, Berlin Heidelberg New York (Intracranial pressure, vol VIII) (in press)
11. Muizelaar JP, Marmarou A, DeSalles AAF, Ward JD, Zimmerman RS, Li Z, Choi SC, Young HF (1989) Cerebral blood flow and metabolism in severely head injured children. I. Relationship with GCS score, outcome, ICP, and PVI. J Neurosurg 71:63–71
12. Nair P, Whalen WJ, Buerk D (1975) PO2 of cat cerebral cortex: response to breathing N2 and 100% O2. Microvasc Res 9:158–165
13. Obrist WD, Langfitt TW, Jaggi JL, Criz J, Gennarelli TA (1984) Cerebral blood flow and metabolism in comatose patients with acute head injury. Relationship to intracranial hypertension. J Neurosurg 61:241–253
14. Robertson CS, Narayan RK, Gokaslan ZL, Pahwa R, Grossman RG, Caram P, Allen E (1989) Cerebral arteriovenous oxygen difference as an estimate of cerebral blood flow in comatose patients. J Neurosurg 70:222–230
15. Smith RH, Guilbeau EJ, Reneau DD (1977) The oxygen tension field with a discret volume of cerebral cortex. Microvasc Res 13:233–240

Cerebral and Tumor Blood Flow in Intracranial Tumors

S. Mirzai[1], M. Tatagiba, D.-K. Böker, and M. Samii

Introduction

It is well known that the regional cerebral blood flow (rCBF) and metabolism in brain tumor patients is abnormal in the tumor area and the surrounding brain tissue [7, 15, 17, 24, 31]. The rCBF in regions remote from the tumor has been found to be altered [9]. Little is known, however, about the regional distribution of such alteration.

The use of chemotherapeutics in tumor tissue depends on tissue blood flow and capillary permeability [23]. The initial access of anticancer agents to tumor cells was partially or completely limited by low blood flow [2, 4]. Also, the effects of irradiation are remarkably affected by tissue oxygen concentration, which is closely related to tissue blood flow and metabolism [23]. Therefore a better knowledge of the basic metabolic and hemodynamic parameters of intracranial tumors and their growth could lead to the design of improved therapy. Various reports have been published on the alteration of CBF in intracranial tumors [1, 6, 20]. Blood flow in tumor tissue as well as in deep-seated brain structures can be estimated by studies using positron emission tomography (PET), single photon emission computed tomography (SPECT), and stable xenon-CT [1, 6, 15, 18, 21, 24].

The aim of the present study was to determine the influence of intracranial tumors on the global CBF and to measure the regional blood flow within the tumor tissue per se and in relation to flow in surrounding nontumor tissue. Together with standard neuroradiological investigations, such as CT and magnetic resonance imaging (MRI), xenon-CT CBF studies were carried out in our clinic in 89 patients with intracranial tumors between 1988 and 1993. This report presents the results of CBF studies in 43 meningiomas and 21 gliomas compared to data from age-matched normal controls.

Material and Methods

This series included 64 patients with benign or malignant intracranial tumors. In all patients the diagnosis was confirmed histologically. The localization and the extent of tumor and the presence of peritumoral edema were determined by CT and MRI.

---

[1] Department of Neurosurgery, Nordstadt Hospital, Haltenhoffstr. 41, 30167 Hannover, Germany.

Advances in Neurosurgery, Vol. 22
B. L. Bauer, M. Brock, M. Klinger (Eds.)

The largest tumor diameter varied between 2.5 and 7 cm. There were 25 men and 39 women, aged from 18 to 78 years. Data were compared with those from 55 normal subjects with a mean age of 47 years.

The rCBF was measured using the stable xenon-CT method. The details of this methodology have been described elsewhere [32]. The method allows the quantitative determination of rCBF. There were no complications. A mixture of 33% stable xenon gas in 67% oxygen was inhaled via face mask for 5 min. For the CBF study 8 or 16 axial slices with 10 mm thickness were performed by CT scanner (80 kV, 200 mA, 4 s, 256 matrix, one- or two-level study). Blood flow was determined in the tumor tissue (TBF), peritumoral area (PTBF), and cerebral hemispheres (hCBF). The rCBF values were analyzed statistically using the unpaired Student's t test. The variables were also analyzed by Spearman's correlation coefficient. A p value of 0.05 or less was considered significant.

Gliomas. There were nine anaplastic astrocytomas, eight glioblastomas, two gliosarcomas, and two benign astrocytomas. All studies presented here were performed before radiation or chemotherapy.

Meningiomas. CBF was studied in 43 cases of intracranial meningiomas. The ages of 26 women and 17 men were 18–78 years. Of the meningiomas 60% were of the meningotheliomatous type.

Volunteers. Measurements of rCBF were made in 55 volunteers. None of the volunteers reported a history of cerebrovascular or cardiovascular disease, hypertension, or diabetes mellitus. There were 37 men and 18 women, aged 21–65 years.

Results

Correlation curves using Spearman's correlation coefficient between peritumoral CBF and ipsilateral hCBF demonstrated a significant positive correlation ($r = 0.7$). There was a negative correlation between hCBF and the size of midline shift.

Gliomas

Table 1 shows the mean CBF values for the whole hemisphere and for the gray and white matter, together with the mean age for glioma patients, compared to data from age-matched healthy volunteers. Comparison with age-matched normal subjects showed that lowered resting flow in the ipsilateral hemisphere was a common finding in glioma patients. The hCBF in glioma patients was significantly lower than in volunteers ($p < 0.01$). In 11 of 21 gliomas the hCBF was even lower than the lowest hCBF in volunteers. This CBF decrease was most marked for white matter flow and less marked for gray matter flow. The presence of a glioma caused in some cases a general decrease in the CBF within the affected hemisphere

Table 1. Regional CBF in patients with malignant gliomas compared to age-matched volunteers

	Age (years)	rCBF (ml/100 g^{-1} min^{-1})		
		CBF_h	CBF_g	CBF_w
Glioma patients	55 ± 14			
Ipsilateral		37 ± 17*	78 ± 29*	9 ± 6*
Contralateral		42 ± 17*	83 ± 31	12 ± 7*
Volunteers	47 ± 8	59 ± 9*	97 ± 13*	27 ± 7*
Significance (p^*)		$p < 0.01$	$p < 0.05$	$p < 0.01$

CBF_h, CBF_g, CBF_w CBF in hemisphere, in gray or white matter.

(Fig. 1). CBF was lower in the ipsilateral hemisphere than in the contralateral. CBF values in peritumoral edematous tissue were significantly lower than the CBF of ipsi- or contralateral hemispheres ($p < 0.01$). CBF in the tumor-free hemisphere within areas corresponding to the tumor location was generally higher (45 ± 25 ml) than that of the tumor (31 ± 16 ml) itself.

TVF averaged 31 ml, lower than hCBF of the ipsilateral hemisphere. There was a positive correlation between TBF and CBF of the ipsilateral hemisphere ($p = 0.002$, $r = 0.65$). TBF was variable, but was lower in the higher grade gliomas. Anaplastic astrocytomas were more perfused (32 ± 18 ml) than glioblastomas (21 ± 7 ml); the differences were not significant. The intratumoral variation of blood flow was more prominent in the larger gliomas. Lower values were generally measured centrally (17 ± 14 ml) in comparison to peripheral tumor regions (36 ± 11 ml). Gliosarcomas showed a homogenously high blood flow; malignant gliomas revealed a heterogeneous TBF with a central area with low flow and a peripheral part with high flow (Fig. 1).

Meningiomas

Meningiomas were significantly more perfused than malignant gliomas (65 ± 25 versus 31 ± 17 ml, $p < 0.01$). Meningiomas revealed two blood flow patterns: frequently a homogeneous pattern showing high tumor blood flow, and in some cases a heterogeneous pattern with high flow at the tumor periphery and a central area of low blood flow. The *average* hCBF values did not differ between the ipsi- and contralateral hemispheres, although in most of the individual cases the ipsilateral hCBF was lower than the contralateral hCBF. In individual cases blood flow values in the peritumoral edematous area were very low (Fig. 2). The minimum CBF values in peritumoral hypodense areas were lower than 15 ml 100 g^{-1} min^{-1}. PTBF correlated with the extent of edema itself. CBF of the affected hemisphere in patients with severe edema was lower than in those with mild edema. PTBF values correlated positively with ipsilateral hCBF values ($p < 0.01$, $r = 0.69$). In contrast,

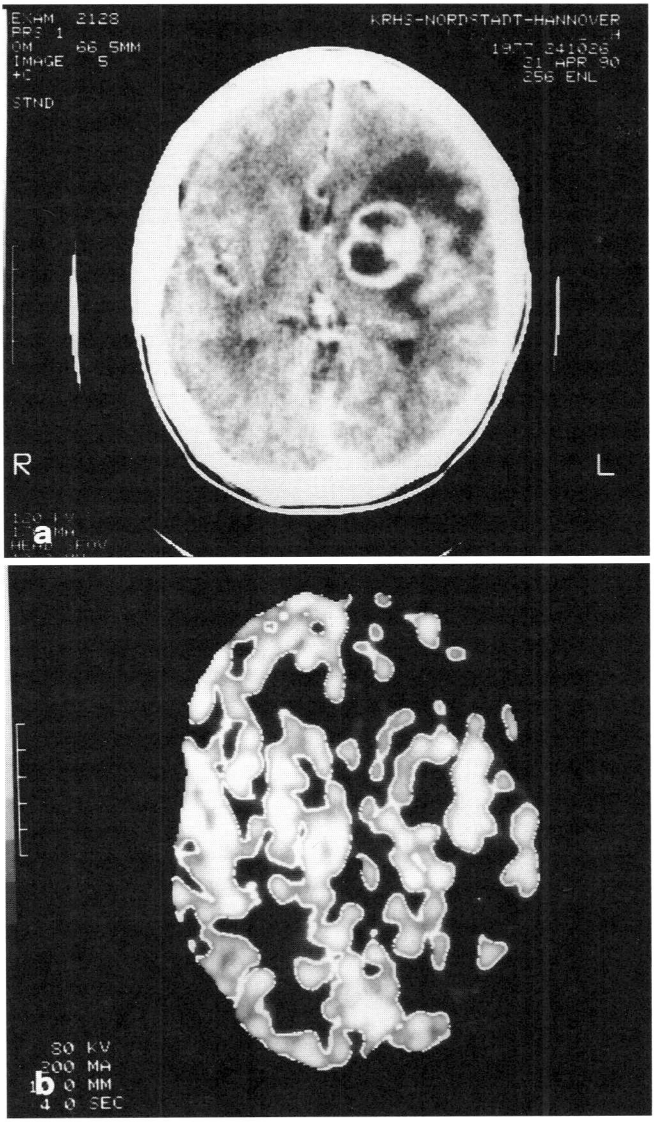

Fig. 1. a Enhanced CT showing a glioblastoma in basal ganglia on the left side (*left*). **b** Xenon-CT showing heterogeneous tumor blood flow with hyperperfusion in the tumor periphery and low flow in central part. Note the global decrease of the ipsilateral hCBF

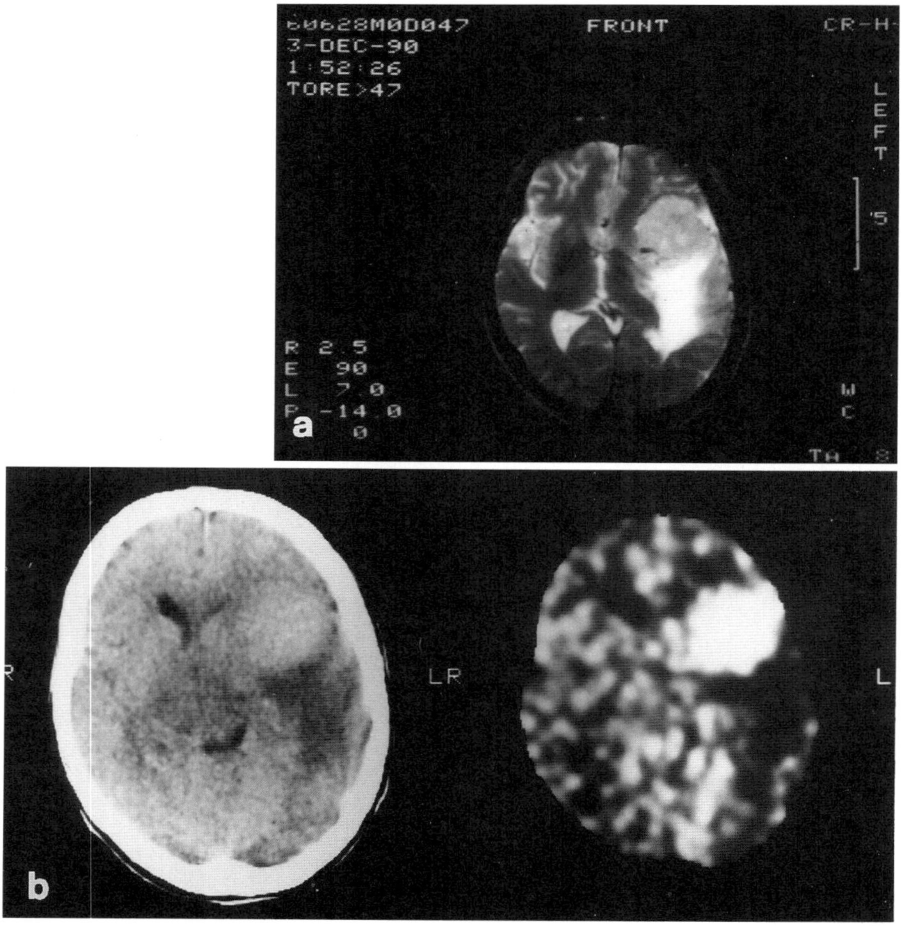

Fig. 2. a T2-weighted MRI (TE = 90, TR = 2.5, 1.0 T) showing a lateral sphenoid ridge meningioma on the left side and the extent of perifocal edema. **b** Native CT showing the slight hyperdense tumor with peritumoral low-density area ("edema") (*left*). Xenon-CT demonstrates high homogenous tumor blood flow pattern; note the reduced cerebral blood flow in the peritumoral low-density area (*right*)

Spearman's correlation coefficient was not significant between PTBF and contralateral hCBF ($p > 0.1$, $r = 0.38$).

Discussion

Cerebral and tumor blood flow and metabolism have important diagnostic and therapeutic implications. DiChiro et al. found that in patients with malignant gliomas the PET results correlated better with length of survival than the histological classification did [7]. Hylton et al. believed that in patients with gliomas a distinction between tumor recurrence and the early transient postirradiation effects can be made using the xenon-133 inhalation technique [14]. PET studies have been used not only to study the response of brain tumors to therapeutic intervention [3]. To improve our understanding of malignant and benign intracranial tumors, more must be known about both qualitative and quantitative differences between normal and neoplastic brain tissue [3]. This knowledge could be of direct relevance in designing therapy regimes. Despite recent advances in therapy regimes survival times remain short for high-grade gliomas [31]. The response of malignant brain tumors to irradiation, chemotherapy, or hyperthermia is influenced largely by the tissue blood flow and metabolism [2, 4, 22, 23].

Some of the main changes in rCBF in cases with intracranial tumors have been reported in previous works in which alteration of both general and local CBF was described [1, 5, 7, 25]. The regional distribution of such changes was, however, not known exactly. Most early works determined blood flow by two-dimensional methods and in experimental models [5, 16, 25]. Many animal experiments show that blood flow in brain tumor varies widely [4, 22]. Different authors have measured CBF in intracranial tumors using stable xenon-CT [1, 24, 27], PET [19–21, 26, 31], or SPECT [8, 20]. It is now generally accepted that rCBF is not evenly distributed throughout the hemispheres in cases of neoplastic brain diseases [9, 12]. Remote rCBF abnormalities have been found in brain tumors [9, 15].

The xenon-CT study provides direct anatomical correlation, relatively high resolution, and quantitative CBF information. The details of this methodology have been described elsewhere [13, 32]. This method has the unique ability to record very low flow values, even in relatively small and centrally located brain regions [13]. Our own clinical experience in more than 1000 studies without serious complications supports the safety of the method.

Gliomas

TBF in gliomas was lower than the ipsilateral hCBF ($p > 0.05$). This result is not in line with those obtained by the xenon-133 clearance method, which found a high blood flow over the tumor [5]. The xenon clearance technique suffers, however, from uncertainties due to physical and geometrical factors [15]. TBF was significantly lower than contralateral hCBF ($p < 0.05$). The hypoperfusion in central parts of tumor is probably due to necrosis or cystic parts. This finding has been also demonstrated in animal studies [4]. As described previously by other authors [31], we found lower TBF values in glioblastomas than in anaplastic astrocytomas. In brain tissue *directly* around the gliomas there was no extremely low CBF value (lower than 5 ml 100 g^{-1} min^{-1}) as seen in meningiomas. Compared to the normal values, gliomas led to a CBF decrease in the ipsilateral hemisphere. This CBF reduction cannot have been caused by tumor compression alone. It must have been due to other secondary effects of the tumor, such as an increase in intracranial pressure or a cytotoxic effect of neoplastic tissue. Increased intracranial pressure has been reported to decrease the CBF [11].

In the present investigation, TBF was found to vary widely irrespective of tumor type and grade of malignancy. Comparison of rCBF in structurally normal brain tissue between patients with gliomas and the volunteers indicated that hCBF values were markedly reduced in the gliomas. This observation is in accord with earlier reports that a focal lesion may cause a general reduction in the CBF [5, 15, 25].

Meningiomas

A close correlation between the extent of cerebral edema and the concurrent decrease in CBF has been reported [11, 30). Our series supports these results. Hino et al. [11] suggested that an increase in mass effect primarily reduces blood flow. Besides true cerebral edema, pressure-induced cerebral atrophy has been suggested as the cause of the hypodense area around meningiomas [29]. Quantification of the PTBF using a region of interest of 1 cm^2 showed peritumoral areas of extremely low blood flow in 15 cases. Flow values near zero have been recorded by the stable xenon-CT method [32]. Also, values less than 12 ml 100 g^{-1} min^{-1} have been accompanied by infarctions defined by CT [32]. We believe that the findings of extremely low PTBF surrounding meningiomas cannot be explained solely by the presence of vasogenic edema [28]. They may support the idea that the peritumoral hypodense areas are in part actual pressure atrophy, which does not respond to corticotherapy and persists after operation [29]. Similar findings were reported by Hino et al. [11] after investigation of peritumoral edema by PET.

There was a homogeneous high blood flow within gliosarcomas and meningiomas. Blood flow was variable within tumor tissue in glioblastomas and anaplastic astrocytomas. Blood flow within the malignant gliomas was consistently higher in the periphery than in the center of the tumor. In the peritumoral region CBF was reduced (especially in white matter), and reduction was lowest around the larger tumors. Correlation curves using Spearman's correlation coefficients between peritumoral CBF and ipsilateral hCBF demonstrated a significant positive correlation. The status of cerebral perfusion positively predicts the blood flow values in the peritumoral area, and possibly influences the grade of ischemia in the peritumoral region.

Although cerebral edema surrounding intracranial tumors is a well-known occurrence, its pathomechanism is not clearly understood [10]. The zone of diminished density surrounding tumors may commonly represent cerebral edema, but areas of necrosis and demyelination may have similar appearances. There are conflicting reports on metabolic dysfunction and alterations of cerebral circulation in peritumoral brain edema [30]. Peritumoral hypodense areas in cranial CT ("edema") may represent primary ischemia caused by chronic mechanical compression by slowly growing benign tumors, for example, meningiomas, and/or primary metabolic suppression in malignant gliomas.

References

1. Aritake K, Segawa H, Yoshimasu N et al. (1985) CBF study in patients with intracranial tumors by CT with stable xenon enhancement. In: Hartmann A, Hoyer S (eds) CBF and Metabolism Measurement. Springer, Berlin Heidelberg New York, pp 350–355
2. Baba T, Fukui M, Sakata et al. (1931) Selective enhancement of intratumoral blood flow in malignant gliomas, experimental study in rats by intracarotid administration of adenosine or adenosine triphosphate. Acta Neurochir 101:66
3. Beaney RP, Brooks DJ, Leenders KL et al. (1985) Blood flow and oxygen utilization in the contralateral cerebral cortex of patients with untreated intracranial tumours as studied by PET, with observations on the effect of decompressive surgery. J Neurol Neurosurg Psychiatry 48:310
4. Blasberg RG, Molnar P, Horowitz M et al. (1983) Regional blood flow in RT-9 brain tumors. J Neurosurg 58:863–873
5. Cronqvist S, Agee F (1968) Regional CBF in intracranial tumours. Acta Radiol 7:393–404
6. Di Chiro G, DeLaPaz RL, Brooks RA et al. (1982) Glucose utilization of cerebral gliomas measured by [F18] fluorodeoxyglucose and PET. Neurology 32:1323–1329
7. Di Chiro G, Hatazawa J, Katz DA et al. (1987) Glucose utilization by intracranial meningiomas as an index of tumor aggressivity and probability of recurrence, a PET study. Radiology 164:521
8. Drayer B, Jaszczak R, Friedman A et al. (1983) In vivo quantitation of rCBF in glioma and cerebral infarction, validation of the HIPDm-SPECT. AJNR Am J Neuroradiol 4:572
9. Endo H, Larsen B, Larssen NA (1977) Regional CBF alterations remote from the site of intracranial tumors. J Neurosurg 46:271–281
10. Go KG, Wilmink JT, Molenaar WM (1988) Peritumoral edema associated with meningiomas. Neurosurgery 23:175–179
11. Hino A, Imahori Y, Tenjin H et al. (1990) Metabolic and hemodynamic aspects of peritumoral low-density areas in human brain tumor. Neurosurgery 26:615–621
12. Hossmann KA, Niebuhr I, Tamura M (1982) Local CBF and glucose consumption of rats with experimental gliomas. J Cereb Blood Flow Metab 2:25
13. Hughes RL, Yonas H, Gur D et al. (1989) Cerebral blood flow determination within the first 8 hours of cerebral infarction using stable xenon-enhanced computed tomography. Stroke 20:754–760
14. Hylton PD, Reichman H, Palutsis R (1987) Monitoring of transient central nervous system postirradiation effects by 133 Xe inhalation rCBF measurements. Neurosurgery 21:843
15. Ito M, Lammertsma AA, Wise RJS et al. (1982) Measurement of rCBF and oxygen utilization in patients with cerebral tumours using 15O and PET, analytical techniques and preliminary results. Neuroradiology 23:63–74
16. Kato A, Sako K, Diksic M et al. (1985) Regional glucose utilization and blood flow in experimental brain tumors studied by double tracer autoradiography. J Neurooncology 3:271
17. Kawase T, Ohira T, Murakami H et al. (1985) Influence of peritumoral edema on rCBF and on cerebral function: analysis by xenon-enhanced CT and EEG topography. In: Inaba Y, Klatzo I, Spatz M (eds) Brain edema. Springer, Berlin Heidelberg New York, pp 484
18. Kohmura E, Gürtner P, Holl K et al. (1986) Erfahrungen mit der Inhalation eines 33%igen Xenon-(stable-)-Sauerstoffgemisches im Zusammenhang mit einer neuen Methode zur lokalen Hirndurchblutungsmessung. Rofo Fortschr Geb Rontgenstr Bildgeb Verfahr 144:531–536

19. Lammertsma AA, Wise RJS, Cox TC et al. (1985) Measurement of blood flow, oxygen utilization, oxygen extraction ratio, and fractional blood volume in human brain tumours and surrounding oedematous tissue. Br J Radiology 58:725
20. Langen KJ, Herzog H, Kuwert T et al. (1988) Tomographic studies of rCBF with 99mTc-HMPAO SPECT in patients with brain tumors, comparison with $C_{15}O_2$ continuous inhalation technique and PET. J Cereb Blood Flow Metab 8:90–94
21. Mineura K, Yasuda T, Kowada M et al. (1986) PET evaluation of histological malignancy in gliomas using oxygen-15 and fluorine-18-fluorodeoxyglucose. Neurol Res 8:164–168
22. Moriyama E (1990) Cerebral blood flow changes during localized hyperthermia. Neurol Med Chir (Tokyo) 30:923
23. Nagashima T, Tamura A, Matsutani M et al. (1983) Regional CBF in experimental brain tumors, comparative study between blood flow and neuropathological characteristics. J Cereb Blood Flow Metab 3[Suppl 1]69–70
24. Nakamura O, Segawa H, Tanaka H et al. (1987) Regional CBF in brain tumours as measured by xenon enhanced CT. Neurol Res 9:24–29
25. Palvölgyi R (1969) Regional CBF in patients with intracranial tumors. J Neurosurg 31:149
26. Rozental JM, Levine RL, Nickels RJ et al. (1990) Cerebral diaschisis in patients with malignant glioma. J Neurooncology 8:153
27. Tachibana H, Meyer JS, Rose JE et al. (1984) Local CBF and partition coefficients measured in cerebral astrocytomas of different grades of malignancy. Surg Neurol 21:125
28. Tatagiba M, Mirzai SH, Samii M (1991) Peritumoral blood flow in intracranial meningiomas. Neurosurgery 28:400
29. Trittmacher S, Traupe H, Schmid A (1988) Pre- and postoperative changes in brain tissue surrounding a meningioma. Neurosurgery 22:882–885
30. Tsubokawa T, Tsukuyama T, Ohta H et al. (1985) Regional metabolism and circulation at peritumoral edema caused by meningioma and malignant glioma. In: Inaba Y, Klatzo I, Spatz M (eds) Brain edema. Springer, Berlin Heidelberg New York, pp 194–199
31. Tyler JL, Diksic M, Villemure JG et al. (1987) Metabolic and hemodynamic evaluation of gliomas using PET. J Nucl Med 28:1123–1133
32. Yonas H, Sekhar L, Johnson DW et al. (1989) Determination of irreversible ischemia by xenon-enhanced computed tomographic monitoring of cerebral blood flow in patients with symptomatic vasospasm. Neurosurgery 24:368–372

Interstitial Immunotherapy of Multicellular Tumor Spheroids Using Liposomes Containing Tumor Necrosis Factor-α

F. Weber[1], M. Klinkhammer[2], B. Rasier[2], J. List[1], T. Höll[1], and M. Brock[1]

Introduction

The effects of immunomodulating cytokines on glial tumor cells can better be investigated in vitro with the aid of a multicellular tumour spheroid (MTS) model rather than in monolayer cultures. Spheroids represent an intermediate level of biological complexity between monolayer cultures in vitro and experimental tumors in vivo. A three-dimensional model is especially appropriate for studying the effect of immunomodulators since their major effects are mediated by the modulated attitude of the malignant transformed cell. The experimental model of glioma used in this work was based on the human glioma cell line A172, derived from a human glioblastoma. This model simulates in vitro the local immunotherapy. In particular, the three-dimensional character of the MTS mimics the in vivo situation when liposomes are administered locally and migrate into the tumor tissue. This contribution describes the preparation of the MTS from A172 cells and their response to empty liposomes, free tumor necrosis factor-α (TNF-α) and TNF-α encapsulated within liposomes.

Materials and Methods

Monolayer cultures. A172 is a cell line derived from a 53-year-old male patient with glioblastoma multiforme; it was obtained from the Tissue Culture Collection of the Department of Experimental Pathology of the German Cancer Research Center (Heidelberg). The cell line was maintained in Ham's F10 medium containing 10% heat-inactivated fetal calf serum (Gibco), glutamine (0.29 mg/ml), and penicillin. Cultures were established at 37 °C in humidified air with 5% CO_2.

Preparation of MTS. The spheroids were cultured in liquid overlay technique [4, 13]. After trypsination from a monolayer culture 10 x 10^6 A172 cells were placed in Ham's F10 medium on a thin layer of agarose (0.5% agarose in distilled water) in six-well plates (Nunc, Roskilde, Denmark) for about 2 weeks.

[1] Department of Neurosurgery, Klinikum Steglitz, Free University of Berlin, Hindenburgdamm 30, 12200 Berlin, Germany.
[2] Department of Neurosurgery, Municipal Hospital of Cologne, Ostmerheimerstr. 200, 51109 Cologne, Germany.

Advances in Neurosurgery, Vol. 22
B. L. Bauer, M. Brock, M. Klinger (Eds.)

Preparation of Multilamellar Liposomes. Multilamellar vesicles (MLV) were prepared from dimyristolylphoshatidyl choline (DMPC) (Nattermann, Cologne, Germany), cholesterol CH (Merck, Darmstadt, Germany), and methylediethanolamine-dipalmitate (MDEAP) in a molar ratio of 50:30:20 (mol/%), respectively. Lipids were dissolved in chloroform in a round-bottomed flask. A thin lipid layer was formed on the inside wall of the flask by removal of the organic solvent through rotary evaporation at reduced pressure. Finally, a phosphate buffer was added, and the dry film was hydrated by shaking overnight. The MLV dispersion was extruded through a polycarbonate filter with well-defined pore sizes which decrease the size and the number of lamellae. The size of the vesicles used in this work was approximately 400 nm (Autosizer II, Malvern, UK).

TNF-α Liposomes. An aliquot of TNF-α solution prepared under sterile conditions (Knoll, Ludwigshafen, Germany) was incubated with empty MLV solution. The optimal lipid concentration for the adsorption of TNF-α was tested before. The vesicle (1 ml) dispersion contained 25 μg TNF-α and 50 mg lipid.

Treatment of the Spheroids with Liposomes. After 7 days of growth, liposomes, free TNF-α, TFN-α-liposomes, and empty liposomes were added. The liposomes were MLV with a size of 400 or 3500 nm. TNF-α was given in concentrations of 100, 200, and 1000 ng/ml. The TNF-α liposomes were added in the following concentrations: 1, 2, and 10 mg/ml. The spheroids were divided into ten groups, each consisting of 50 spheroids. Three groups were treated with increasing doses of TNF-α (100, 200, 1000 ng/ml) and three groups with corresponding doses of TNF-α encapsulated in MLV. Groups 7, 8, and 9 were treated with empty MLV, receiving the same concentrations of liposomes in order to estimate effects due purely to the liposomes. Group 10, which received no treatment, served as the control.

Determination of MTS Growth Characteristics. The diameter of the MTS was measured by means of an ocular scale, manipulated by a micrometer screw in an inverted microscope (Zeiss) for 50 spheroids of each therapeutic group on each day. The mean value of each group and day were compared to each other using Student's *t* test.

Electron Microscopy. The migration of liposomes into the spheroid and the direct interaction with the tumor cells were studied using transmission electron microscopy and light microscopy. After incubation for 48 h the spheroids were isolated from the pellets, washed by sedimentation, and fixed in 2% glutaraldehyde (cacodylate buffer) for 90 min. They were then washed in the buffer, postfixed with 1% osmium tetroxide in the buffer, dehydrated in graded alcohols, and embedded in araldite mixed with metacrylate. The block was trimmed so that ultrathin sections extended inward from the surface of the spheroid to a depth of about 500 μm at the approximate equatorial plane. Thin sections were cut in a Leica Ultracut ultramicrotome, stained with uranyl acetate and lead citrate, and examined with a Zeiss EM 902 transmission electron microscope. Sections for light microscopy were cut at 1 μm and stained with toluidine blue.

Results

Growth Delay of the Spheroids. To initiate MTS growth, 1 x 10^6 cells trypsinated from a monolayer culture were placed in agarose-coated six-well plates. Spheroids were detectable after only 1 day (Fig. 1).

No significant difference among the groups which had been treated with three different concentrations of TNF-α (Fig. 2) was observed. There was a significant difference in growth ($p < 0.001$) between spheroids treated with TNF-α and those coincubated with empty liposomes. The difference correlated with the dosage of liposomes. A similar significant difference ($p < 0.001$) was observed between the "free" TNF-α groups and those which had received liposomes loaded with TNF-α. A significant growth delay was found in the MTS treated with empty liposomes ($p < 0.001$) and in those incubated with TNF loaded liposomes ($p < 0.001$; Figs. 3, 4). Comparison of the "empty-liposome" groups to the "loaded-liposome" groups revealed that the TNF-α had a stronger growth-inhibiting effect, which, however, was not significant. These results indicate that the growth-inhibiting effect was mediated mainly by the liposomes. TNF-α had no significant growth-inhibiting effect on MTS of the cell line A172. The results of the statistical analysis (*t* test) are summarized in Table 1.

Electron Microscopy. Transmission electron microscopy revealed that MLV liposomes were located intracellularly. The liposomes showed the capablility to migrate into the MTS, even where cells were tightly attached to adjacent cells (Fig. 5 a). The MLV liposomes are located intracellularly around the nucleus (Fig. 5 b). This picture demonstrates the fact that liposomes invade glioma cells even in a

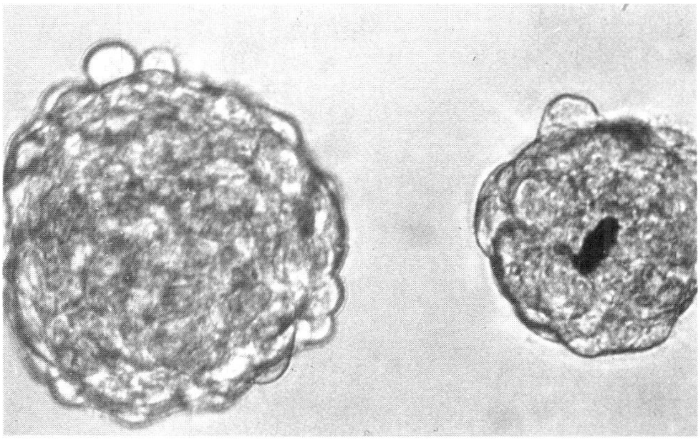

Fig. 1. Light microscopic picture of a MTS (A172) 4 days after onset of growth from single cells. Original magnification x 10

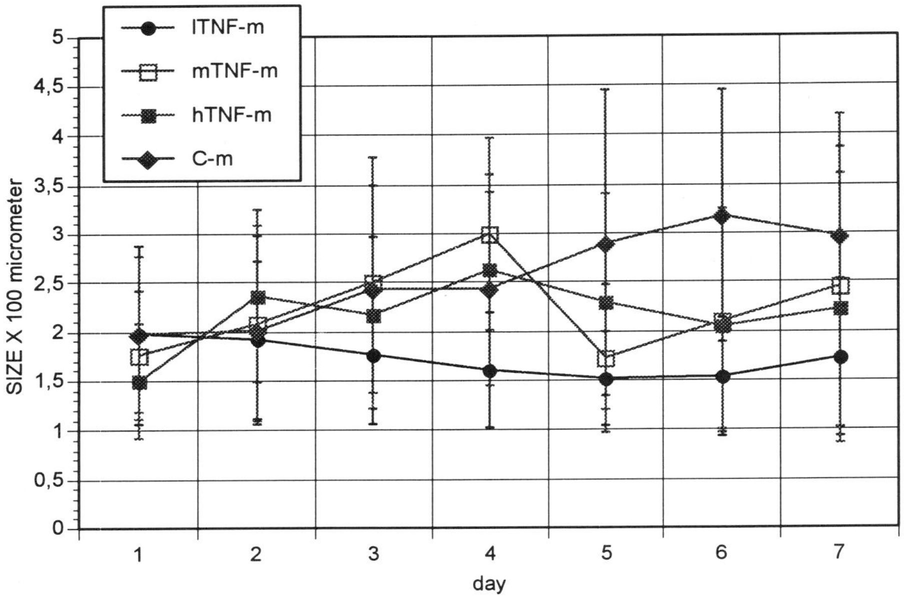

Fig. 2. Growth curves for A172 MTS treated with TNF-α. The three administered doses were 100 (low), 200 (medium), and 1000 ng/ml (high). Each *point* represents the mean of a group of 50 MTS. There was no significant growth delay attributable to TNF-α. *lTNF-m*, Mean size of the spheroids treated with TNF (low concentration); *mTNF-m*, mean size of the spheroids treated with TNF (medium concentration); *hTNF-m*, mean size of the spheroids treated with TNF (high concentration); *C-m*, mean values of the control

three-dimensional cell aggregation. These findings suggest that liposomes are appropriate vesicles to transport TNF α into the cell.

Discussion

This study investigated the direct cytotoxic effect of TNF-α on the tumor cell line A172. To augment the activity of TNF-α, its administration was tested in combination with liposomes (MLV) as carrier vehicles. Although the mechanism for resistance to cytotoxicity is unknown, it cannot be due only to differences in the type and/or number of cell surface receptors for TNF-α since resistant cells can bind TNF-α without undergoing lysis [10]. The internalization of TNF-α is necessary to achieve a cytotoxic effect since agents that disrupt the cytoskeleton or inhibit lysomal activity inhibit TNF-α cytotoxicity. The fact that inhibition of protein synthesis sensitizes cells to the cytotoxic action of TFN-a suggests that cells synthesize proteins that actively protect them from TNF-α cytotoxicity.

It is hypothesized that the release of free radicals is one of the mechanisms by which this occurs [6–8, 13, 15]. It is not known whether TNF-α mediates an in-

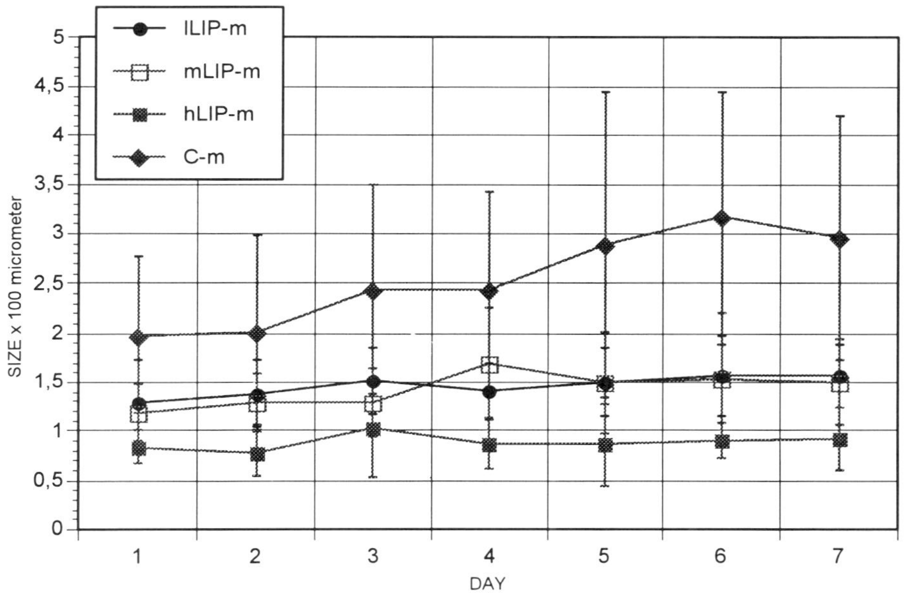

Fig. 3. Growth curves for A172 MTS treated with "empty liposomes." The three administrated dosages were 1, 2, and 10 mg/ml. Each point represents the mean of a group of 50 MTS. There was significant growth delay related to the liposomes (Table 1). *lLIP-m*, Mean size of the spheroids treated with liposomes (low concentration); *mLIP-m*, mean size of the spheroids treated with liposomes (medium concentration); *hLIP-m*, mean size of the spheroids treated with liposomes (high concentration); *C-m*, mean values of the control

creased release of O_2^- from mitochondria. Manganese superoxide dismutase reduces O_2^- to H_2O_2 and decreases the release of free radicals due to the effect of TNF-α. In the presence of an appropriate metal chelate O_2^- and H_2O_2 can react to form highly reactive oxidants that can cause damage to cellular proteins, lipids, and macromolecules and thus mediate TNF-α cytotoxicity [2, 3, 10]. The fact that several glial tumor model systems [4, 8, 9, 12] are resistant to TNF-α cytotoxicity may be related to increased manganese superoxide dismutase activity.

The fact that the major growth-inhibiting effect is mediated by liposomes might be due to methylediethanolamine-dipalmitate, which is positively loaded. The effect of these positively loaded molecules on cell membranes is still unclear. Stearylamine, another positively loaded component of liposomes, shows even stronger growth-inhibiting effects. Our reports show that the direct cytotoxic effect of TFN-α is insufficient for effective cytoreduction. Most research work has been perfomed using monolayer cultures [1, 2]. A difference in growth of the cell line A172 was found by Chen [1] in terms of whether they grew under confluent or subconfluent conditions. Confluently growing cells showed a much lower amount of proliferating cells (% KI-67 positive cells), indicating that cell to cell interaction

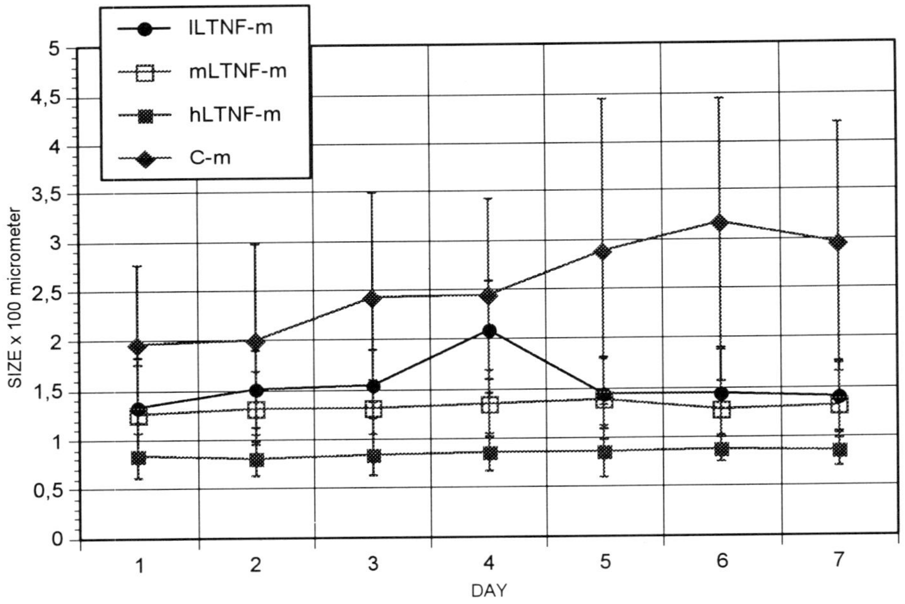

Fig. 4. Growth curves for A172 MTS treated with TNF-α liposomes in doses of 0.2, 0.4 (lipid/medium), and 2 mg/ml (lipid/medium); 500 ng TNF-α was absorbed to 1 mg lipid. Adminstered doses were 1, 2, and 10 mg/ml, whereby 1 mg contained 100 ng, 2 mg 200 ng, and 10 mg 1000 ng TNF-α. Each *point* represents the mean of a group of 50 MTS. There was a significant growth delay related to the liposomes (Table 1). *lTNF-m*, Mean size of the spheroids treated with "TNF-loaded" liposomes (low concentration); *mTNF-m*, mean size of the spheroids treated with "TNF-loaded" liposomes (medium concentration); *hTNF-m*, mean size of the spheroids treated with "TNF-loaded" liposomes (high concentration); *C-m*, mean values of the control

can modulate the effects of TFN-α on tumor cells. Recording such effects might be more pronounced in a three-dimensional MTS model.

Conclusion

Summarizing these findings with respect to the results of Del Maestro [2] and Chen [1], the effects of TNF-α on tumor cells are very complex and variable, and probably depend on the growth condition of the cells as well as several autocrine and/or paracrine processes during cell growth. The direct cytotoxic effect which can be achieved by local administration of pure TNF-α is insufficient. Liposomes seem an appropriate carrier system to prolong and enforce the effects of biological response modifier after local administration. Nonetheless, lioposomes invade tumor cells and transport substances into the cell. Problems regarding liposomal cytotoxicity arise which must be examined in in vivo models.

Table 1. Significance levels of correlations (each p value represents the mean of 50 spheroids)

	l-TNF	m-TNF	h-TNF	l-LIP	m-LIP	h-LIP	l-LTNF	m-LTNF	h-LTNF	Control
Day 1										
l-TNF		< 0.21	< 0.003	> 0.0001	< 0.0001	< 0.0001	< 0.0001	< 0.0001	< 0.0001	< 0.97
m-TNF			< 0.029	< 0.0001	< 0.0001	< 0.0001	< 0.0001	< 0.0001	< 0.0001	< 0.17
h-TNF				< 0.0001	< 0.0001	< 0.0001	< 0.0001	< 0.0001	< 0.0001	< 0.001
l-LIP					< 0.53	< 0.0001	< 0.588	< 0.534	< 0.0001	< 0.0001
m-LIP						< 0.0001	< 0.0002	< 0.27	< 0.0001	< 0.0001
h-LIP							< 0.0001	< 0.0001	< 0.88	< 0.0001
l-LTNF								< 0.2029	< 0.0001	< 0.0001
m-LTNF									< 0.0001	< 0.0001
h-LTNF										< 0.0001
Day 2										
l-TNF		< 0.014	< 0.009	> 0.0001	< 0.0001	< 0.0001	< 0.0001	< 0.0001	< 0.0001	< 0.588
m-TNF			< 0.138	< 0.0001	< 0.0001	< 0.0001	< 0.0001	< 0.0001	< 0.0001	< 0.721
h-TNF				< 0.0001	< 0.0001	< 0.0001	< 0.0001	< 0.0001	< 0.0001	< 0.059
l-LIP					< 0.014	< 0.01	< 0.0883	< 0.0001	< 0.0001	< 0.0001
m-LIP						< 0.01	< 0.0001	< 0.6107	< 0.0001	< 0.0001
h-LIP							< 0.0001	< 0.0001	< 0.4897	< 0.0001
l-LTNF								< 0.1432	< 0.0018	< 0.0001
m-LTNF									< 0.0001	< 0.0001
h-LTNF										< 0.0001
Day 3										
l-TNF		< 0.0001	< 0.0090	> 0.0001	< 0.0001	< 0.0001	< 0.0008	< 0.0001	< 0.0001	< 0.0057
m-TNF			< 0.013	< 0.0001	< 0.0001	< 0.0001	< 0.0001	< 0.0001	< 0.0001	< 0.7922
h-TNF				< 0.0001	< 0.0001	< 0.0001	< 0.0001	< 0.0001	< 0.0001	< 0.1530

Table 1 (continued)

	l-TNF	m-TNF	h-TNF	l-LIP	m-LIP	h-LIP	l-LTNF	m-LTNF	h-LTNF	Control
Day 3										
l-LIP					< 0.0004	< 0.0006	< 0.0412	< 0.0001	< 0.0001	< 0.0001
m-LIP						< 0.0491	< 0.0001	< 0.0337	< 0.0001	< 0.0001
h-LIP							< 0.0001	< 0.0001	< 0.0003	< 0.0001
l-LTNF								< 0.0001	< 0.0001	< 0.0001
m-LTNF									< 0.0001	< 0.0001
h-LTNF										< 0.0001
Day 4										
l-TNF		< 0.0003	< 0.0003	> 0.0001	< 0.0002	< 0.0001	< 0.0001	< 0.0001	< 0.0001	< 0.0003
m-TNF			< 0.0634	< 0.0001	< 0.0001	< 0.0001	< 0.0001	< 0.0001	< 0.0001	< 0.0064
h-TNF				< 0.0001	< 0.0001	< 0.0001	< 0.0001	< 0.0001	< 0.0001	< 0.3632
l-LIP					< 0.0001	< 0.0001	< 0.0002	< 0.0027	< 0.0001	< 0.0001
m-LIP						< 0.0001	< 0.0001	< 0.0007	< 0.0001	< 0.0001
h-LIP							< 0.0001	< 0.0001	< 0.0001	< 0.0001
l-LTNF								< 0.0001	< 0.0001	< 0.0001
m-LTNF									< 0.0001	< 0.0001
h-LTNF										< 0.0001
Day 5										
l-TNF		< 0.0015	< 0.0001	> 0.3954	< 0.3188	< 0.0001	< 0.488	< 0.0001	< 0.0001	< 0.0001
m-TNF			< 0.0001	< 0.0106	< 0.0001	< 0.0001	< 0.0001	< 0.008	< 0.0001	< 0.0001
h-TNF				< 0.0001	< 0.0001	< 0.0001	< 0.0001	< 0.0001	< 0.0001	< 0.0163
l-LIP					< 0.4866	< 0.0215	< 0.4538	< 0.0001	< 0.0001	< 0.0001
m-LIP						< 0.0016	< 0.1273	< 0.2756	< 0.0001	< 0.0001
h-LIP							< 0.0001	< 0.0001	< 0.0009	< 0.0001

l-LTNF							< 0.0123	< 0.0001	< 0.0001
m-LTNF								< 0.0001	< 0.0001
h-LTNF									< 0.0001
Day 6									
l-TNF	< 0.0001	< 0.0001	> 0.3856	< 0.9443	< 0.0001	< 0.0139	< 0.0001	< 0.0001	< 0.0001
m-TNF		< 0.8054	< 0.0001	< 0.0001	< 0.0001	< 0.0001	< 0.0002	< 0.0001	< 0.0001
h-TNF			< 0.0001	< 0.0001	< 0.0001	< 0.0001	< 0.0001	< 0.0001	< 0.0001
l-LIP				< 0.0021	< 0.0001	< 0.1767	< 0.0001	< 0.0001	< 0.0001
m-LIP					< 0.0001	< 0.0135	< 0.0001	< 0.0001	< 0.0001
h-LIP						< 0.0001	< 0.0001	< 0.0294	< 0.0001
l-LTNF							< 0.0017	< 0.0001	< 0.0001
m-LTNF								< 0.0001	< 0.0001
h-LTNF									< 0.0001
Day 7									
l-TNF	< 0.0001	< 0.0003	> 0.0001	< 0.0001	< 0.0001	< 0.0001	< 0.0001	< 0.0001	< 0.0032
m-TNF		< 0.4526	< 0.0001	< 0.0001	< 0.0001	< 0.0001	< 0.0001	< 0.0001	< 0.0549
h-TNF			< 0.0001	< 0.0001	< 0.0001	< 0.0001	< 0.0001	< 0.0001	< 0.0062
l-LIP				< 0.1919	< 0.0001	< 0.0196	< 0.0001	< 0.0001	< 0.0001
m-LIP					< 0.0001	< 0.0001	< 0.0222	< 0.0001	< 0.0001
h-LIP						< 0.0001	< 0.0001	< 0.0001	< 0.0001
l-LTNF							< 0.0309	< 0.0001	< 0.0001
m-LTNF								< 0.0227	< 0.0001
h-LTNF									< 0.0001

TNF, Spheroids treated with tumor necrosis factor; LIP, spheroids treated with liposomes; LTNF, spheroids treated with tumor necrosis factor loaded liposomes; *l*-, low concentration, *m*-, medium concentration, *h*-, high concentration.

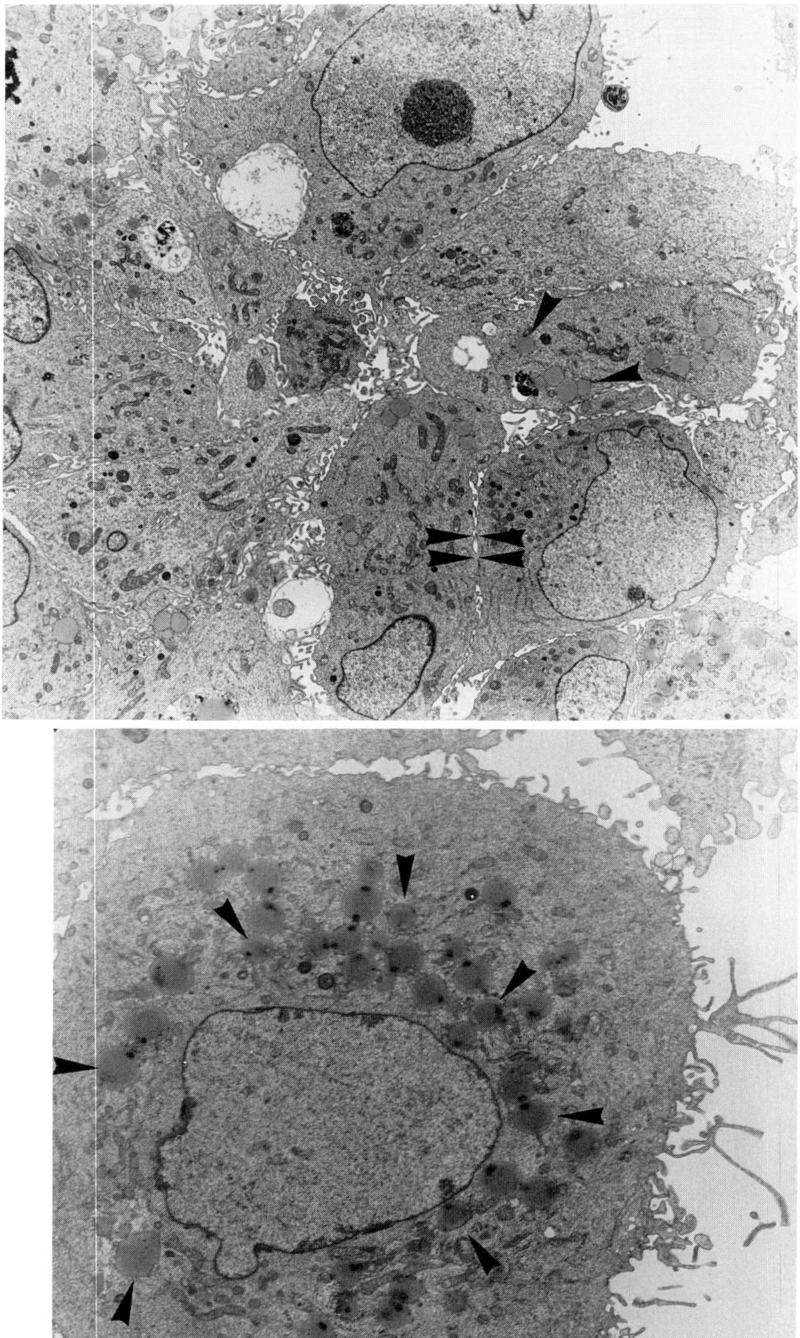

a

b

References

1. Chen TC, Hinton DR, Apuzzo MLJ, Hofman FM (1993) Differential effects of tumor necrosis factor-alpha on proliferation, cell surface antigen expression, and cytokine interactions in malignant gliomas. Neurosurgery 32(1):85–94
2. Del Maestro RF (1980) An approach to free radicals in medicine and biology. Acta Physiol Scand [Suppl] 492:153–168
3. Del Maestro RF (1991) Free radicals as mediators of tissue injury. In: Dreoti I (ed) Micronutrients and free radicals. Humana, Clifton, pp 25–51
4. Del Maestro RF, Lopez-Torres M, McDonald WB, Stroude EC, Vaithilingam IS (1992) The effect of tumor necrosis factor-α on human malignant glial cells. J Neurosurg 76:652–659
5. Haji-Karim M, Carlsson J (1978) Proliferation and viability in cellular spheroids of human origin. Cancer Res 38:1457–1464
6. Larrick JW, Wright SC (1990) Cytotoxic mechanism of tumor necrosis factor-α. FASEB J 4:3215–3223
7. McCord J, Fridovich I (1969) Superoxide dismutase. An enzymatic function for erythrocuprein (hemocuprein). J Biol Chem 244:6049–6055
8. Oberley LW, Buettner GR (1979) Role of superoxide dismutase in cancer: a review. Cancer Res 39:1141–1149
9. Oberley LW, Oberley TD, Buettner GR (1980) Cell differentiation, ageing and cancer: the possible roles of superoxide and superoxide dismutases. Med Hypotheses 6:249–268
10. Tsujimoto M, Yip YK, Vilcek J (1985) Tumor necrosis factor: specific binding and internalization in sensitive and resistant cells. Proc Natl Acad Sci USA 82:7626–7630
11. Tsujimoto M, Yokota S, Vilcek J (1986) Tumor necrosis factor provokes superoxide antigen generation from neutrophils. Biochem Biophys Res Commun 137:1094–1100
12. Wong GHW, Elwell JH, Oberley LW (1989) Manganese superoxide dismutase is essential for cellular resistance to cytotoxicity of tumor necrosis factor. Cell 58:923–931
13. Yamauchi N, Kuriyama H, Watanabe N (1989) Intracellular hydroxyl radical production induced by recombinant human tumor necrosis factor and its a implication in the killing of tumor cells in vitro. Cancer Res 49:1671–1675
14. Yuhas JM, Li AP, Martinez AO, Ladman AJ (1977) A simplified method for production and growth of multicellular tumour spheroids. Cancer Res 37:3639–3643
15. Zimmerman RJ, Chan A, Leadon SA (1989) Oxidative damage in murine tumor cells treated in vitro by recombinant tumor necrosis factor. Cancer Res 49:1644–1648

Fig. 5 a. Ultrastructure of the A172 MTS 3 days after growth onset from single cells. The MLV liposomes are intracellular (*single arrow*). Cells are tightly attached to adjacent cells (*two arrows*). Transmission electron microscopy, original magnification x 3000. **b** Ultrastructure of a single cell of an A172 MTS 3 days after growth onset from single cells. The MLV liposomes surround the nucleus (*single arrow*). This picture demonstrates the fact that liposomes invade glioma cells even in three-dimensional aggregation. Transmission electron microscopy, original magnification x 4000

Cavernomas and Developmental Venous Anomalies: Diagnosis and Therapy

E. Donauer[1], J. R. Moringlane[1], J. Reif[1], G. Huber[2], and W. Feiden[3]

Introduction

In comparison to angiographically apparent vascular malformations (AVMs) little is known about the incidence and impact of hemorrhages from angiographically occult vascular malformations (AOVMs) [1, 4, 9, 10, 13, 14]. However, with the widespread availability of magnetic resonance imaging it has become considerably easier to identify AOVMs [3, 8, 12]. From our evaluation of more than 2500 angiograms the incidence rate of developmental venous anomalies (DVAs) and the rate of their coincidence with cavernomas were determined retrospectively. The clinical symptoms and complications of these lesions were also evaluated. Apart from this retrospective neuroradiological examination the therapeutic strategy and operative results are demonstrated in 33 patients with cavernoma. For deep lesions the significance of a combined stereotactical-microsurgical approach is illustrated.

Materials and Methods

More than 3500 angiographic examinations performed at the Department of Neuroradiology, University Clinic in Homburg/Saar, between 1982 and 1991 were evaluated retrospectively [3]. A total of 35 cases of DVA were found; for the present analysis these are divided into two groups. Group I comprises the 18 patients (10 male, 8 female; ages 5–66 years, mean 32) who presented with DVA only [7]. Group 2 includes the 17 patients (12 male, 5 female, ages 8–62 years, mean 29) who presented with a cavernous hemangioma in the immediate vicinity of the DVA (two aneurysms, one fistula of the dura). In addition, the follow-up data were analyzed for a third group of 33 patients (19 male, 14 female; ages 4–75 years, mean 30) diagnosed as having a cavernoma (three multiple, one orbital) and treated at the Department of Neurosurgery between 1986 and 1992. The localization of hematomas in the three groups is presented in Table 1.

---

[1] Department of Neurosurgery, University of the Saarland, 66421 Homburg/Saar, Germany.
[2] Department of Neuroradiology, University of the Saarland, 66421 Homburg/Saar, Germany.
[3] Department of Neuropathology, University of the Saarland, 66421 Homburg/Saar, Germany.

Advances in Neurosurgery, Vol. 22
B. L. Bauer, M. Brock, M. Klinger (Eds.)

Table 1. Localization of hematomas

Group	Anomaly/ malformation	*n*	Frontal	Temporal/ parietal	Occipital	Basal ganglia	Posterior fossa
1	DVA	18	7	5	1	1	4
2	DVA and cavernoma	17	9	2	0	3	3
3	Cavernoma	33	7	12	1	5	5
Total		68	23	19	2	9	12

Results

Table 2 shows the neurological symptoms of the three patient groups. In group 1 ($n = 18$) no hemorrhages were found, and 13 patients had no neurological symptoms. In group 2 ($n = 17$) two cases of hemorrhage were observed (Fig. 1). In group 3 ($n = 33$) 24 patients experienced hemorrhage, 15 epileptic seizures, and 2 patients remained asymptomatic. Seven patients in group 3 were treated conservatively; three improved and three remained clinically unchanged (Table 3). In three patients of group 3 the contents of the hematoma was aspirated under stereotactic conditions alone; two showed very satisfactory clinical recovery and the third remained unchanged. Seven patients received a combination of microsurgical and stereotactic treatment; these lesions were small and situated deep within the parenchyma. It was possible to localize the lesion via a stereotactic trajectory and simultaneously to obtain biopsy material for histopathological examination (Fig. 1). Subseqently, the cavernoma was removed microsurgically through a small incision following the stereotactic trajectory. Two of these seven patients remained clinically unchanged, four improved, and in one case of a centrally localized cavernoma transient arm paresis occurred. In 16 cases the cavernoma was removed by microsurgical intervention alone. Postoperatively, two

Table 2. Neurological symptoms

Group	Anomaly/ malformation	*n*	Acute bleeding	Epileptic seizures	Hemiparesis	Dysphasia	Visual disturbances	Other	Without clinical symptoms
1	DVA	18	0	2	2 (2)	1 (1)		1	13
2	DVA and cavernoma	17	2	3	3 (2)	2 (2)	1	1	9
3	cavernoma[a]	33	24	15	12 (6)	6 (4)	5 (2)	4 (2)	2

Parentheses, transient neurological disturbances.
[a] 14 patients suffered intermittent headaches.

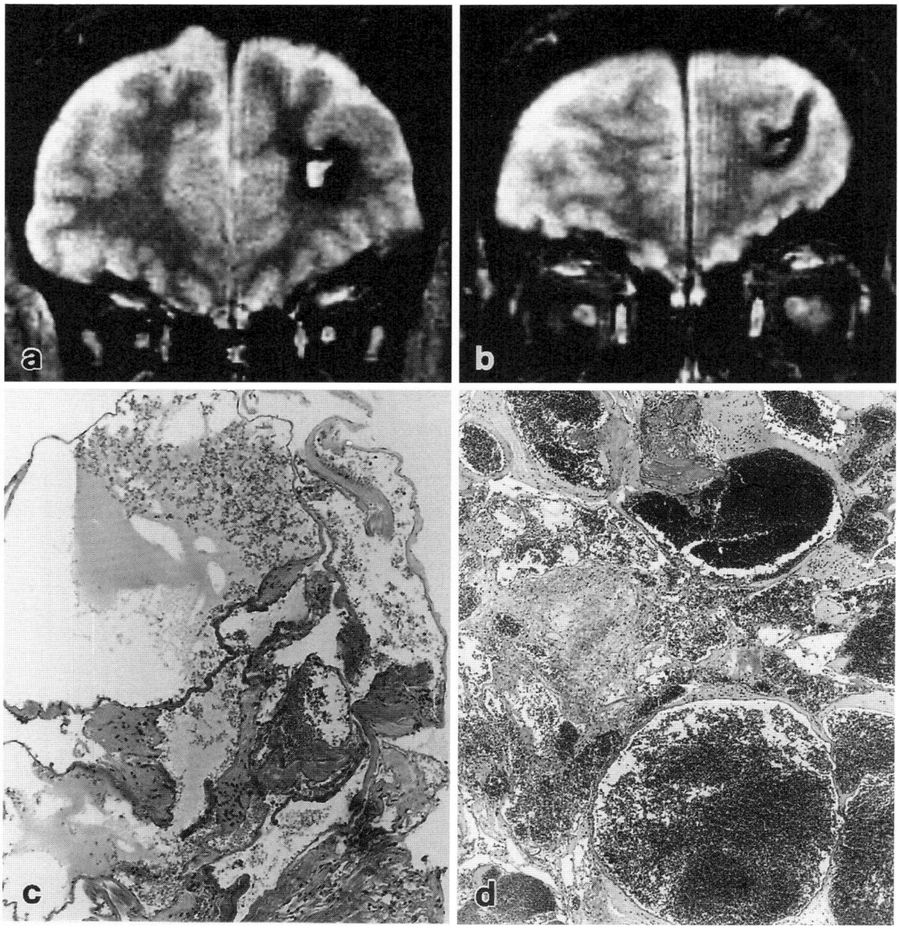

Fig. 1. **a** Acute bleeding in a frontal cavernoma. **b** Note venous drainage; DVA diagnosis suspected. **c** Stereotactic biopsy shows typical cavernous hemangioma. x 120. **d** Stereotactically guided resection; histology of the resectate. x 35

of these 16 patients remained unchanged and 13 improved considerably. One patient who had experienced intraventricular bleeding showed functional disturbances. Interestingly, four patients with a cavernoma who had experienced hemorrhage suffered from particularly severe epileptic seizures. These patients profited considerably from operative treatment. In two patients the seizures subsided after the operation.

Table 3. Treatment outcome in 33 patients with cavernomas (group 3)

Treatment	*n*	Improved	Unchanged	Fair
Conservative	7	3	4	
Stereotactic	3	2	1	
Stereotactic and microsurgical	7	4	2	1 (transient paresis of the arm)
Microsurgical	16	13	2	1 with IVH (dysphasia and dyscalculia)

IVH, intraventricular hemorrhage.

Discussion

Isolated DVAs rarely become symptomatic. In our group 1, only 5 of the 18 patients showed symptoms; three showed signs of ischemia. No hemorrhages occurred in this group. In comparison, DVAs combined with a cavernoma more often became symptomatic (8 of 17). Fourteen patients in group 2 (DVA combined with a cavernoma) showed calcifications on the neuroradiological images, and in two cases residual acute bleeding was discovered. Of the 33 neurosurgically treated patients 24 suffered hemorrhage prior to admittance. According to a study by Lobato et al. the incidence of bleeding is approximately 60%–65% in both AOVMs and AVMs [8]. However, the bleeding in AOVMs is less severe.

Operative resection of cavernomas appears to be an adequate treatment strategy for removing the source of epilepsy with the surrounding hemosiderin-stained tissue margin, reducing the mass effect in cases of extensive hemorrhage, minimizing the risk of rebleeding. These goals can be reached, however, only by total resection, which is not always possible, such as in cavernomas situated in the brainstem or in speech regions of the brain. It must also be considered that neurological symptoms may be only temporary and can sometimes subside even under conservative treatment alone. For this reason the risk of the operation and the possible benefits must be weighed carefully [2, 4, 6, 11, 14]. Our best clinical results were in five cases of cavernomas with two consecutive extensive bleeding episodes. Excellent clinical recovery occurred following operative resection of the cavernoma and stopping the hemorrhage. Superficially situated cavernomas and superficial brainstem cavernomas are best suited for microsurgical treatment. Deep-seated lesions, especially when located in speech areas, should be removed with a combined stereotactic-microsurgical approach. Cavernomas localized deep within the brainstem or in the speech center should be removed only in cases of extensive hemorrhage. In these cases a conservative approach seems justified. Recently, radiosurgical approaches to AVMs have been recommended [5].

When performing magnetic resonance imaging or highly selective digital subtraction angiography, great care should be taken in cases of cavernous hemangiomas not to overlook possible additional DVAs [7, 11]. The presence of a DVA must be taken into consideration when planing the operative strategy. Intraoperatively it must be ensured that the venous drainage of the DVA is not damaged as the DVA serves locally as the only venous drainage [7]. Typically, the DVA is situated as a large venous drainage deeply within the parenchyma [3, 14] and can, when occluded, lead to hemorrhagic infarction.

References

1. Donauer E, Faubert C (1992) Management of spontaneous intracerebral and cerebellar hemorrhage. In: Kaufmann HH (ed) Intracerebral hematomas. Raven, New York, pp 211–227
2. Fahlbusch R, Strauss C, Huk W, Röckelein G, Kompf D, Ruprecht KW (1990) Surgical removal of pontomesencephalic cavernous hemangiomas. Neurosurgery 26:449–457
3. Huber G, Hermes M, Henkes H, Piepgras U (1992) Assoziation der zerebralen sog. venösen Angiome mit kryptischen Gefässmalformationen. Klin Neuroradiol 2:148–156
4. Kashiwagi S, Loveren HR, Tew JM, Wiot JG, Weil SM, Lukin RA (1990) Diagnosis and treatment of vascular brain stem malformations. J Neurosurg 72:27–34
5. Konziolka D, Lunsford LD, Coffey RJ, Bissonette DJ, Flickinger JC (1990) Stereotactic radiosurgery of angiographically occult vascular malformations: indications and preliminary experience. Neurosurgery 27:892–900
6. Konvalov AN, Spallone A, Makhmudow UB, Kuhlajeva JA, Ozerova VI (1990) Surgical management of hematomas of the brain stem. J Neurosurg 73:181–186
7. Lasjaunias P, Burrow S, Platelet C (1986) Developmental venous anomalies (DVA). The so-called venous angioma. Neurosurg Rev 9:233
8. Lobato RD, Rivas JJ, Gomez PA, Cabrera A, Sarabia R, Lamas E (1992) Comparison of the clinical presentation of symptomatic arteriovenous malformations (angiographically visualized) and occult vascular malformations. Neurosurgery 31:391–397
9. Moringlane JR, Ramina R (1984) Angiographically occult vascular in functional areas of the brain. Zentralbl Neurochir 45:268–272
10. Ondra SL, Troupp H, George ED, Schwab K (1990) The natural history of symptomatic arteriovenous malformations of the brain: a 24-year follow-up assessment. J Neurosurg 73:387–391
11. Rigamonti D, Spetzler RF (1988) The association of venous and cavernous malformations. Report of four cases and discussion of the pathophysiological, diagnostic and therapeutic implications. Acta Neurochir (Wien) 92:100–105
12. Roda JM, Alvarez F, Isla A, Blazquez MG (1990) Thalamic cavernous malformation. J Neurosurg 72:647–649
13. Scott MR, Barnes P, Kupsky W, Adelman LS (1992) Cavernous angiomas of the central nervous system in children. J Neurosurg 76:38–46
14. Tung H, Gianotta ST, Chandrasoma PT, Zee CH (1990) Recurrent intraparenchymal hemorrhages from angiographically occult malformations. J Neurosurg 73:1764

Results of Proton Beam Radiosurgery in Cerebral Arteriovenous Malformations

D. Stolke[1], V. Seifert[1], H. M. Mehdorn[2], and B. Hoffmann[2]

Introduction

The routine use of microneurosurgical techniques has dramatically reduced the peri- and postoperative morbidity and mortality of patients harboring an arteriovenous malformation (AVM) of the brain [6, 18]. However, AVMs located in speech or deep areas of the brain or with a large size and/or high blood flow through the AVM nidus still represent a formidable challenge for the treating neurosurgeon. Stereotactic proton beam radiosurgery has been advocated for the treatment of AVMs of the brain that are considered to be of high surgical risk either due to their location in speech or deep areas of the brain or to their size [3, 4]. Because of excellent results of proton beam radiosurgery reported in the literature in the early 1980s [3], a group of 68 patients harboring high-risk cerebral AVMs were referred from our Department to a major radiosurgical center in the United States over a period of 10 years. However, intermediate and long-term follow-up revealed that in the vast majority of these patients the dimension of the AVM after radiation therapy remained virtually unchanged [11]. Additionally, the clinical symptoms present prior to radiation therapy did not show amelioration after radiosurgery in more than half of the patients, while deterioration due to hemorrhage from the radiated AVM, increased seizure frequency, progressive neurological deficits or as the result of radiation-induced leukencephalopathy developed in a considerable percentage of the patients. Therefore, it was decided to perform the following retrospective study to define the long-term results of radiosurgery using stereotactic Bragg-peak proton beam therapy in patients with cerebral AVMs.

Materials and Methods

Over a period of almost 10 years (October 1980 to May 1990) a total of 68 patients with cerebral AVMs were referred to a radiosurgical center in the United States for stereotactic Bragg-peak proton beam therapy. Radiosurgery was chosen as an alternative treatment, either because these AVMs, due to their size and/or location, were considered to be of such a high surgical risk that the possible benefits of surgery were outweighed by the high possibility of major postoperative neurological

---

[1] Neurosurgical Clinic, University of Essen, Essen, Germany.
[2] Neurosurgical Clinic, University of Kiel, Kiel, Germany.

Advances in Neurosurgery, Vol. 22
B. L. Bauer, M. Brock, M. Klinger (Eds.)

deficits, or because the patients refused surgery. The patient group consisted of 38 women and 30 men, with an age distribution ranging from 14 to 60 years and a mean age of 32.8 years. Of these, 28 AVMs (41.2%) were located in the centroparietal region on the left or right side, 15 (22%) in the left temporal region, 6 (8.8%) in the left frontal region, 5 (7.4%) in the area calcarina and the basal ganglia, and 3 (4.4%) in the brain stem, corpus callosum, and cerebellar peduncle. In regard to their size, 17 AVMs (35%) were up to 3 cm in diameter, 41 (60.3%) between 3 and 6 cm, and 10 (14.7%) larger than 6 cm. When the AVMs were graded according to the Spetzler-Martin grading scale [14], the following distribution was found: 3 (4.4%) were of grade I, 4 (5.9%) of grade II, 29 (42.6%) of grade III, 25 (36.8%) of grade IV, 2 (2.9%) of grade V, and 5 (7.4%) of grade 6. The patients became symptomatic due to the following initial symptoms (some appearing in combination): seizures in 39 patients, hemorrhage in 32, progressive neurological deficits in 16, and headache in 9. In three the AVM was found incidentally.

Results

Five patients were lost to follow-up. In the remaining 63 patients (92.6%) complete clinical and radiological follow-up examinations were available. Clinical work-up consisted of clinical and neurological examination which was performed at least at yearly intervals after proton beam therapy. Radiological examination consisted of a first angiogram 2 years after radiation therapy. The angiogram was repeated in 62 patients at irregular intervals ranging from 28 months to 9 years after radiation treatment. In one patient with severe postradiation encephalopathy, magnetic resonance imaging as follow-up examination was performed instead. A number of patients were examined angiographically more than twice, either because postradiation complications had occurred, or because endovascular embolization was performed, mostly prior to planned microsurgical angioma extirpation. The time of postradiation follow-up in the whole cohort of 63 patients ranged from 30 months to 12 years.

In regard to their preradiation neurological symptoms, 28 patients (44.4%) were improved, in 17 (27%) the symptoms were the same as before, and in 18 (28.6%) the symptoms had become worse after proton beam therapy. In 7 of these 18 patients (38.9%) deterioration was the result of an increased seizure frequency. In 5 patients (27.8%) hemorrhage from the radiated AVM occurred, which was fatal in 2. Progressive neurological deficits were seen in 2 patients (11.1%), and 4 (22.2%) developed progressive neurological deterioration due to radiation-induced leukencephalopathy. In 12 of these 18 patients (66.7%) clinical worsening occurred after a postradiation period of more than 2 years. When the postradiation *clinical course* of the patients was correlated to the *size of the malformations*, the following results were found: of 17 patients harboring an AVM of up to 3 cm in size, 13 (76.4%) had improved after proton therapy, 2 (11.8%) remained the same, and 2 (11.8%) had become worse; of 37 patients with an AVM between 3 and 6 cm, 12 (32.4%) had clinically improved, 13 (35.2%) remained the same, and 12 (32.4%) had be-

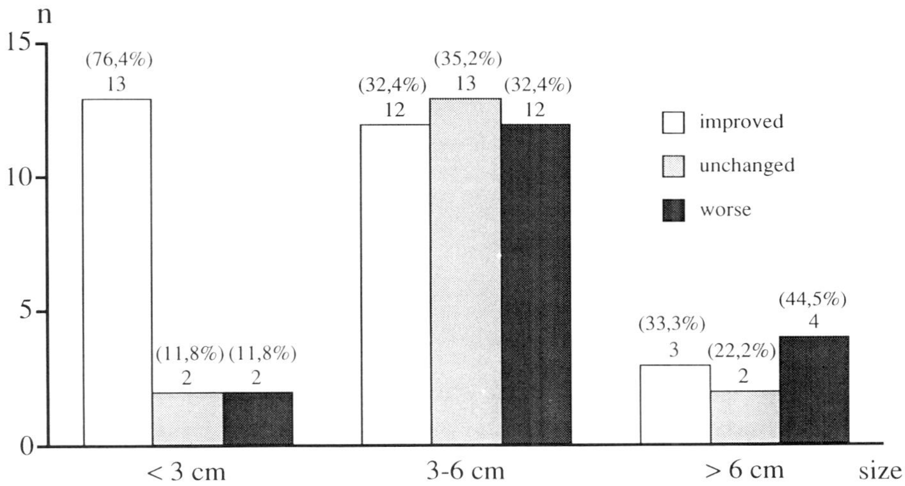

Fig. 1. Results of postradiation clinical follow-up correlated to size of AVM

come worse; of 9 with an AVM larger than 6 cm, 3 (33.3%) had improved, 2 (22.2%) remained the same, and 4 (44.5%) had become worse (Fig. 1). Correlation of *clinical outcome* with the *Spetzler-Martin grading scale* showed the following results: of 7 patients in grades I and II, 6 (85.7%) improved after proton beam therapy and 1 (14.3%) remained the same; of 24 patients in grade III, 13 (54.2%) improved, 9 (37.5%) remained the same, and 2 (8.3%) became worse; of 25 patients in grade IV, 6 (24%) improved, 5 (20%) were the same, and 14 (56%) became worse; of the 2 patients in grade V, both (100%) remained the same after proton

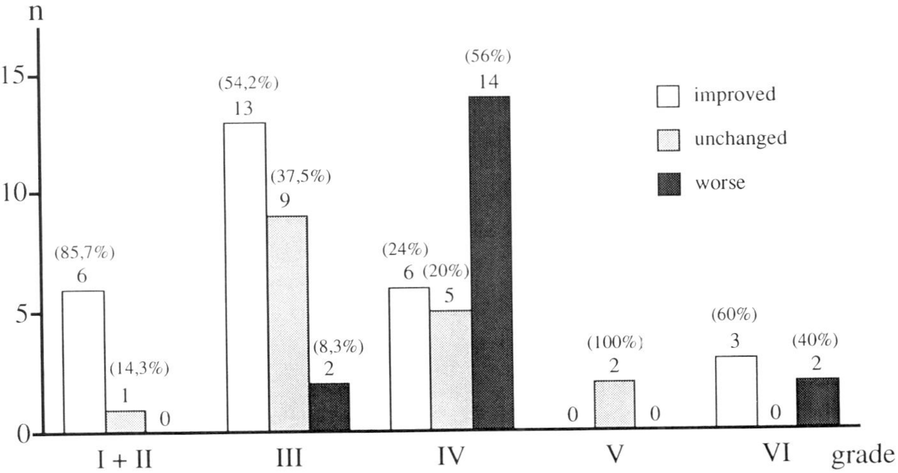

Fig. 2. Results of postradiation clinical follow-up correlated to grading of AVM (Spetzler-Martin scale)

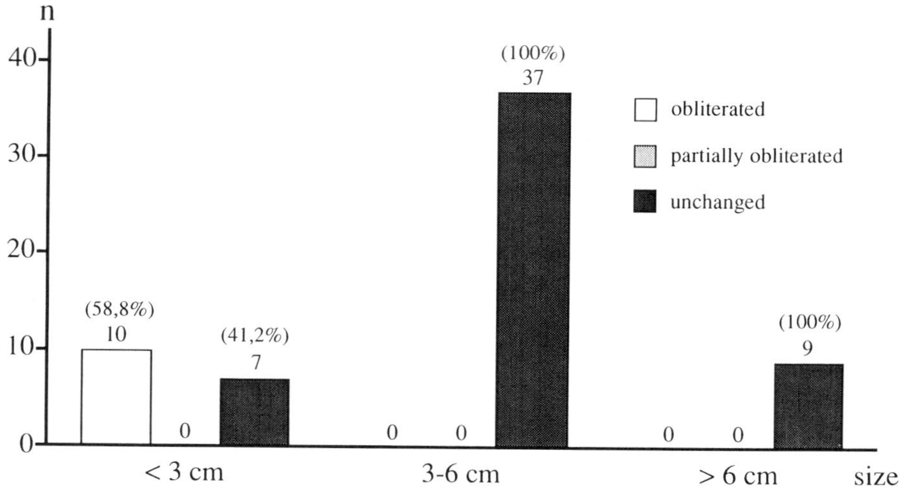

Fig. 3. Results of postradiation radiological follow-up correlated to size of AVM

treatment; and of 5 patients in grade VI, 3 (60%) improved, and 2 (40%) became worse (Fig. 2). When the results of the radiological *follow-up examinations* were correlated with the *size of the AVM*, the following results were found: of the 17 patients with an AVM smaller than 3 cm, 10 (58.8%) were completely obliterated, none showed partial obliteration, and 7 (41.2%) showed no change in their angiographic appearance; of the 37 malformations 3–6 cm in size, none was partially obliterated, and none was completely obliterated; of the 9 larger than 6 cm, none was partially obliterated, and none was completely obliterated. In summary, of 63

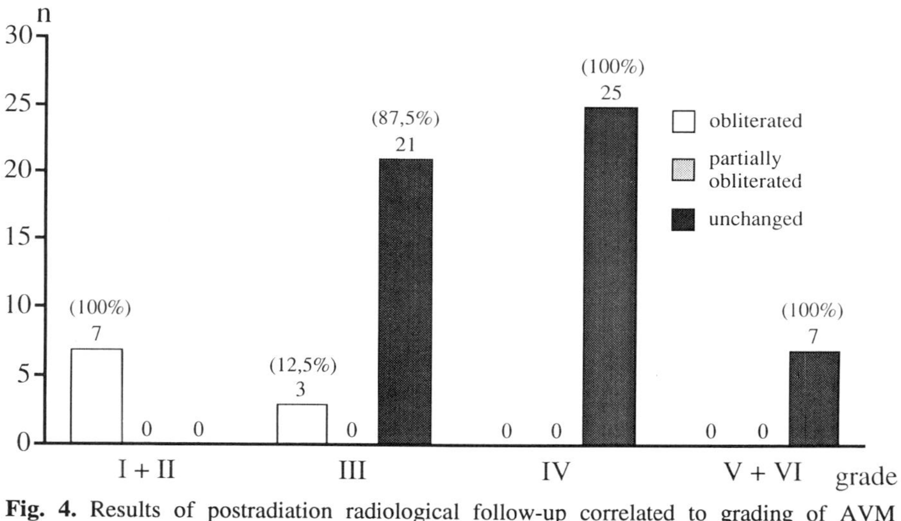

Fig. 4. Results of postradiation radiological follow-up correlated to grading of AVM (Spetzler-Martin scale)

radiated AVMs available for radiological follow-up, 10 (15.9%) were completely obliterated, all of which were smaller than 3 cm. There were 53 malformations (84.1%) that showed no change in their radiological follow-up appearance (Fig. 3). When the radiological follow-up results were correlated to the Spetzler-Martin grading scale, the following results were found: in all 7 patients in grade I or II the AVM was completely obliterated by proton beam therapy; of 24 with an grade III, complete obliteration was achieved in 3 (12.5%), while 21 (87.5%) showed no change in the radiological appearance of their AVM; of 25 in grade IV, none was partially or completely obliterated; of 7 harboring an AVM of grade V or VI none was partially or completely obliterated (Fig. 4).

Discussion

Although a combination of presurgical endovascular embolization and microsurgery is increasingly used by many neurosurgeons for the treatment of high-risk AVMs with good to excellent results [7, 12, 15], stereotactic radiosurgery has been advocated as an effective and safe alternative treatment for those AVMs considered to be of high or unacceptable surgical risk. The term radiosurgery was coined by Leksell in the early 1950s [8, 9] to describe the technique of closed-skull destruction of a predetermined intracranial target by a single-fraction treatment of a high dose of radiation, using the precision of a stereotactic apparatus. Since that time a broad spectrum of intracranial diseases has been treated by radiosurgery, for which currently three different types of penetrating radiation are in use. These are protons or helium ions produced by a cyclotron or a synchrotron [3, 4, 5, 16], Y-rays delivered by a cobalt^{-60} source such as in the gamma-knife unit [10, 17] and X-rays produced by a linear accelerator [1, 2]. All three sources of high-dose radiation have been used extensively for the treatment of AVMs; however, the results reported in this study are derived from AVM treatment by Bragg–peak proton beam radiation. The first detailed study on a larger group of patients harboring an AVM and treated by stereotactic proton beam radiation was presented by Kjellberg and coworkers in 1983 [3]. They reported on 75 consecutive patients with AVMs who were followed up for a period of 2–16 years. Radiation-induced complications occurred in eight patients – four with postradiation hemiparesis and two with high-grade hydrocephalus and hemianopsia. Follow-up arteriograms were obtained in 62 of the 75 patients. In 20% of the patients, the AVM was totally obliterated, in 56% the AVM was reduced in size by 50% or more, and in 13% the malformations were unchanged. However, no information in regard to the size of the AVM or percentage of obliteration were given. In 1988 Kjellberg reported his results in 717 procedures for the treatment of AVMs in 709 patients using stereotactic proton beam therapy [4], with 92% of the patients followed up for more than 2 years. In regard to the arteriographic findings after radiation therapy, surprisingly, the distribution of radiological treatment results were virtually identical to those reported 5 years earlier; 20% total obliteration, 56% with obliteration of 50% or more, and 13% unchanged.

Unfortunately, we have not been able to repeat these results on the basis of our own retrospective analysis. The results of stereotactic proton beam therapy in our study have been equally disapointing in terms of clinical outcome and in terms of radiological results. More than half of our patients did not profit clinically from the radiation treatment or showed substantial clinical deterioration. In more than 77% of those with postradiation worsening of clinical symptoms deterioration was due to complications such as increased frequency of seizures or hemorrhage from the radiated AVM, of which two were fatal. Moreover, four patients developed severe radiation-induced leukencephalopathy. In regard to the relationship between the size of the AVM or its grading (Spetzler-Martin scale) and the clinical outcome, the results of radiation therapy were better the smaller or less complex the AVM was. With increasing size or higher grade on the Spetzler-Martin scale, the clinical results of proton beam therapy become progessively worse. Of 37 patients with an AVM diameter of 3–6 cm only one-third showed amelioration of their clinical symptoms, while two-thirds remained the same or even deteriorated after radiation treatment. The same results apply to patients with very large AVMs, of whom, again, only one-third profited from proton therapy. While 85.7% of patients in Spetzler-Martin grade I or II showed postradiation amelioration of their clinical symptoms, the figure was only 54.2% of those in grade III, and only of those 24% in grade IV. Complete angiographic obliteration of the AVM was detectable in only 10 patients, or 15.9%, which is less than one-sixth of the whole group of 63 patients. This means that almost 85% of the patients treated by stereotactic proton beam therapy showed no angiographically detectable change in the radiological appearance of their radiated AVM during follow-up. Of those 10 AVMs obliterated by radiation treatment all were smaller than 3 cm in diameter [1, 2, 5, 10, 16, 17].

We conclude from these findings that stereotacitc proton beam therapy should not be recommended to patients harboring an AVM larger than 3 cm in size and is best restricted to AVMs with difficult access or those smaller than 3 cm in size. However, as a recent study by Stein's group has shown [13], even in these patients microsurgical removal of small AVMs results in a higher cure rate and lower morbidity than radiosurgery.

Acknowledgments. We are indebted to Prof. Löhr, Department of Radiology, University of Essen, and to Prof. Kühne, Department of Radiology, Alfried Krupp-Hospital, Essen, for performing the radiological examinations in the large part of the patients.

References

1. Colombo F, Benedetti A, Pozzi F et al. (1989) Linear accelerator radiosurgery for cerebral arteriovenous malformations. Neurosurgery 24:833–840
2. Friedman WA (1992) Linear accelerator radiosurgery. Clin Neurosurg 38:445–471
3. Kjellberg RN, Hanamura T, Davis KR et al. (1982) Bragg-peak proton beam therapy for arteriovenous malformations of the brain. N Engl J Med 309:269–274

4. Kjellberg RN (1988) Proton beam therapy for arteriovenous malformations of the brain. In: Schmidek HH, Sweet WH (eds) Operative neurosurgical techniques. Grune and Stratton, New York, pp 911–915
5. Fabrikant JI, Levy RP, Steinberg GK et al. (1992) Stereotactic charged-particle radiosurgery: clinical results of treatment of 1200 patients with intracranial arteriovenous malformations and pituitary disorders. Clin Neurosurg 38:472–492
6. Heros RC, Korosue D, Diebold PM (1990) Surgical excision of cerebral arteriovenous malformations: late results. Neurosurgery 26:570–576
7. Jafar JJ, Adam JD, Berenstien A et al. (1993) The effect of embolization with N. butyl cyanoacrylate prior to surgical resection of cerebral arteriovenous malformations. J Neurosurg 79:60–69
8. Leksell L (1949) A sterotaxic apparatus for intracerebral surgery. Acta Chri Scand 99:231
9. Leksell L (1951) The stereotaxic method and radiosurgery of the brain. Acta Chir Scand 102:316–319
10. Lunsford LD, Kondziolka D, Flickinger JC (1991) Stereotactic radiosurgery for arteriovenous malformations of the brain. J Neurosurg 75:512–524
11. Mehdorn HM, Müller SP, Koch D, Grote W (1991) Follow-up after treatment for intracranial arteriovenous malformations. Adv Neurosurg 19:74–80
12. Pasqualin A, Scienza R, Cioffi F et al. (1991) Treatment of cerebral arteriovenous malformations with a combination of preoperative embolization and surgery. Neurosurgery 29:358–368
13. Sisti MB, Kader A, Stein BM (1992) Comparison between microsurgery and radiosurgery in the treatment of small AVM's. 1993 annual meeting of the American Association of Neurological Surgeons (abstract). J Neurosurg 78:342A
14. Spetzler RF, Martin NA (1986) A proposed grading system for arteriovenous malformations. J Neurosurg 65:476–483
15. Spetzler FR, Martin NA, Carter LP et al. (1987) Surgical management of large AVM's by staged embolization and operative excision. J Neurosurg 67:17–28
16. Steinberg GK, Fabrikant JI, Marks MP et al. (1990) Stereotacitc heavy-charged-particle Bragg-peak radiation for intracranial arteriovenous malformations. N Engl J Med 323:96–101
17. Steiner L, Lindquist C, Adler JR et al. (1992) Clinical outcome of radiosurgery for cerebral arteriovenous malformations. J Neurosurg 77:1–8
18. Yasargil MG (1987) Summary of operative results. In: Yasargil MG (ed) Microneurosurgery, vol 33. Thieme, Stuttgart, pp 369–392

Spontaneous Intracerebral Hemorrhage due to Sinus Venous Thrombosis

F. Erbguth[1], W. Huk[2], M. Winterholler[1], D. Claus[1], and B. Neundörfer[1]

Introduction

Thrombosis of cortical veins and sinuses in the past has been associated with a high mortality [1, 5, 12]. Due to its varied and nonspecific clinical manifestations, this condition is often misdiagnosed, or the diagnosis is delayed. Therefore the frequency of aseptic sinus venous thrombosis (SVT) is probably underestimated. The introduction of computed tomography (CT) has made radiological diagnosis easier by providing clues such as "empty delta sign" or "cord sign" [4, 9, 10, 16]. Intracerebral hemorrhage (ICH) is more frequently seen in other cerebral diseases and considered to be less indicative of SVT. However, one of the most frequent complications of cerebral venous obstruction is hemorrhagic infarction or massive parenchymal hemorrhage, either unilaterally or bilaterally [1, 2, 5, 12]. When Toffol et al. studied the diagnostic value of arteriography in nontraumatic ICH, they found 3 thromboses of the superior sagittal sinus (SSS) among 102 hypertensive and nonhypertensive patients [19]. We report on the diagnosis and treatment of 22 patients with confirmed aseptic sinovenous occlusion, in whom the initial CT revealed ICH. Three exemplary case reports illustrate this condition.

Case Reports

Case 1. A 38-year-old woman had undergone varicotomy on her leg. After the operation she developed headache. Three days later she had a sudden onset of vomiting and right hemiparesis. CT revealed a left frontoparietal hemorrhage (Fig. 1 a). The patient was transferred to our department. During preparation for angiography she became tetraplegic and comatose. Repeated CT showed an additional right fronto-parietal hemorrhage (Fig. 1 b). Angiography and magnetic resonance imaging confirmed a thrombosis of the SSS. In spite of hematoma the woman intravenously received 25 000–35 000 IU heparin daily (target partial thromboplastin time 80 s), which was switched to phenprocoumon after 4 weeks. No cerebral hemorrhagic complication occurred during the favorable clinical course. The patient was transferred to a rehabilitation unit with mild cognitive deficits.

---

[1] Department of Neurology, Friedrich-Alexander University of Erlangen-Nürnberg, Schwabachanlage 6, 91054 Erlangen, Germany.
[2] Department of Neuroradiology, Friedrich-Alexander University of Erlangen-Nürnberg, Schwabachanlage 6, 91054 Erlangen, Germany.

Advances in Neurosurgery, Vol. 22
B. L. Bauer, M. Brock, M. Klinger (Eds.)

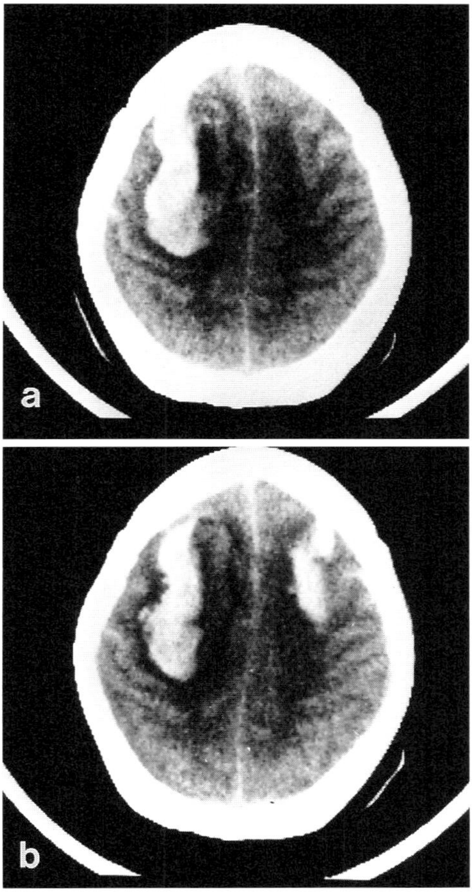

Fig. 1. Case 1. **a** Left hemorrhage on admission. **b** Bilateral hemorrhage 24 h later

Case 2. A 59-year-old woman was admitted to a district hospital after a sudden onset of right hemiparesis and obtundation. CT revealed a left thalamic hemorrhage, which was related to her arterial hypertension (Fig. 2 a). After admission to our department she required an external ventricular drainage, due to occlusive hydrocephalus. After she developed tetraparesis and coma, repeated CT demonstrated bilateral hemorrhagic infarctions, which were indicative of thrombosis of the internal cerebral veins. MRI and angiography confirmed the diagnosis of thrombosis of the galenic venous system (Fig. 2 b). Protein S deficiency was found to be responsible for the hypercoagulability. The patient received 25 00–40 000 IU heparin per day intravenously. She recovered slowly, but after 1 year of rehabilitation she was able to walk, although with severe cognitive deficits. No bleeding complication had occurred during treatment.

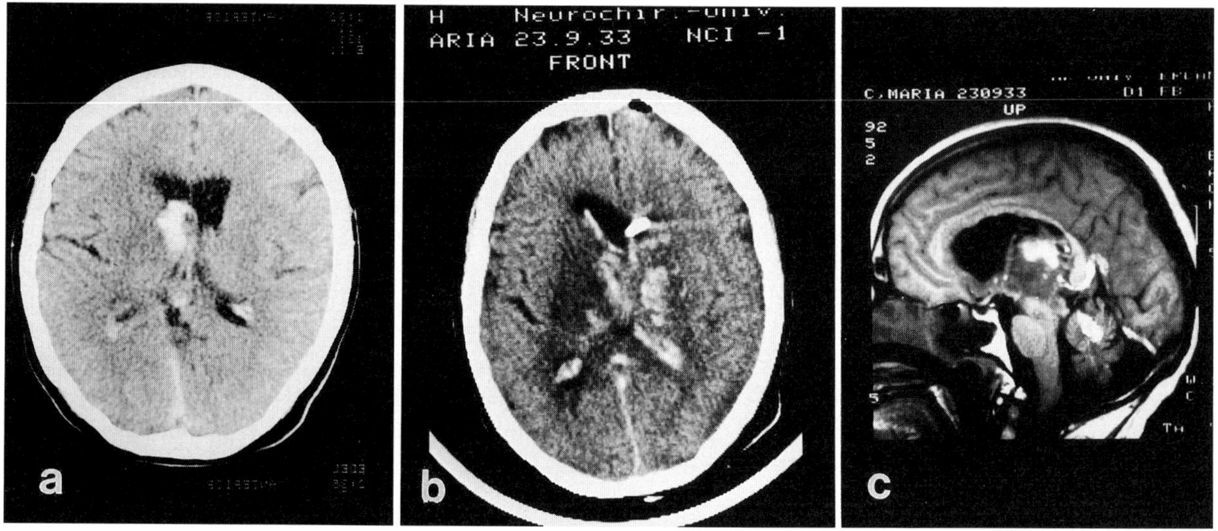

Fig. 2. Case 2. **a** Left hemorrhage of nucleus caudatus and thalamus. **b** Bilateral thalamic hemorrhagic infarction after 3 days. **c** Hyperintense visualization of thrombosis in the straight sinus and great cerebral vein of Galen on MRI

Case 3. A 33-year-old teacher with a history of repeated phlebothromboses broke down after 3 days of headache. Aphasia and right hemiparesis were found. CT was performed in a district hospital and revealed a temporal hemorrhage, which was suspected to be of traumatic origin (Fig. 3 a). After transferral to our department, he showed rapid deterioration with a fixed pupil on the right and coma. Angiography showed occlusion of the left straight sinus and the vein of Labbe. Thrombosis was caused by protein S deficiency. Due to the threat of transtentorial herniation, surgically the hemorrhage was treated (Fig. 3 b). Afterwards the patient received intravenously 25 000–35 000 IU heparin daily. No bleeding complications occurred. After clinical improvement within 8 weeks the patient returned home with mild aphasia. For anticoagulation phenprocoumon therapy was given instead of heparin.

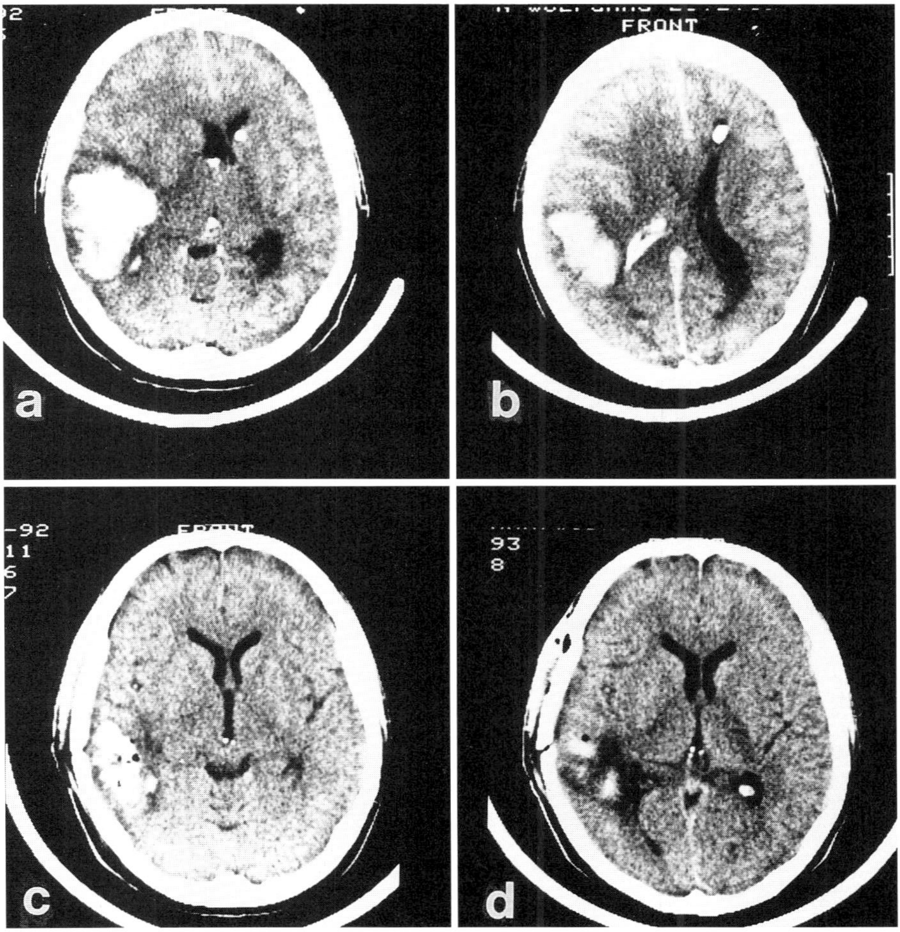

Fig. 3. Case 3. **a** Left temporal hemorrhage on admission. **b** Increase in midline shift after 1 day; fixed pupil. **c** CT 6 h after surgical removal of hematoma. **d** CT 3 weeks after operation

Patients and Results

Between 1983 and 1993 we diagnosed thrombosis of the intracranial venous system in 39 patients (25 women, 14 men; mean age 45.3 years, range 16–79). In all patients cranial CT was performed; the diagnosis was verified by transfemoral angiography and/or by MRI. In 22 patients, the initial CT revealed different types of intracerebral hemorrhage.

Clinical Symptoms. The most frequent neurological features were headache, papilledema, hemiparesis, altered level of consciousness, and seizures. At the beginning of treatment patients had a mean severity score of 4.6 (hemorrhagic patients 4.9, nonhemorrhagic patients 4.2) on the SVT severity scale (0 = no symptoms, 9 = death) of Einhäupl et al. [7].

Site of Hemorrhage and Thrombosis. In 9 cases CT demonstrated hypodense areas with spotted hyperdensities indicating hemorrhagic infarction. In 13 other cases solid masses of blood were found, indicating "parenchymatous hemorrhage". Localization was unilateral in 12, bilateral in 7, and multifocal in 3 cases (Table 1). Hemorrhages of parietal, frontoparietal and parieto-occupital site correlated with thrombosis of the SSS and/or cortical veins; temporal hemorrhage was related to thrombosis of the straight sinus and/or vein of Galen, and bilateral basal ganglia and thalamic hemorrhage was found in thrombosis or the galenic venous system (straight sinus, great vein of Galen, internal cerebral veins).

Neuroradiology. In 12 cases hemorrhage was diagnosed prior to admission to our department: in 7 of them a possible etiology of hemorrhage was suspected, but in only one case was it diagnosed correctly; in 6 cases cause of hemorrhage was misdiagnosed: 3 were suspected as hypertensive, 2 as probable vascular malformation, 1 as posttraumatic. In 13 of 22 cases diagnosis was confirmed by angiography only, in 4 cases by MRI only, and in 5 cases by the combination of MRI and angiography. The advantage of MRI lies in the better visualization of the stage of thrombosis; on the other hand, angiography is better in demonstrating thrombosis of single veins.

Table 1. Localization and type of hemorrhage: hemorrhagic infarction (HI) versus parenchymatous hemorrhage (PH)

Localization	Unilateral (n = 12)			Bilateral (n = 7)			Multifocal (n = 3)		
	Total	HI	PH	Total	HI	PH	Total	HI	PH
Parietal	2	1	1	2	1	1	3	2	1
Frontoparietal	2	1	1	1	0	1	0	0	0
Parieto-occipital	2	0	2	1	1	0	0	0	0
Temporal	6	1	5	0	0	0	0	0	0
Basal ganglia/ thalamic	0	0	0	3	2	1	0	0	0

Table 2. Predisposing factors for SVT

Cause of thrombosis	All (n = 39)	Hemorrhage (n = 22)
Oral contraceptives	3	1
Oral contraceptices + smoking	3	2
Postpartum status	3	2
Protein S deficiency	2	2
Protein C deficiency	1	1
Angiotensin-III deficiency	2	1
Posttraumatic	1	0
Unknown	24	13

Causes of Thrombosis. They are listed in Table 2.

Treatment and Outcome. All 39 patients (with and without hemorrhage) were treated with dose-adjusted heparin; the dose ranged between 25 000 and 45 000 IU/day by continuous intravenous infusion. The dose was adjusted to 1.5–2 times the normal partial thromboplastin time and should not exceed 100 s. Coagulation parameters were measured twice a day. In 33 patients no bleeding complications occurred during treatment. In four cases extracranial bleeding occurred. In two patients preexisting hemorrhage increased during treatment; both patients had been comatose at time of admission and had had a delay of diagnosis of 21 and 35 days, respectively. Both patients died. One patient without hemorrhage died of general brain edema, one other of complications of ileus. All other patients had a favorable clinical course, and the mean severity score of all patients after 1 year was 1.2 (1.3 in patients with hemorrhage, 1.1 in patients without hemorrhage).

Discussion

Most case reports and series of SVT mention ICH as a frequent complication [1–5, 12]. In 20%–60% of patients there was hemorrhagic transformation of the venous infarction at time of admission [7]. However, differential diagnosis of ICH often does not take SVT adequately into account. Only Beal et al. report on the differential diagnosis of ICH in cases of cerebral vein thrombosis [2]. In our series, 56% of patients showed intracerebral bleeding on the inital CT. Even solid masses of blood without a visible infarction area may be caused by SVT. Especially thrombosis of the straight sinus frequently correlates with temporal hemorrhage [11]. Hemorrhage of basal ganglia and thalamus may be due to an occlusion of the galenic venous system, but may be misdiagnosed as "hypertensive" [8]. Therefore, hemorrhagic infarctions or parenchymatous hemorrhages may indeed be of venous etiology, particularly when they do not correspond to territories of arterial supply. Traditional radiological diagnosis of SVT has relied heavily on the use of cerebral angiography [21]. With MRI the diagnosis is made by demonstrating a lack of flow void normally present within venous structures. Macchi et al. divide venous thrombosis into initial, intermediate, and late stages based on signal intensity on T1- and T2-weighted spin-echo images [13]. The technique of magnetic resonance angiography has also shown its value in detecting venous thrombosis [14, 17].

Treatment of SVT has always been controversial. Although heparin has been used successfully for this condition [3], most authors have strongly opposed its use because of the frequent occurrence of intracranial hemorrhage during the natural course of the disease. Preexisting ICH in particular was regarded as a strict contraindication for anticoagulation treatment. Most neurology textbooks reject heparin in case of preexisting hemorrhage. However, heparin is potentially beneficial since it can prevent extension of thrombosis and allows collateral circulation to develop. Our experience from this uncontrolled series suggests that heparin treatment is not associated with a high risk of promoting intracerebral bleeding in SVT. Recently Einhäupl et al. demonstrated the beneficial effect of heparin in a prospective, randomized, double-blind, placebo-controlled study in 20 patients [7]: among the ten without heparin three cerebral bleeding complications occurred whereas in the ten with heparin no bleeding was observed. In a retrospecitve analysis of the study, 33 of 34 nonheparin patients developed ICH but only 2 of 56 patients with high-dose heparin.

We conclude that anticoagulation with heparin is the treatment of choice in SVT. This strategy does not promote ICH and therefore ICH is not a contraindica for heparin treatment. Surgical removal of blood masses can be beneficial in cases with elevated intracranial pressure and threat of transtentorial herniation. Only in rapidly progressing thrombosis, where heparin may be ineffective, may thrombolytic therapy be useful either intravenously or by local administration [6, 15, 18, 20]. However, preexisting ICH is a definite contraindication for thrombolysis.

The favorable treatment of SVT with heparin makes early and accurate diagnosis of this condition necessary. Therefore, differential diagnosis of ICH must take SVT into consideration.

References

1. Averback P (1978) Primary cerebral venous thrombosis in young adults: the diverse manifestations of an underrecognized disease. Ann Neurol 3:81–83
2. Beal MF, Wechsler LR, Davies KR (1982) Cerebral vein thrombosis and multiple intracranial hemorrhages by computed tomography. Arch Neurol 39:437–438
3. Bousser MG, Chiras J, Bories J, Castaigne P (1985) Cerebral venous thrombosis – a review of 38 cases. Stroke 16:199–213
4. Chiras J, Bousser MG, Meder JF, Koussa A, Bories J (1985) CT in cerebral thrombophlebitis. Neuroradiology 27:145–154
5. Chiras J, Dubs M, Bories J (1985) Venous infarctions. Neuroradiology 27:593–600
6. Di Rocco C, Iannelli A, Leone G, Moschini M, Valori VM (1981) Heparin-urokinase treatment of aseptic dural sinus thrombosis. Arch Neurol 38:431–435
7. Einhäupl KM, Villringer A, Meister W, Mehraein S, Garner C, Pellkofer M, Haberl RL, Pfister HW, Schmiedeck P (1991) Heparin treatment in sinus venous thrombosis. Lancet 338:597–600

8. Erbguth F, Brenner P, Schuierer G, Druschky KF, Neundörfer B (1991) Diagnosis and treatment of deep cerebral vein thrombosis. Neurosurg Rev 14:145–148
9. Gabrielsen TO, Seeger JF, Knake JE, Stilwill EW (1981) Radiology of cerebral vein occlusion without dural sinus occlusion. Radiology 140:403–408
10. Goldenberg AL, Rosenbaun AE, Wang HE, Kim WS, Lewis VL, Hanley DL (1986) Computed tomography of dural sinus thrombosis. J Comput Assist Tomogr 10:16–20
11. Isensee C, Reul J, Thron A (1992) Thrombose des Sinus transversus als Ursache temporaler Blutungen. Stellenwert von MRT und Angiographie. Aktuel Neurol 19:78–81
12. Krayenbühl HA (1967) Cerebral venous and sinus thrombosis. Clin Neurosurg 14:1–24
13. Macchi PJ, Grossmann RI, Gomori JM, Goldberg HI, Zimmermann RA, Bilaniuk LT (1986) High field MR imaging of cerebral venous thrombosis. J Comput Assist Tomogr 10:10–15
14. Mattle HP, Wentz K, Edelmann RR, Wallner B, NN JP, Barnes P, Atkinson B, Kleefield J, Hoogewoud HM (1991) Cerebral venography with MR. Radiology 178:453–458
15. Persson L, Lilja A (1990) Extensive dural sinus thrombosis treated by surgical removal and local streptokinase infusion. Neurosurgery 26:117–120
16. Rao KCVG, Knipp HC, Wagner EJ (1981) Computed tomographic findings in cerebral sinus and venous thrombosis. Radiology 140:391–398
17. Rippe DJ, Boyko OB, Spritzer CE, Meisler WJ, Dumoulin CL, Souza SP, Heinz ER (1990) Demonstration of dural sinus occlusion by the use of MR angiography. AJNR 11:199–201
18. Scott JA, Pascuzzi RM, Hall PV, Becker GJ (1988) Treatment of dural sinus thrombosis with local urokinase infusion. Case report. J Neurosurg 68:284–287
19. Toffol GJ, Biller J, Adams HP, Smoker WRK (1986) The predicted value of arteriography in nontraumatic intracerebral hemorrhage. Stroke 17:881–883
20. Tsai FY, Higashida RT, Matovich V, Alfieri K (1991) Acute thrombosis of the intracranial dural sinus: direct thrombolytic treatment. AJNR 13:1137–1141
21. Vines FS, Davis DO (1971) Clinical-radiological correlation in cerebral venous occlusive disease. Radiology 98:9–11

Endovascular Treatment of Intracranial Aneurysms with Electrically Detachable Coils

M. Schumacher[1], A. K. Wakhloo[1], W. Radü[2], A. Hammen[3], and W. Seeger[4]

Introduction

The recent development of electrically detachable coils by Guglielmi [2] has given a new perspective to the treatment of aneurysms. It has extended and improved previously used occlusion techniques with detachable balloons or freely removable coils through two essential advantages: (a) the direct current applied for detachment induces an intra-aneurysmic electrothrombosis, and (b) the placement of the coils in the aneurysm is reversible through angiographic control, at any time until the actual detachment. Because variable sizes (3–12 mm) and lengths (8–20 cm) of coils can be selected, this system can be utilized for extreme aneurysm sizes, from giant ones down to microaneurysms with a diameter of 3 mm. This brief report summarizes our initial experience with the Guglielmi detachable coil (GBC) in endovascular approach of experimentally created aneurysms and in the first 18 patients.

Materials and Methods

The experimental aneurysms were created in Labrador dogs by anastomosing the common carotid artery and the external jugular vein side to side. The jugular vein was ligated proximally and distally, and the arterial wall was punched at the anastomosis, creating one giant aneurysm (20 x 60 mm) and another medium-sized aneurysm (5 x 15 mm). Endovascular treatment was achieved by a microcatheter (Tracker 18), which was placed close to the aneurysmal dome (Fig. 1). Complete occlusion of the giant aneurysm was achieved by the insertion of three platinum coils each with a spiral diameter of 8 mm and a length of 40 cm (Fig. 2). For occlusion of the medium-sized aneurysm four coils, each with 6 mm memory and 20 cm in length, were sufficient.

During the last 1.5 years 18 patients with aneurysms (varying in size from 3 x 5 to 2 x 2.5 cm) were treated with the GDC system. The mean age of the patients (5

---

[1] Section of Neuradiology, University Hospital, Hauptstr. 5, 79104 Freiburg, Germany.
[2] Department of Neuradiology, Kantonsspital Basel, Petersgraben 4, 4031 Basel, Switzerland.
[3] Department of Neuropathology, University of Freiburg, Alberstr. 19, 79104 Freiburg, Germany.
[4] Neurosurgical Clinic, University Hospital, Hugstetter Str. 56, 79106 Freiburg, Germany.

Advances in Neurosurgery, Vol. 22
B. L. Bauer, M. Brock, M. Klinger (Eds.)

1 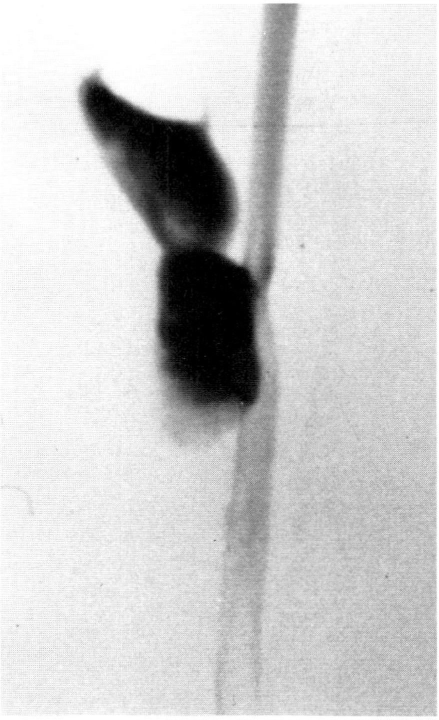 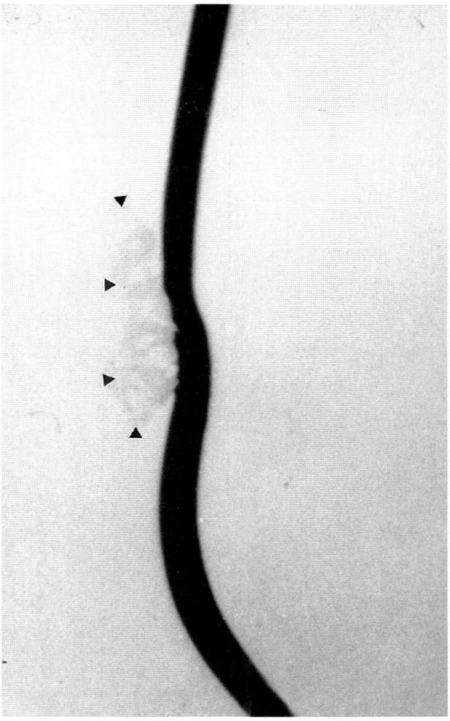 2

Fig. 1. Experimentally constructed giant aneurysm of the common carotid artery in dog created by side-to-side anastomosis before treatment

Fig. 2. Follow-up angiogram 6 months after treatment with electrically detachable coils demonstrating complete occlusion of the aneurysm. Coils in the aneurysm sack *(arrowheads)*. Some irregularities at the wall of the parent vessel

men, 13 women) ranged from 25 to 70 years. Only those patients were included in the study who were considered to be at high surgical risk or who presented with aneurysms in locations difficult to surgical approach. The largest treated group consisted of precavernous and cavernous carotid aneurysms (nine patients), or basilar artery aneurysms (eight patients) frequently located at the tip of the basilar artery and involving the origin of the posterior inferior cerebellar artery in one case.

The tip of the microcatheter was placed close to the aneurysmal dome so that the aneurysm could be filled from distal toward the neck. Coils of different memory and various lengths up to a maximum of 140 cm were used. Control angiography was performed to evaluate the patency of the parent artery before the final detachment of the coils. Electrolyt detachment was accomplished using 0.5 or 1.0 mA in an average detachment time of 8 min. All procedures were performed under full heparinization with 7500 U heparin as bolus under anticoagulant therapy monitoring.

Results

The experimental aneurysms were completely occluded. Follow-up angiography after 8 weeks and 6 months showed minor surface irregularities on the previous origin of the aneurysm (Fig. 2). The histology (Fig. 3) showed a regular configuration of the vessel wall with endothelialization having already set in, as well as a fibrocellular proliferation at the origin of the aneurysm and inside the aneurysmal sack. Although tightly packed, the coils did not occupy more than about 30% of the total volume.

As listed in Table 1, a complete endovascular occlusion of the aneurysm was achieved in 10 of 18 patients. In one of these patients occlusion of a parent vessel occurred at the same time (internal carotid artery). However, this remained asymptomatic thanks to a good interhemispheric collateral circulation. In 2/18 patients a subtotal occlusion was achieved with still patent neck remnant (10%–20% of total aneurysm volume). In three patients either only a partial occlusion was possible, or it was impossible to place to the coil in the aneurysm because a broad communication existed between it and the parent vessel so that a sufficiently reliable detachment of the coil did not appear attainable. The clinical follow-up showed improvement of the neurological deficit, predominantly involving the

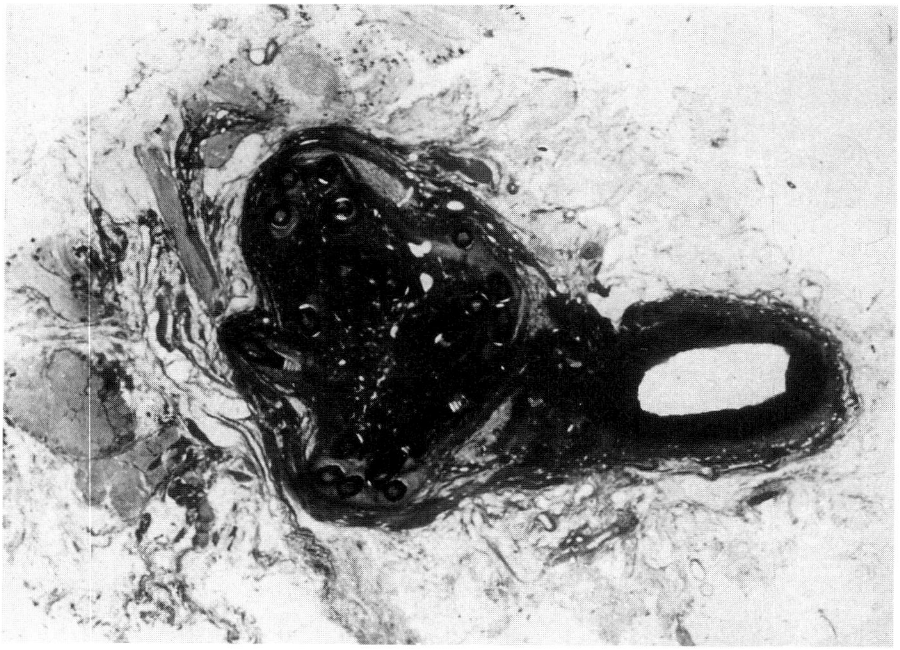

Fig. 3. Histological cross-section of the thrombosed aneurysm. Thrombosis and fibrocellular proliferation between coils, which do not occupy more than 30% of the whole aneurysmal volume. The right side demonstrates the smooth parent vessel wall. Richardson a. Leveletzkostaining, x 15

Table 1. Aneurysms treated with GDC coils (18 patients, 15 definitively treated)

	Occlusion			
	100%	80%–90%	≤ 70%	Coil not to place
Basilar artery ($n = 8$)	5	1	0	2
Posterior inferior cerebellar artery ($n = 1$)	1	0	0	0
Internal carotid artery ($n = 9$)	4	1	3	1
Total	10	2	3	3

neuro-ophthamological symptoms in 5/15 patients (in 3 patients coils were not detached). A deterioration occurred in 3/15 patients, 2 of whom had a giant cavernous carotid aneurysm. Small and medium-sized aneurysms at this location (Fig. 4) did not show any clinical worsening. In 10/15 patients there was no change in the neurological status, 6 of these patients having also had a normal neurological finding before treatment.

Discussion

Since the introduction of electrolytically detachable coils by Guglielmi [2] a large number of treatments for aneurysms have been performed worldwide, and now the first results of multicenter studies are available [3]. The technical principle is the detachment of the coils attached to the end of a guide wire by direct current which

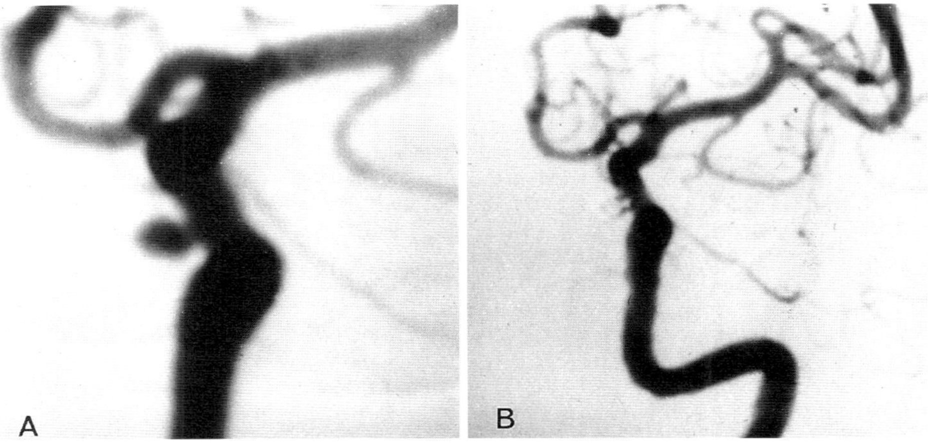

Fig. 4. Aneurysm of the cavernous portion of the internal carotid artery (3 x 5 mm) before (**A**) and after treatment (**B**) with the GDC system (3 x 15 mm)

releases free Fe^{2+} metal ions at the joint between the coil and the guide wire, thereby detaching the coil. The positive charge of the coils during application of the current has been shown to induce electrothrombosis by attracting negatively charged, corpuscular blood components (erythrocytes, leukocytes, and thrombocytes) and fibrinogen. In addition, the thrombus formation may stabilize the detached coils from floating out of the aneurysm.

The selection of patients at the present time is based on neurosurgical criteria. Consequently those patients are preferred for endovascular treatment in whom surgical access to aneurysms is difficult and those who are at high surgical risk. Obviously, the results from these studies are biased. In comparison, the results of endovascular treatment with detachable coils appears to be more effective and safer than treatment with detachable balloons [4, 7, 9] or surgical clipping [1, 5]. For the evaluation of the results of the treatment and the rate of complications, it must be taken into account that in most cases a selected group of high-risk patients is involved. However, long-term follow-up of aneurysms treated with the GDC device is required to exclude recurrence and delayed aneurysmal rupture before this technique is routinely used.

Acknowledgments. We thank Mrs. A Lindner and Dr. H. Nagursky, Clinical-Chemical Laboratory of the ZMK, University Hospital, Freiburg, for preparation of the cuts.

References

1. Fox AJ, Drake CHG (1990) Endovascular therapy of intracranial aneurysms. AJNR 11:641–642
2. Guglielmi G, Vinuela F, Sepetka E, Macellare V (1991) Electrothrombosis of saccular aneurysms via endovascular approach. I. Electrochemical basis, technique and experimental results. J Neurosurg 75:1–7
3. Guglielmi G, Vinuela F, Duckwiler G et al. (1992) Endovascular treatment of posterior circulation aneurysms by electrothrombosis using electrically detachable coils. J Neurosurg 77:515–524
4. Higashida RT, Halbach VV, Barnwell ST, Dowd CH, Dorndandy B, Bell J, Hieshima GB (1990) Treatment of intracranial aneurysms with preservation of the parent vessel: results of percutaneous ballon embolisation in 84 patients. AJNR 11:633–640
5. Kassell NF, Torner JC, Jane JA et al. (1990) The international cooperative study on the timing of aneurysm surgery. II. Surgical Results. J Neurosurg 73:730–740
6. Lin T, Fox AJ, Drake CG (1989) Regrowth of aneurysm sacs from residual neck following aneurysm clipping. J Neurosurg 70:556–560
7. Radü W, Schumacher M, Mader I (1992) Type, incidence and treatment of neurological complications during neuroradiologic interventions. In: Steinbrich W, Gross-Fengels W (eds) Interventional radiology: adjunctive medication and monitoring. Springer, Berlin Heidelberg New York, pp 213–232
8. Schumacher M, Radü W (1992) Endovascular treatment of basilar bifurcation aneurysms. In: Piscol K, Klinger N, Brock M (eds) Advances in neurosurgery. Springer, Berlin Heidelberg New York, pp 52–57

Cysticercosis Cerebri: Experiences from an Endemic Area

V. Tronnier[1] and J. H. Neal[2]

Introduction

Cysticercosis is the most common parasitosis affecting the central nervous system in many developing countries. Although it is not yet a severe problem in Western Europe, there is a growing incidence of the disease which can be attributed to immigration from developing countries and an increasing number of tourists traveling to developing countries. Cysticercosis is endemic in rural parts of Latin America, Asia, Africa, and Southeastern Europe. Today, Southern California can be considered an endemic area because of a high precentage of hispanic inhabitants. In 1989 cysticercosis became a reportable disease in California. A total of 134 cases of cysticercosis were reported to the California Department of Health Services during the first year, 92% of the patients being of hispanic origin [4]. Clinical and surgical experiences relating to the treatment of neurocysticercosis are presented below.

Clinical Symptoms and Diagnostic Measures

Neurocysticercosis is produced by the infection of the larval form (cysticercus) of *Taenia solium*, the pork tapeworm. In contrast to human taeniasis, where humans are the definitive hosts infected by eating undercooked pork contaminated with cysticerci, cysticercosis is acquired by ingesting taenia eggs shed in the feces of the human carrier of tapeworms, or by regurgitation of proglottids from the intestine into the stomach. A third means of infection is ano-oral autoinfection.

The larval tape worm (oncosphere) penetrates the intestinal wall and enters the bloodstream. Although the larval tapeworm may localize throughout the body, there is a preference for striated muscles, heart, eye, and the central nervous system. The oncosphere encysts forming a cysticercus. The development period from infection to a cysticercus cyst lasts about 60–70 days.

The clinical manifestations depend on the localization of the cysts. Most common are seizures (77%–96%), elevated intracranial pressure due to a mass lession (9%–55%), and hydrocephalus (7%–16%) [7, 8, 10]; meningitis (11%–15%) and strokes resulting from vasculitis (1.5%) [12, 2, 16] have also been reported. In ad-

[1] Neurochirurgische Universitätsklinik Heidelberg, Im Neuenheimer Feld 400, 69120 Heidelberg, Germany.
[2] Department of Neurosurgery, University of California Medical Center, 101 City Drive South, Orange, CA 92668, USA.

Advances in Neurosurgery, Vol. 22
B. L. Bauer, M. Brock, M. Klinger (Eds.)

dition to localization, other factors including size, the number of cysts, and patient immune response may play a crucial role. Asymptomatic cases are reported in the literature as ranging between 6% and 38% [7, 8]. Cysticerci can be located in the brain parenchyma (*Cysticercus cellulosae*; 30%–63%); or the basal cisterns (*Cysticercus racemosus*; 27%–56%); or be intraventricular (10%–12%) or intraspinal (< 1%). Various combinations of localization are common (23%).

Diagnostic measures include computed tomography (CT), magnetic resonance imaging (MRI), and serologic tests. In order to rule out retinal involvement funduscopic examination is strongly recommended before starting medical treatment. The general clinical examination should also include a search for palpable cysticerci in the muscles, ova or proglottids in stool, and calcified lesions in the skull X-ray. CT criteria for a suspected cysticercosis infection consist of the following: (a) three or more calcified spotty lesions in cortical areas, (b) a combination of cystic and calcified lesions (Fig. 1), (c) a single cyst or calcification with typical calcifications in the muscle, (d) cyst(s) which respond to a specific therapy, and (e) cystic lesions and positive serologic tests. MRI provides greater specificity of cysticercosis than CT. Intraparenchymal active lesions show a cyst with low intensity and a hyperintense scolex on T1-weighted images. When degeneration of the cyst starts to occur, either spontaneous or secondary to medical treatment, an inflammatory reaction with disturbance of the blood-brain barrier is visible as a hyperintense ring around the cystic lesion (Fig. 2). This stage may be accompanied by

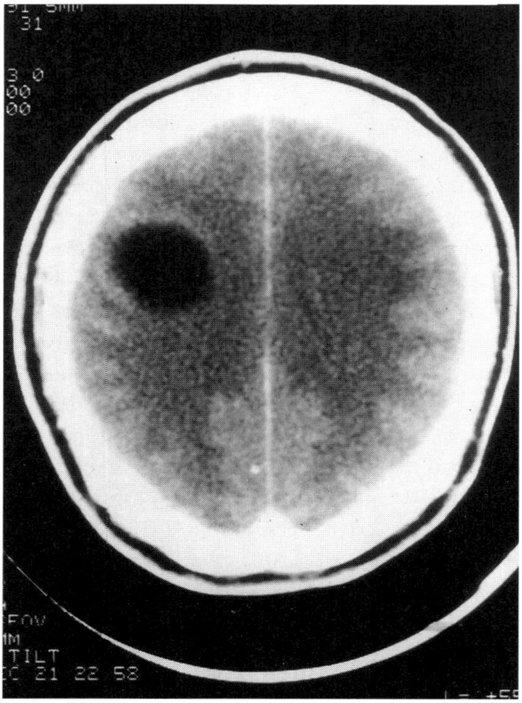

Fig. 1. A noncontrast CT scan showing a hypodense cyst and a calcified lesion typical for neurocysticercosis

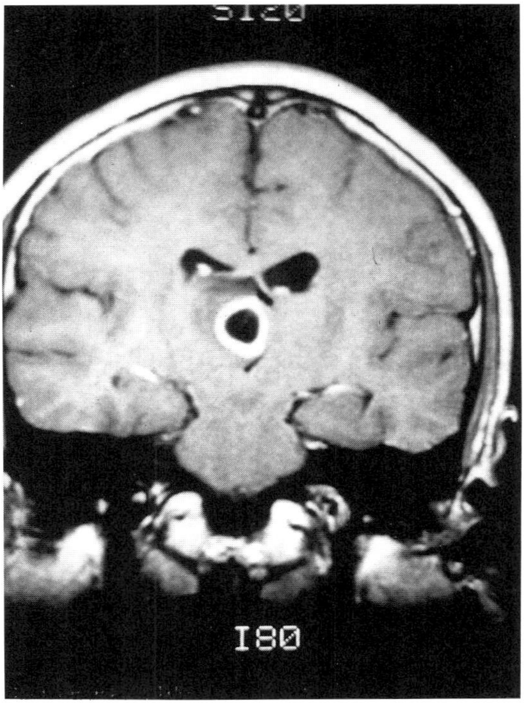

Fig. 2. A T1-weighted image with enhancement of Gd-DTPA showing a hyperintense scolex within a hypointense cystic lesion surrounded by an inflammatory reaction

surrounding edema. After the death of the cysticercus, the calcified lesion appears as a hypointense lesion on T1-weighted images. T2-weighted images do not contribute very much to the diagosis of a cysticercus cyst.

Complement fixation tests were originally used as serologic tests for the diagnosis of neurocysticercosis [9]. Today the enzyme-linked immunosorbent assay (ELISA), the enzyme-linked immunoelectrotransfer blot, and the indirect hemagglutination assay (IHA) are the most common serologic tests. Titers of 1:64 in serum and 1:8 in cerebrospinal fluid (CSF) are considered to be positive for the ELISA (1:128 and 1:8 for the IHA, respectively). The sensitivity of ELISA in active forms, according to Rosas et al. [11], is 50% in serum and 87% in CSF and the specificity 70% in serum and 95% in CSF. These titers have been confirmed by other authors [6]. Cross-reactivity between antibodies in different forms of parasitosis may occur. The low sensitivity in serum may be due to the fact that cysticercosis in the brain causes merely a local inflammatory reaction without circulating antibodies in the bloodstream.

Therapy

Primary treatment and therapeutic strategies for neurocysticercosis depend on the localization:

- Racemose form: medical treatment not successful, surgical treatment, if mass effect.
- Parenchymatous form: medical treatment is treatment of choice; surgery if mass effect exists or develops.
- Intraventricular form: surgical treatment.
- Spinal form: surgical treatment.

In general, surgery never provides a cure of the infectious disease. It can only be accomplished by an accompanying medical treatment. Praziquantel (Biltricide, Bayer; Cysticide, Merck) is widely used for the medical treatment of neurocysticercosis. The recommended dose is 50 mg/kg for 15 days [12, 13, 17, 18]. Albendazole (Eskazole, Smith Kline Beecham) is a newer drug which has also been shown effective in the treatment of cysticercosis. The originally recommended dose of 15 mg/kg albendazole taken for 1 month [15] can be shortened to 1 week [14]. With this regimen the number of cysts documented on CT has been reduced by 97% after 3 months. A marked improvement in the associated seizure disorder after medical treatment has also been reported [3, 18]. The death of the cysticercus is usually accompanied by an inflammatory reaction. Therefore, additional corticosteroid therapy may be beneficial. The racemose and intraventricular forms of neurocysticercosis do not respond as well as the parenchymatous lesions to medical treatment. In these cases and in the compression of the spinal cord surgical removal is the treatment of choice. The surgical indications in patients with neurocysticercosis can be summarized as follows:

- Single viable parenchymatous cyst (2 cm or larger in diameter) producing focal neurologic symptoms or mass effect after failure of medical treatment or when medical treatment increases the mass effect.
- Intraventricular lesions causing hydrocephalus. Removal under endoscopic control is possible (Fig. 3 a). Caution should be used because these cysts are usually mobile and not easy to grasp. Transaqueductal migration is described [5] and occurred in one of our cases (Fig. 3).
- Spinal lesions with compression of roots and cord.
- Racemose lesions with mass effect. In contrast to hydatid cysts the cyst contents are not antigenic and usually consist of only one scolex. Spillage of cyst fluid is not dangerous, and specific surgical maneuvers such as the Arana-Iniguez or Dowling technique are unnecessary.

Acknowledgments. This research was made possible by a grant of the Deutsche Forschungsgemeinschaft and the Wilhelm-Toennis-Foundation of the German Society of Neurosurgery.

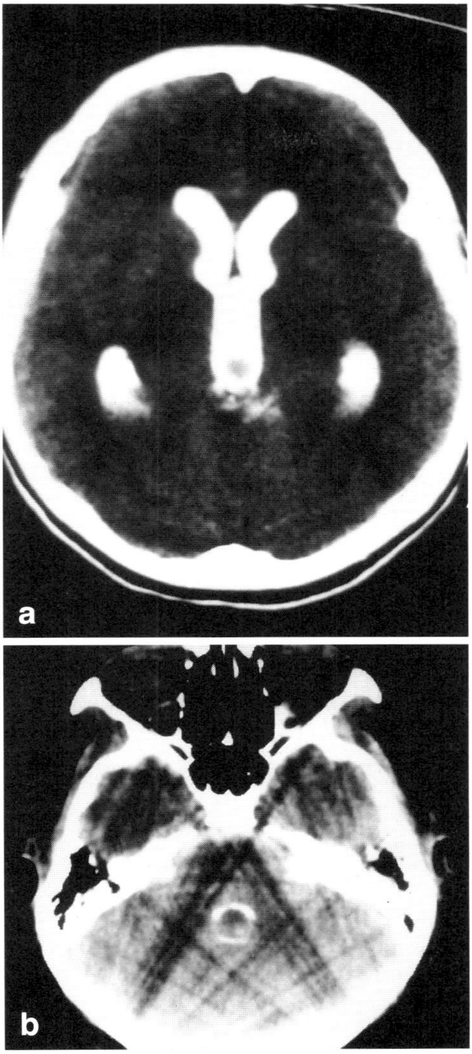

Fig. 3 a, b. Intraventricular cyst migrating from the third to the fourth ventricle

References

1. Alarcon G, Hidalgo F, Moncayo J, Vinan I, Duenas G (1992) Cerebral cysticercosis and stroke. Stroke 23:224–228
2. Del Brutto O (1992) Cysticercosis and cerebrovascular disease: a review. J Neurol Neurosurg Psychiatr 55:252–254
3. Del Brutto OH, Santibanez R, Noboa CA, Aguirre R, Diaz E, Alarcon TA (1992) Epilepsy due to neurocysticercosis: analysis of 203 patients. Neurology 42:389–392
4. Ehnert KL, Roberto RR, Barett L, Sorvillo FJ, Rutherford GW (1992) Cysticercosis: first 12 months of reporting in California. Bull Pan Am Health Organ 26:165–172

5. Kramer J, Carrazana EJ, Cosgrove GR, Kleefield J, Edlmann R (1992) Transaqueductal migration of a cysticercus cyst. J Neurosurg 77:956–958
6. Leblanc R, Knowles KF, Melanson D, Maclean JD, Rouleau G, Famer J.-P. (1986) Neurocysticercosis: surgical and medical management with praziquantel. Neurosurgery 18:419–427
7. McCormick GF, Zee CS, Heide J (1982) Cysticercosis cerebri. Review of 127 cases. Arch Neurol 39:534–539
8. Monteiro L, Coelho T, Stocker A (1992) Neurocysticercosis. A review of 231 cases. Infection 20:61–65
9. Nieto C (1956) Cysticercosis of the nervous system. Diagnosis by means of the spinal fluid complement fixation test. Neurology 6:725–738
10. Puri V, Sharma DK, Kumar S, Choudhury V, Gupta RK, Khalil A (1991) Neurocysticercosis in children. Indian Pediatr 28:1309–1317
11. Rosas N, Sotelo J, Nieto D (1986) ELISA in the diagnosis of neurocysticercosis. Arch Neurol 43:353–356
12. Sotelo J, Escobedo F, Rodriquez-Carbajal J, Torres B, Rubio-Donnadieu F (1984) Therapy of parenchymal brain cysticercosis with praziquantel. N Engl J Med 310:1001–1007
13. Sotelo J, Escobedo F, Rodriquez-Carbajal J (1985) Praziquantel in the treatment of neurocysticercosis: long-term follow-up. Neurology 35:752–755
14. Sotelo J, Penagos P, Escobedo F, Del Brutto O (1988) Short course of albendazole therapy for neurocysticercosis. Arch Neurol 45:1130–1133
15. Sotelo J, Escobedo F, Penagos P (1988) Albendazole vs praziquantel for therapy for neurocysticercosis. Arch Neurol 45:532–534
16. terPenning B, Litchman CD, Heier L (1992) Bilateral middle cerebral artery occlusions in neurocysticercosis. Stroke 23:280–283
17. Vanijanonta S, Bunnag D, Riganti M (1992) The treatment of neurocysticercosis with praziquantel. Southeast Asian J Trop Med Public Health [Suppl] 22:275–278
18. Vasquez V, Sotelo J (1992) The course of seizures after treatment for cerebral cysticercosis. N Engl J Med 327:696–701

Head Injuries from Bicycle Accidents

J. Zentner[1], G. Naujocks[1], H. Franken[1], and J. Schramm[1]

Introduction

In the interests of both health and economy, bicycling has enjoyed increasing popularity in recent decades. In 1990 the German Federal Office for Statistics in Wiesbaden counted 29 294 bicycle accidents in the country. Of the injured riders 908 (1.3%) died of their injuries [12]. Recent studies have shown that head injuries account for 70%–85% of deaths and serious morbidity in bicycle-related injuries [6, 13, 18]. Children and young adults seem to be at greatest risk, and cycling is now a leading cause of head injury in childhood [1, 3, 4, 7, 10, 11]. In the light of these statistics this study was undertaken to define the severity and types of bicycle-related head injuries in a German community.

Patients and Methods

From January 1987 to December 1992 a total of 116 victims of bicycle accidents were treated as inpatients for head injuries at the Department of Neurosurgery, University of Bonn. There were 89 men and 27 women, aged 3 months–78 years (mean 43 years); the distribution by age and sex is presented in Fig. 1. Medical charts of the 116 patients were reviewed retrospectively. Data evaluated included details on the accident, severity of head injury, treatment modalities, and outcome. Data collection and evaluation were computerized (dBase+++). To standardize severity of head injury the Abbreviated Injury Scale (AIS) was used [2]. The outcome was evaluated according to the Glasgow Outcome Scale [8]. Long-term results were obtained by questionnaires. Observation time ranged from 1 to 72 months and averaged 36 months.

Results

Most injuries were sustained by children and young adults aged between 11 and 20 years (Fig. 1). Of the 116 patients 27 (23.3%) suffered mild injuries (AIS 0, 1), 40 (34.5%) moderate injuries (AIS 2, 3), and 49 (42.2%) severe injuries (AIS 4, 5; Table 1). Craniofacial soft tissue injuries were observed in 48 cases (41.4%), skull

[1] Department of Neurosurgery, University Bonn, Sigmund-Freud-Str. 25, 53105 Bonn, Germany.

Advances in Neurosurgery, Vol. 22
B. L. Bauer, M. Brock, M. Klinger (Eds.)

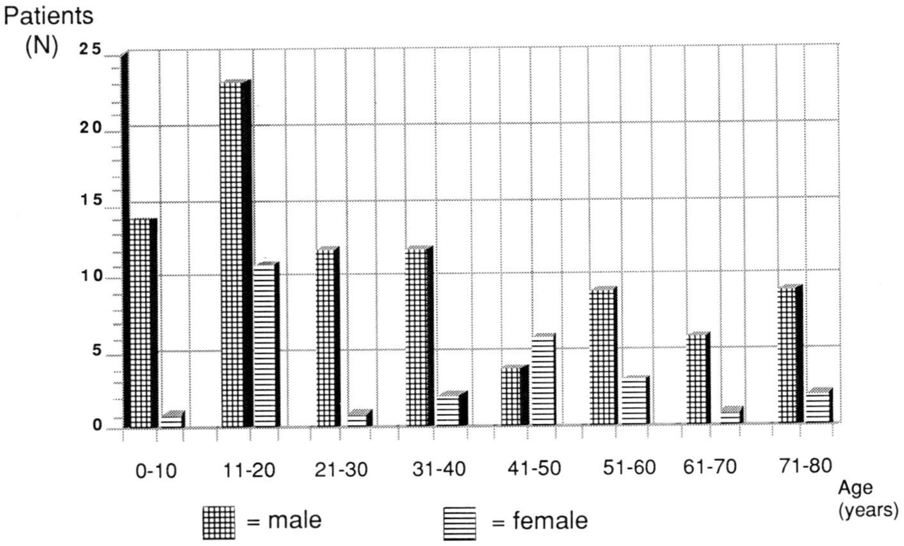

Fig. 1. Age and sex distribution of 116 head-injured patients

and/or midface fractures in 74 (63.8%), brain contusions in 37 (31.9%), and extracerebral hematomas in 48 (41.4%).

Neurosurgical operations were performed in 53 patients (45.7%; Table 2). Most of these operations were related to the evacuation of an extracerebral hematoma (36 cases, 31.0%). One patient (0.9%) was operated on for intracerebral hematoma, three (2.6%) for impression fractures, and two (1.7%) for rhinoliquorrhea. In 11 cases (9.5%) ventriculostomy was performed for measurement and control of intracranial pressure (Table 3).

Of the 116 victims 76 (65.5%) had a good recovery (GOS 5) on follow-up. Moderate disability (GOS 4) was encountered in eight (6.9%) and severe disability (GOS 4) in two (1.7%). One patient (0.9%) survived in a vegetative state, and 24

Table 1. Severity of head injuries on the Abbreviated Injury Score

	n	%
0 Soft tissue injury	12	10.3
1 Concussion, amnesia	15	12.9
2 Unconsciousness ≤ 15 min	23	19.8
3 Unconsciousness ≤ 1 h	17	14.7
4 Unconsciousness 1–24 h	22	19.0
5 Unconsciousness > 24 h	27	23.3
Total	116	100.0

Table 2. Neurosurgical procedures in 116 patients

	n	%
Epidural hematoma	22	19.0
Subdural hematoma	14	12.1
Intracerebral hematoma	1	0.9
Impression fracture	3	2.6
Rhinoliquorrhea	2	1.7
Ventriculostomy	11	9.5
Total	53	100.0

Table 3. Outcome of 116 patients on the Glasgow Outcome Scale

	n	%
1 Death	24	20.7
2 Vegetative state	1	0.9
3 Severe disability	2	1.7
4 Moderate disability	8	6.9
5 Good recovery	76	65.5
Unknown	5	4.3
Total	116	100.0

patients (20.7%) had died. In five cases (4.3%) the outcome remained unknown (Table 3).

Discussion

Head injuries from bicycling are an important problem and one that grows as cycling continues to increase in popularity. Our results clearly indicate that bicycle victims requiring neurosurgical care suffer serious head trauma in a large percentage of cases. The severity of injuries is reflected in the high mortality rate (20.7%). The majority of our patients were young, with a male predominance. Obviously, our data do not reflect the true incidence of different head-injury patterns since there is an unknown number of patients who have been treated either as outpatients or in other emergency rooms. Assuming that victims primarily undergoing neurosurgical care as inpatients have probably experienced a major head trauma, our figures certainly overestimate the real situation. However, we can state that bicycling today considerably contributes to morbidity and mortality in consequence of road accidents.

Various recommendations have been made to reduce both the risk of accident and the risk of injury. Active measures to prevent accidents include enforcement of traffic regulations, education of riders, and the creation of bicycling lanes [6, 9, 14,

15, 19]. Passive security may be increased by improved design of vehicles and wearing of protective helmets. Wassermann et al. [17] found that helmet wearers experience significantly fewer skull fractures (1% versus 11%) and soft tissue injuries (5% versus 18%) than those not wearing helmets. From the analysis of 235 cases of head injuries, Thompson et al. [16] concluded that safety helmets reduce the risk of head injury by 85% and that of brain injury by 78%. In other words, riders who not wear helmets appear to be at a 6.6-fold greater risk of head injury and a 8.3-fold greater risk of brain injury than riders who do. Similar results have been obtained by others [5, 17, 20]. It has been suggested that hard-shell helmets with a complete or almost complete inner lining afford much better head protection than do hairnet helmets [5]. Although these reports must be interpreted with caution due to essential methodological limitations, the literature provides convincing evidence of the effectiveness of bicycle helmets in preventing injury.

References

1. Armson CJ, Pollard CW (1986) Child cyclist injuries: a prospective study. Med J Aust 144:144–146
2. Baker SP, O'Neill B, Haddon J et al. (1976) The Injury Severity Score: a method for describing patients with multiple injuries and evaluating medical care. J Trauma 16:882
3. Brown B, Farley C (1989) The pertinence of promoting the use of bicycle helmets for 8 to 12 year old children. Chron Dis Can 10:92–95
4. Cushman RA, Down J, MacMillan N, Waclawik H (1990) Bicycle helmets use in Ottawa. Can Fam Physician 36:697–700
5. Dorsch MM, Woodward AJ, Somers RL (1987) Do bicycle safety helmets reduce severity of head injury in real crashes? Accid Anal Prev 19:183–190
6. Friede AM, Azzara CV, Gallagher SS, Guyer B (19859 The epidemiology of injuries to bicycle riders. Pediatr Clin North Am 32:141–151
7. Ivan LP, Choo SH, Ventureyra EC (1983) Head injuries in childhood: a 2-year survey. Can Med Assoc J 128:281–284
8. Jennet B, Bond M (1975) Assessment of outcome after severe brain damage, a practical scale. Lancet 1:480–484
9. Kruse DL, McBeath AA (1980) Bicycle accidents and injuries. A random survey of a college population. Am J Sports Med 8:342–344
10. Lapner M, Leslie PI (1981) Bicycle injuries in children. Can Med Assoc J 125:132
11. O'Rourke NA, Costello F, Yelland JD, Stuart GG (1987) Head injuries to children riding bicycles. Med J Aust 146:619–621
12. Otte D (1981) Unfall- und Sicherheitsforschung im Straßenverkehr. Bundesanstalt für Straßenwesen 82:115–123
13. Reynolds R, Cohen D (1987) Children, bicycles and head injuries. Med J Aust 146:615
14. Scaglione NA, Suljaga-Petchel K, Frankel VH (1983) Bicycle-related accidents and injuries in a population of urban cyclists. Bull Hosp Joint Dis 2:80–89
15. Simpson W, Unwin PS, Nelson IWC (1988) Head injuries, helmets, cycle lanes, and cyclists. Br Med J 296:1161–1162
16. Thompson RS, Rivara FP, Thompson DC (1989) A case-control study of the effectiveness of bicycle safety helmets. N Engl J Med 320:1361–1367
17. Wassermann RC, Waller JA, Monty MJ, Emery AB, Robinson DR (1988) Bicyclists, helmets and head injuries: a rider-based study of helmet use and effectiveness. Am J Public Health 78:1120–1121

18. Weiss BD (1987) Childhood bicycle injuries, what can we do? Am J Dis Child 141:135–136
19. Williams AF (1976) Factors in the initiation of bicycle-motor vehicle collisions. Am J Dis Child 130:370–377
20. Worrell J (1987) Head injuries in pedal cyclists: how much will protection help? Injury 18:5–6

Clinical Applicability of Laser Doppler Flowmetry in Neurosurgery

R. Steinmeier[1], A. Dötterl[1], I. Bondar[1], and R. Fahlbusch[1]

Introduction

Different methods for the measurement of cerebral perfusion must be distinguished: methods for *discontinuous* measurement of regional cerebral perfusion and methods for *continuous* measurement of microflow. Only thermoclearance and laser Doppler flowmetry (LDF) can be used during surgery or in critically ill patients on the intensive care unit, and both provide real-time, online results of microflow estimation [1–3, 6]. LDF was established in the 1970 by Nielsson and Bonner and Nossal.

The LDF device generates a monochromatic laser beam with a wavelength of 780 nm. The photons are reflected in tissue by stationary and moving tissue structures. Moving tissue structures generate a Doppler shift, and stationary structures reflect the light without Doppler shift. Thus, the signal consists of a stationary DC part and a frequency-modulated AC part. When the number of moving particles compared to the number of nonmoving structures increases, the amplitude of the AC signal increases; this ratio AC/DC is called *volume*. When the velocity of moving particles increases, the frequency of the AC part increases by Doppler shift, which is proportional to the mean *velocity* of moving structures per volume. Tissue perfusion or microflow is calculated as the scaled product of velocity and volume and is called *flux* or *flow*.

Because of inherent difficulties with calibration we and most other groups use arbitrary units. Nevertheless, these arbitrary units correlate well with the physical units of perfusion (ml 100 g^{-1} tissue min^{-1}) [4]. The sample volume of LDF is about 1 mm^3.

Methods

A digital data acquisition system was used for data sampling, and the three LDF signals were continuously monitored: the mean *velocity* of red blood cells (kHz), the proportion of moving to nonmoving cells in tissue, *volume*, and the product of both signals, *flux*. ECG, arterial blood pressure and endexpiratory pCO_2 were monitored simultaneously by the same data acquisition system.

---

[1] Neurochirurgische Klinik, Universität Erlangen-Nürnberg, Schwabachanlage 6, 91054 Erlangen, Germany.

Advances in Neurosurgery, Vol. 22
B. L. Bauer, M. Brock, M. Klinger (Eds.)

Results

Three examples for applications of LDF technology in neurosurgery are presented below.

Experimental Evaluation of Spatial Microvascular Heterogeneity

The aim of these studies was to evaluate spatial microvascular heterogeneity as measured by LDF. Investigations were performed in animals (New Zealand rabbits). After trephination and opening of the dura, artificial CSF was filled in a glass cylinder fixed to the bone. The LDF probe was positioned at different matrix points on the brain surface by a stepper motor driver, three-dimensional micromanipulator. At each measurement point, the LDF probe was stopped, and after 1 s (to allow stabilization of the probe holder) the measurement was started, and the LDF signals were averaged over a time period of 10 s. When performed in the horizontal plane, the procedure is called scanning or mapping, and this is completely controlled by a personal computer with adjustment of all steps in vertical and horizontal planes. In each of the ten animal experiments, an area of 3.5 x 4.5 mm was scanned; the distance between each point was 250 mm. The total time for scanning the complete area with 252 points lasted about 45 min. Vascular structures larger than 200 or 300 mm cause an increase in the velocity signal. A comparison between the scanned brain area and the LDF contour plots reveals large similitarities between the microvascular anatomy and results of LDF measurement.

LDF Measurement in the ICU

Two LDF probes were introduced through a frontal burr hole placed for routine external ventricular drainage implantation. The probes were gently pushed forward and placed subdurally over the frontopolar and frontolateral pial cortical surface. To prevent undesired displacements, the probes were secured with sutures to the skin. Following study completion, the probes were removed in the ICU through the scalp incision. The studies were performed in eight comatose patients with severe head injury or higher grade subarachnoid hemorrhage. Systemic and local physiological parameters were monitored three times a day over a period of up to several hours; the entire study lasted maximally 5 days.

A preliminary analysis of the simultaneous measurements of systemic and local physiological parameters in comatose patients often revealed well-known and therefore expected, predictable, and explainable interdependencies between these parameters. However, a closer look at the LDF signals showed some types of highly unexpected and seemingly "paradox", but perhaps explainable, patterns of the LDF signals, which we tentatively subdivided into three distinct categories. (a) Rather frequently, "spontaneous", abrupt fluctuations of the LDF signals without any simultaneous or shortly preceding change of other monitored parameters were observed. These unpredictable "LDF signal drifts" were probably due to slight displacements of the LDF probe over the cerebral cortex, causing a change in the distance between the LDF probe and the brain surface and thus of the signal intensity. (b) "Paradox" patterns with the LDF signals out of phase could often be discerned. The "spontaneous" change of the first signal in one direction was associated with a marked change of the corresponding second signal in the opposite direction, suggesting spatial heterogeneity of functional response of the cerebral microvascular bed. (c) Another striking feature was the onset of signal changes during CO_2 tests in the expected direction but at different points in time, suggesting additional temporal heterogeneity of functional response of the cerebral microvascular bed.

LDF Measurement During Transsphenoidal Microsurgery

All patients ($n = 96$) who underwent transsphenoidal microsurgery for intra-/supra/ parasellar adenomas were included in this series (between January 1990 and May 1991), irrespective of the endocrinological activity or pharmacological pretreatment (bromocriptine, octreotide) in cases of prolactinoma or acromegaly. In this total group 52 were systematically analyzed [5]. Significant differences for the nonpulsatile LDF signals were found between the anterior (AL) and posterior lobe (PL). Mean AL microflow and velocity were 27.4 ± 2.7 (flux) and 0.81 ± 0.12 (kHz), while mean PL microflow and velocity were 177.7 ± 12.7 (flux) and 4.35 ± 0.27 (kHz). No difference was found between LDF fractional volume in the AL [0.73 ± 0.06] and PL [$0.77 \pm 0,07$].

Pulsatile Pattern of LDF Signals. All LDF signals (microflow, velocity, and volume) exhibit pulsatile fluctuations. The major part of these fluctuations can obviously be attributed to blood pressure pulsatility. In addition, other factors such as central venous pressure and ventilation pressure influence these pulsatile variations, especially the LDF volume signal. Pulsatile LDF signal patterns are seen in both AL and PL, and amplitude increases depending on the mean value of each LDF signal.

Discussion

Continuous monitoring of global, regional, and local cerebral blood flow in comatose patients with severe head injury, higher grade subarachnoid hemorrhage, and other conditions leading to diffuse or focal brain damage, raised intracranial pressure, and impaired cerebral circulation would be of paramount importance in improving treatment strategies and consequently clinical outcome in these patients. Unfortunately, despite various technological advances in recent decades there is still no straightforward approach to a simple, reliable, and continuous assessment of global and regional changes of the brain macro- and microcirculation.

In our opinion, the "inconsistent" LDF signal patterns are probably caused by three main sources of "bias": (a) specific properties of the LDF measurement system as applied in the described clinical setting lead to slight displacements of the LDF probe and consequently to more less marked and abrupt changes of the LDF signals. Despite several efforts to improve the stability of the probe position, we could not manage to avoid this major source of error for longer measurements. More important, the data strongly suggest the presence of (b) spatial and (c) temporal heterogeneity of functional responses of the microvascular bed, which was demonstrated in our experimental investigations on spatial heterogeneity. These properties inherent in the measurement setup and physiological system investigated severely compromise a straightforward and unequivocal interpretation of the information provided by LDF measurements of local cerebral perfusion. Therefore, the establishment of LDF as a valuable tool to understand the pathophysiology and improve the management of comatose patients will require a great amount of further experimental and clinical investigations as well as theoretical reflection to improve understanding of the complex system involved both in the regulation of cerebral hemodynamics and in the interaction between the LDF device and brain tissue.

Application of the LDF technology during transphenoidal microsurgery is rather helpful, since the pituitary PL can easily be identified by the much higher flow in the anterior lobe of the adenoma. A study to discriminate between AL and adenoma with LDF flow characteristics is in progress.

Conclusions

The handling of commercial LDF devices is rather simple; however, one must acknowledge the following points: (a) LDF is very sensitive to motion artifacts (relative motion between probe and tissue). (b) The LDF sample volume is small (approximately 1 mm^3), and due to the spatial heterogeneity of cerebral microflow single measurements cannot be extrapolated to larger tissue volumes. (c) Heterogeneity of pituitary microflow is low, and pituitary compartments can be identified by LDF due to their different levels of microflow.

References

1. Arbit E, Di Resta GR, Bedford RF, Shah NK, Galicich JH (1989) Intraoperative measurement of cerebral and tumor blood flow with laser-Doppler flowmetry. Neurosurgery 24:166–170
2. Eyre JA, Essex TJH, Flecknell PA, Bartholomew PH, Sinclair JI (1988) A comparison oby, J, and Yonas H (1991): Acute regional cerebral blood flow changes caused by severe head injuries. J Neurosurg 74:407–414
3. Meyerson BA, Gunasekera L, Linderoth B, Gazelius B (1991) Bedside monitoring of regional cortical blood flow in comatose patients using laser Doppler flowmetry. Neurosurgery 29:750–755

4. Skarphedinsson JO, Hårding H, Thorén P (1988) Repeated measurements of cerebral blood flow in rats. Comparisons between the hydrogen clearance method and laser Doppler flowmetry. Acta Physiol Scand 134:133–142
5. Steinmeier R, Fahlbusch R, Powers AD, Dötterl A, Buchfelder M (1991) Pituitary microcirculation: physiological aspects and clinical implications. A laser-Doppler flow study during transsphenoidal adenomectomy. Neurosurgery 29:47–54
6. Tenjin H, Hirakawa K, Mizukawa N, Yano I, Ohta T, Uchibori M, Hino A (1988) Dysautoregulation in patients with ruptured aneurysms: cerebral blood flow measurements obtained during surgery by a temperature-controlled thermoelectrical method. Neurosurgery 23:705–709

Neurosurgery of the Spine

Microsurgery in Intervertebral Disc Disease: Whom Does It Benefit?

W. A. Dauch[1] and S. Murrish[1]

Introduction

Whether or not microsurgical techniques improve outcome after operation for intervertebral disc disease is still a matter of discussion [6, 9]. Since randomization is difficult and therapist blinding not possible, results of microsurgery are usually compared to "conventionally" operated historical control groups, and thus subject to the hazard of serious bias [5]. To yield meaningful results, this kind of trial must be meticulously controlled for baseline conditions with regard to both patients and adjuvant treatment.

Patients and Methods

When we changed the mode of our operative treatment of lumbar intervertebral disc disease from conventional [8] to microsurgical [2, 7] techniques, we made use of this historical opportunity and initiated a prospective clinical trial, comparing treatment results of the last 100 patients operated on conventionally to those of 100 consecutive, microsurgically treated patients who were operated on by the same three neurosurgeons after 3 months of microsurgical training. We replaced the "Mecca" position by the prone position of the patient, introduced preoperative X-rays for segment localization, used a speculum instead of retractors, new microsurgical tools, and, of course, the microscope itself from the beginning of yellow ligament opening until control of hemostasis. The patient's mobilization starts on the first postoperative day, as had also been the custom with conventional surgery. To create a rather homogeneous study population, we excluded patients with root compression due to spondylosis, a narrow spinal canal, and spinal instability and those who had previous lumbar operations.

Follow-up examinations were performed in our neurosurgical outpatient department 33–39 months after the operation by a single member of the staff who had not been involved in the surgical treatment of the patients. Success of treatment was judged according to 16 parameters. Four of these refer to posture and mobility of the lumbar spine, four to neurological findings, one to postoperative pain in general, and seven to pain in distinct situations (walking, standing, sitting, lifting, working, sleeping, and with personal hygiene). With every pain item the

[1] Neurochirurgische Klinik, Philipps-Universität, Baldingerstr., 35033 Marburg, Germany.

Advances in Neurosurgery, Vol. 22
B. L. Bauer, M. Brock, M. Klinger (Eds.)

Table 1. Pre- and intraoperative characteristics of treatment groups undergoing conventional ($n = 72$) or microsurgical ($n = 74$) lumbar disc operations and complete follow-up 3 years later

	Conventional	Microsurgical
Male: female ratio	69%:31%	53%:47%
Age		
< 40 years	39%	39%
40–59 years	50%	50%
> 59 years	11%	11%
Segment		
LW5/SW1	49%	49%
LW4/5	46%	43%
LW3/4	3%	1%
Multiple	3%	7%
Duration of illness		
> 6 months	22%	24%
6–18 months	24%	19%
> 18 months	54%	57%
Lasegue's sign positive	81%	91%
Hyp-/anesthesia	79%	57%
Paresis	36%	37%
Perforation of PLL	74%	54%

patient had to choose one out of six preformulated statements indicating levels of increasing pain sensation from pain-free to pain-related impossibility of action. These eight pain items were derived from a questionnaire developed by the Mainz Pain Center (Mainz, Germany).

As expected, the two study groups differed from each other with respect to some parameters (Table 1). Two of these were regarded as relevant: sex and intraoperative findings (perforation versus no perforation of the posterior longitudinal ligament, PLL). Consequently, statistical analysis was performed after stratification for these two parameters, using the Mantel-Haenszel test. While 6 months after operation follow-up was complete in 96% of patients, this number dropped to 73% after 3 years, but it was almost equal in both groups. In this paper, we report the 3-year results.

Results

Early complications of treatment were rare (such as deep vein thrombosis in four patients, wound healing disturbances in seven) and occurred in both groups or were not observed at all (for instance CSF fistula, spondylitis, pulmonary embolism). After 3 years, there were no significant differences between the treatment groups with respect to posture and mobility of the lumbar spine, Lasegue's sign, or

Table 2. Treatment results 3 years after conventional or microsurgical operation for herniated lumbar disc

	Conventional	Microsurgical	p^a
Reduced lordosis	2%	3%	NS
Scoliosis	0%	0%	NS
Minimal FTFD > 40 cm	8%	8%	NS
Schober's Index < 12 cm	4%	8%	NS
Laseque's sign positive	22%	20%	NS
Valleix' point sensitive	19%	12%	NS
Hypesthesia	33%	15%	0.01
Paresis	18%	3%	0.003
Pain			
Global rating > 2/6	51%	32%	0.04
Standing	43%	31%	NS
Walking	55%	42%	NS
Sitting	24%	21%	NS
Working	55%	35%	NS
Lifting	73%	62%	NS
At personal hygiene	18%	7%	NS
At work	55%	35%	NS

[a] FTFD, Fingertip-to-floor distance. Mantel-Haenszel Test after stratification for sex and PLL perforation.

pain sensation with pressure at Valleix' points (Table 2). Postoperative hypesthesia was observed in fewer patients in the microsurgical group (15%) than in the conventional group (33%), which was significantly different ($p = 0.03$) even when the unequal preoperative sensibility findings in both groups were taken into account. Paresis was of equal frequency in both groups preoperatively (36% prior to conventional operation and 37% before microsurgery) but not postoperatively (18% after conventional and 3% after microsurgical treatment, $p = 0.006$). This surprisingly large difference was due to a combination of (a) better recovery from preoperative paresis in the microsurgical group, (b) less perioperative deterioration, and (c) the delayed development of paresis in the second or third postoperative year which was observed in three patients after conventional surgery but in one after microsurgery. Regarding postoperative pain, the global index was slightly better after microsurgery ($p = 0.04$), but in the seven subitems there was no significant difference. Interestingly, after resolving stratification, some of these pain items (pain at night, at work, with personal hygiene, and the global index) turned out to be significantly different between the treatment groups only in women (indicating some benefit from microsurgery) but not in men. With the other four pain items (pain at walking, standing, sitting, and lifting), in neither men nor women was a relationship found between treatment result and surgical technique. Superiority of microsurgery with respect to paresis and global pain was not related to the intraoperative finding of PLL rupture.

Discussion and Conclusions

Microsurgery has found its way into the treatment of intervertebral disc disease in many centers in recent years. However, there is a lack of definitive confirmation of its superiority over conventional technique. There may be several reasons, for this, for instance, the virtual impossibility of performing a randomized clinical trial. The only realistic option seems to be a controlled sequential study design, using historic control groups. This has been carried out in some instances [1, 3, 4, 6, 9, 10] but has yielded contradictory results. Nevertheless, this kind of study is capable of giving useful insights when properly performed and carefully evaluated.

Since we intended to observe the late results of treatment, we performed follow-up examinations about 3 years after the operation, facing the problem of incompleteness of data. After 6 months we had a follow-up rate of 96%, but this figure dropped to 73% after 33–39 months; however, this was almost equal in both groups. Regarding the differences in patient characteristics between the study groups with respect to sex and intraoperative finding of PLL perforation, we could find no systematic explanation and attributed them to chance and handled them statistically by stratification. We observed one major influence of operative technique on late results: neurological deficits, paresis, and hypesthesia were observed less often after microsurgery than after conventional operation. A variety of factors may have contributed to this finding, including gentle retraction, more subtle hemostasis, better illumination, and smaller instruments, but this issue remains subject to discussion. Spinal stability and function do not seem to be influenced by the operative technique, while with pain assessment some distinct differences between treatment groups were observed. Nevertheless, the restriction of these differences to four out of eight pain items and to women indicates complex relationships. They require further investigations to determine the way in which patients benefit from microsurgery.

References

1. Barrios C, Ahmed M, Arrótegui J, Björnsson A, Gillström G (1990) Microsurgery versus standard removal of the herniated lumbar disc. A 3-year comparison in 150 cases. Acta Orthop Scand 61:399–403
2. Caspar W (1977) A new surgical procedure for lumbar disc herniation causing less tissue damage through a microsurgical approach. Adv Neurosurg 4:74–80
3. Caspar W, Campbell B, Barbier DD, Kretschmmer R, Gotfried Y (1991) The Caspar microsurgical discectomy and comparison with a conventional standard lumbar disc procedure. Neurosurgery 28:78–87
4. Dauch WA (1985) Infection of the intervertebral space following conventional and microsurgical operation on the herniated lumbar intervertebral disc. Acta Neurochir (Wien) 82:43–49
5. Elwood JM (1988) Causal relationships in medicine. Oxford University Press, Oxford
6. Kho HC, Steudel WI (1986) Vergleich der mikrochirurgischen lumbalen Bandscheibenoperation mit der konventionellen Technik beim frei sequestrierten Bandscheibenvorfall. Eine retrospektive Studie anhand von 267 Fällen. Neurochirurgia (Stuttg) 29:181–185

7. Loew F, Caspar W (1978) Surgical approach to lumbar disc herniation. In: Krayenbühl H (ed) Advances and technical standards in neurosurgery, vol 5. Springer, Vienna New York, pp 153–175
8. Love JG (1939) Protruded intervertebral disks. JAMA 113:2029–2034
9. Nyström B (1987) Experience of microsurgical compared with conventional technique in lumbar disc operations. Acta Neurol Scand 76:129–141
10. Probst C (1989) Lumbale Diskushernien: Mikrochirurgie – Ja oder Nein? Neurochirurgia (Stuttg) 32:172–176

The European Myelopathy Score

J. Herdmann[1], M. Linzbach[1], M. Krzan[2], J. Dvorák[3], and W. J. Bock[1]

Introduction

In 1975 the Japanese Orthopedic Association (JOA) introduced a score for the clinical neurological judgment of *cervical myelopathy*. In Japan and other Oriental countries this so-called *JOA score* is especially popular for judging the clinical progression of a disease known as ossification of the posterior longitudinal ligament (OPLL), which is very common in Japan. Attempts to apply the JOA score to European, i.e. Western, patients have been disappointing because of cultural differences between Orientals and Westerners: the first criterion on the JOA score rates the ability to eat with chopsticks, which would leave most Westerners with a distinct impairment of upper limb function as a sign of cervical myelopathy. In particular, the JOA score does not take into account the four major neural systems, the impairment of which contributes to the clinical picture of cervical myelopathy: (a) the upper motor neuron with signs of spasticity as well as bladder and bowel malfunction, (b) the lower motor neuron with impairment of hand function, (c) the posterior roots with upper limb radicular deficits and paresthesias, and (d) the posterior columns with proprioceptive sensory loss, disturbed coordination, and ataxia. In order to close this gap a *European Myelopathy Score* was developed which rates these systems in a simple and concise manner.

Integration of Pathoanatomical and Functional Aspects in Cervical Myelopathy

The European Myelopathy Score has five subscores (Table 1). The significance of each subscore is weighed by the maximal number of points that is achieved if the subscore is normal. All of these subscores are functional criteria that do not require formal testing. They can be obtained only by taking the patient history or even by questionnaires filled in by the patients themselves.

The *upper motor neuron* is critical in the control of lower limb function. Gait is of major importance for judgment of cervical myelopathy. It is the only subscore

[1] Department of Neurosurgery, Heinrich-Heine University, Moorenstr. 5, 40225 Düsseldorf, Germany.
[2] Department of Clinical Neurophysiology, University Clinical Center, Zaloska 7, 61000 Ljubljana, Slovenia.
[3] Spine Unit, W. Schulthess Klinik, Neumünsterallee 3, 8008 Zürich, Switzerland.

Advances in Neurosurgery, Vol. 22
B. L. Bauer, M. Brock, M. Klinger (Eds.)

Table 1. The European Myelopathy Score

Upper motor neuron function (gait)	Points
Unable to walk, wheelchair	1
Walking on flat ground only with cane or aid	2
Climbing stairs only with aid	3
Gait clumsy, but no aid necessary	4
Normal walking and climbing stairs	5
Upper motor neuron function (bladder and bowel function)	
Retention, no control over bladder and/or bowel function	1
Inadequate micturition and urinary frequency	2
Normal bladder and bowel function	3
Lower motor neuron function (hand function)	
Handwriting and eating with knife and fork impossible	1
Handwriting and eating with knife and fork impaired	2
Handwriting, tying shoe laces or a tie clumsy	3
Normal handwriting	4
Posterior column function (proprioception and coordination)	
Getting dressed only with aid	1
Getting dressed clumsily and slowly	2
Getting dressed normally	3
Posterior cervical roots (paresthesias and dysesthesia)	
Disabling sensations disturbing all daily activities	1
Tolerable sensations	2
No paresthesia or dysesthesia	3

that can reach 5 points. *Bladder and bowel function* (3 points) depends on both motor and sensory integrity. In cervical myelopathy, however, bladder or bowel dysfunction is caused primarily by a bilateral upper motor neuron lesion. Cervical myelopathy is generally due to degenerative changes of the middle and lower cervical spine. Therefore impairment of hand function can be attributed mainly to a *lower motor neuron function* (4 points) although similar disturbances of precision movements are also seen in upper motor neuron function or cortical lesions. Proprioception and coordination depend on *posterior column function* (3 points). Posterior column function was included in the European Myelopathy Score instead of the JOA subscores for sensory function, a disturbance of which is very difficult to classify in categories. Pain is not a major symptom in cervical myelopathy. Nevertheless, unpleasant sensations such as paresthesia or dysesthesia are often reported and are mostly caused by a mechanical irritation of the afferent *posterior cervical roots* (3 points). The maximum number of points a normal subject can reach is 18 points.

Borrowing from the Glasgow Coma Scale, the worst result is rated with one point for each subscore. The minimum score is therefore five. Depending on the sum reached in the score, cervical myelopathy is classified in three grades: grade III, 5–8 points; grade II, 9–12 points; and grade I, 13–16 points. Subjects with 17 or 18 points are considered free of signs of cervical myelopathy.

Application of the European Myelopathy Score in 186 Patients with Cervical Myelopathy

A total of 186 patients aged 20–86 years (mean 56 ± 13) have been judged according to the European Myelopathy Score. There were 131 men and 55 women. Of these, 76% suffered from degenerative cervical spine disease and 16% from cervical spine trauma. The lower cervical spine was affected in 68% and the middle cervical spine in 21%. Preoperatively more than 40% of patients were classified as having a grade I cervical myelopathy, with a mean European Myelopathy Score of 13 ± 3 points. Six months after decompressive surgery (in most cases an anterior approach according to Smith-Robinson) 60% of patients had an unchanged or improved myelopathy grade. A further 45% of patients were now classified as having a grade II myelopathy, with a mean European Myelopathy Score of 11.5 ± 3 points. The recovery rate for those patients who showed an overall improvement was 35%; this was calculated as follows: (postoperative score – preoperative score)/(maximum score [18] – preoperative score) x 100. These figures show how useful such a score is for grouping and comparing patients.

Discussion and Conclusions

The functional character of the criteria used in the European Myelopathy Score allows a critical evaluation of cervical myelopathy from different centers and different countries. The European Myelopathy Score helps to judge the natural course of the disease and to determine the timing of surgery. It also allows a more objective control of postoperative outcome. The European Myelopathy Score is a valuable tool for the evaluation of all conditions involving cervical myelopathy. It will also allow for rapid communication when comparing radiological findings or neurophysiological results in patients with cervical myelopathy.

Spinal Hamartomas in Adulthood

J. Klekamp[1], M. Samii[1], and A. J. Raimondi[1]

Introduction

The natural history of spinal dysraphism has not been determined precisely. According to many authors only about one-half of patients eventually become symptomatic [9, 27–29]. Therefore, the indication for and timing of surgical procedures in asymptomatic children with dysraphic malformations is very controversial. We have undertaken a retrospective analysis of spinal hamartomas associated with spinal dysraphism in patients who became symptomatic in adulthood to describe clinical features and results of treatment and to help to define guidelines for the treatment of children.

Patients and Methods

A total of 19 patients with onset of symptoms of spinal hamartoma malformations in adult life were identified between 1977 and 1992. Case records, operation notes, and radiographs were evaluated, and follow-up examinations were performed. Spinal hamartomas consisted of either lipomatous or dermal hamartomas [19] and one neurenteric cyst. Only patients with progressive neurological disease were operated on. Surgery consisted of laminectomy, tumor removal, and dissection of arachnoid adhesions if feasible. The filum terminale was not cut in every instance. For monitoring of the postoperative course a grading system was used for each individual symptom: gait ataxia, motor weakness, sensory deficits, dysesthesias, pain, and bladder and bowel function [11]. Patients were also graded according to the Karnofsky score. For tests of statistical significance Student's *t*-test was employed. The rates of recurrence were determined by Kaplan-Meier analysis [10]. A recurrence was defined as reonset of neurological progression. Surgical morbidity was defined as a new, permanent, postoperative deficit or the permanent aggravation of a preexisting deficit. For Kaplan-Meier analysis these cases were classified as a recurrence on the day of surgery.

[1] Neurochirurgische Klinik, Nordstadt Krankenhaus, Haltenhoffstr. 41, 30167 Hannover, Germany.

Advances in Neurosurgery, Vol. 22
B. L. Bauer, M. Brock, M. Klinger (Eds.)

Results

Of 19 patients presenting at our hospital, 16 showed signs of neurological progession and were operated on. The remaining three did not show neurological progression and continue to be observed clinically. Table 1 gives an overview of sex distribution, mean age, length of history and follow-up, and radiological features. According to their main symptom the patients were divided into two groups: paraparesis (group A; $n = 8$) and pain (group B; $n = 11$). In both groups the ratio between intra- and extramedullary tumors was 2:1. In general, dysraphic malformations were more complex in group B. They were more likely to have an additional dermal sinus or diastematomyelia. The most prominent difference was the higher proportion of patients with a tethered cord and spina bifida occulta compared to group A (Table 1). Furthermore, the spinal level tended to be lower. Syringomyelia and arachnoid adhesions were seen in equal proportions in both groups.

Analysis of the postoperative course revealed that the majority of patients in group A benefited from operation. Dysesthesias, motor weakness, and gait ataxia improved, whereas sensory deficits, pain, and bladder and bowel dysfunction increased slightly. Overall, the Karnofsky score remained unchanged. In group B pain improved postoperatively but tended to increase again after 6 months so that most of the benefit was lost again within 1 year. Similarly, we observed a tendency for deterioration in sensory deficits, dysesthesias, and motor weakness starting 6–12 months after surgery. Gait ataxia and bladder and bowel dysfunction continued to progress despite surgery. The Karnofsky score decreased postoperatively. Kaplan-Meier analysis revealed a higher rate of recurrence for group B patients compared to those in group A. We observed no surgical morbidity in group A but 10% in group B. The subsequent rates of recurrence were 25% and 47%, respectively. No recurrences were observed later than 12 months postoperatively (Fig. 1).

Table 1. Characteristics of patients with spinal hamartomas

	Total	Paresis group	Pain group
Number	19	8	11
Male/female ratio	8/11	4/4	4/7
Age (years)	39 ± 14	37 ± 15	41 ± 14
History (months)	101 ± 112	81 ± 111	116 ± 113
Follow-Up (months)	14 ± 17	15 ± 15	14 ± 19
Spina bifida occulta	9	2	7
Tethered cord	10	1	9
Diastematomyelia	4	1	3
Dermal sinus	3	1	2
Syringomyelia	6	4	2
Arachnoid scars	10	4	6
Surgery	16	8	8

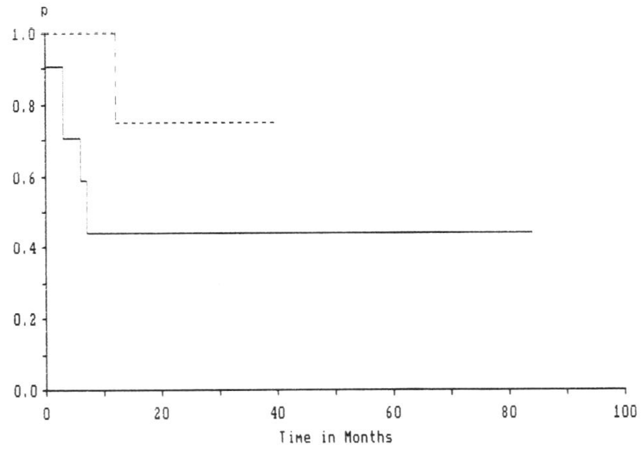

Fig. 1. Postoperative reonset of neurological deterioration. Kaplan-Meier analysis for patients with spinal hamartomas and surgical treatment. ——, Pain group; ----, paresis group

Discussion

The results of surgery in this study are somewhat less favorable than those reported in the literature [12, 14, 16, 30]. However, exact data on the length of follow-up were not given in these publications. A number of case reports have claimed postoperative improvements, but follow-up information for at least 12 months postoperatively is not available [2, 6, 21]. Similarly to our findings, reports about children with spinal dysraphism and follow-up information over several years state that stabilization of the disease process was achieved after a variable degree of early but transient postoperative improvements [8, 13, 17, 22, 25, 30].

In our study every recurrence was marked by reappearance of back pain with radiation into sacral dermatomes. Magnetic resonance imaging in these patients did not disclose regrowth of the partially removed hamartoma but extensive arachnoid scarring at the level of operation. In general, we observed that spinal hamartomas are associated with more severe postoperative arachnoid scarring than other spinal processes [1, 3, 5, 23]. Therefore we consider the aggravation of arachnoid scarring as a major cause for the reappearance of pain and failure of surgery.

Every patient with a recurrence also had a spina bifida occulta. Orthopedic problems due to the bony anomaly may have contributed to the recurrence of pain as well [24].

Among different authors there is general agreement that the filum terminale should be cut if a tethered cord is present. However, the rate of retethering due to postoperative arachnoid scars is generally believed to be very high [4, 7, 26]. Furthermore, several reports mention that arachnoid scars may render surgery extremely difficult in adults [6, 26], raising the probability of retethering even further. Nevertheless, we recommend untethering the spinal cord and cutting the filum terminale whenever a tethered cord is present; this can be done safely, although our results do not allow a final conclusion as to whether untethering in every instance would have improved postoperative outcome.

In comparison to children adult patients present with pain more often rather than bladder dysfunction [16, 18, 20, 29, 30], presumably due to the higher spinal level and degenerative changes of the spine in adults. Therefore conclusions for the treatment of children can be drawn only with caution. Lagae et al. [13] compared 20 children with release of the tethered cord to 21 with known tethered cord but without surgery. Surgery achieved stabilization of neurological signs and symptoms but did not improve deficits. In the nonsurgical group only two children showed neurological progression during a follow-up period of 8 months–13 years. Oi et al. [15] have shown that patients without a tethered cord are not at significant risk for neurological deterioration.

Conclusion

Our retrospective analysis shows that a considerable number of patients with occult dysraphism reach adulthood or even old age before becoming symptomatic. This suggests that not every dysraphic process inevitably leads to progressive neurological problems. We consider it justified to delay surgery in children if no progression of symptoms occurs – particularly in patients without a tethered cord. The risk of causing a neurological deficit or exacerbation of arachnoid scarring should be weighed carefully when prophylactic surgery is considered. Adults and children should be operated on as soon as neurological symptoms appear or progress because only a stabilization of the disease is achieved in the majority of cases.

References

1. Anderson FM (1975) Occult spinal dysraphism: a series of 73 cases. Pediatrics 55:826–835
2. Balagura S (1984) Late neurological dysfunction in adult lumbosacral lipoma with tethered cord. Neurosurgery 15:724–726
3. English JE, Maltby GL (1967) Diastematomyelia in adults. J Neurosurg 27:260–264
4. Epstein F (1983) Meningomyelocele: "pitfalls" in early and late management. Clin Neurosurg 30:366–284
5. Fain B, Vellet D, Hertzanu Y (1985) Adult tethered cord syndrome. A case report. S Afr Med J 67:985–986
6. Freeman LW (1961) Late symptoms from diastematomyelia. J Neurosurg 18:538–541
7. Heinz ER, Rosenbaum AE, Scarff TB, Reigel DH, Drayer BP (1979) Tethered spinal cord following myelomeningocele repair. Radiology 131:153–160
8. HogenEsch R, Zeilstra DJ, Breukers SME, Wiertsema GPA, Begeer JH, Ter Weeme CA (1990) Tethered cord syndrome following spina bifida aperta. Adv Neurosurg 18:158–162
9. Humphreys RP (1991) Current trends in spinal dysraphism. Paraplegia 29:79–83
10. Kaplan EL, Meier P (1958) Nonparametric estimation from incomplete observations. J Am Stat Assoc 53:457–481

11. Klekamp J, Samii M (in press) Introduction of a score system for the clinical evaluation of patients with spinal processes. Acta Neurochir Suppl (Wien)
12. Kondo A, Kato K, Kanai S, Skakibara T (1986) Bladder dysfunction secondary to tethered cord syndrome in adults: is it curable? J Urol 135:313–316
13. Lagae L, Verpoorten C, Casaer P, Vereecken R, Fabry G, Plets C (1990) Conservative versus neurosurgical treatment of tethered cord patients. Z Kinderchir 45 [Suppl 1]:16–17
14. Lesoin F, Petit H, Destee A, Rousseaux M, Julliot JP, Jomin M (1984) Spinal dysraphia and elongated spinal cord in adults. Surg Neurol 21:119–124
15. Oi S, Yamada H, Matsumoto S (1990) Tethered cord syndrome versus low-placed conus medullaris in an over-distended spinal cord following initial repair for myelodysplasia. Childs Nerv Syst 6:264–269
16. Pang D, Wilberger JE Jr (1982) Tethered cord syndrome in adults. J Neurosurg 57:32–47
17. Peter JC (1992) Occult dysraphism of the spine. A retrospective analysis of 88 operative cases, 1979–1989. S Afr Med J 81:351–354
18. Pierre-Kahn A, Lacombe J, Pichon J, Giudicelli Y, Renier D, Sainte-Rose C, Perrigot M, Hirsch JF (1986) Intraspinal lipomas with spina bifida. Prognosis and treatment in 73 cases. J Neurosurg 65:756–761
19. Raimonde AJ (1987) Pediatric neurosurgery. Springer, Berlin Heidelberg New York
20. Reuter I (1987) Das Tethered Cord Syndrom. Möglichkeiten der Diagnose durch klinische Untersuchung und Kernspintomographie. Medical dissertation University of Frankfurt
21. Salvati M, Orlando Ramundo E, Artico M, Martini S, Caruso R, Fortuns A (1990) The tethered cord syndrome in the adult. Report of three cases and review of the literature. Zentralbl Neurochir 51:91–93
22. Schmidt DM, Robinson B, Jones D (1990) The tethered spinal cord. Etiology and clinical manifestations. Orthop Rev 19:870–876
23. Shikata J, Yamamuro T, Mikawa Y, Kotoura Y (1988) Intraspinal epidermoid and dermoid cysts. Surgical results of seven cases. Arch Orthop Trauma Surg 107:105–109
24. Sostrin RD, Thompson JR, Rouhe SA, Hasso AN (1977) Occult spinal dysraphism in the geriatric patient. Radiology 125:165–169
25. Stolke D, Zumkeller M, Seifert V (1988) Intraspinal lipomas in infancy and childhood causing a tethered cord syndrome. Neurosurg Rev 11:59–65
26. Tamaki N, Shirataki K, Kojima N, Shouse Y, Matsumoto S (1988) Tethered cord syndrome of delayed onset following repair of myelomeingocele. J Neurosurg 69:393–398
27. Tani S, Yamada S, Knighton RS (1987) Extensibility of the lumbar and sacral cord. Pathophysiology of the tethered spinal cord in cats. J Neurosurg 66:116–123
28. Vogel S, Neumaerker K, Klepel K (1990) The optimal time for operative treatment of the tethered cord syndrome. Adv Neurosurg 18:155–157
29. Yamada S, Knierim O, Yonekawa M, Schultz R, Maeda G (1983) Tethered cord syndrome. J Am Paraplegia Soc 6:58–61
30. Zumkeller M, Stolke D, Dietz H (1990) Intraspinal lipomas with tethered cord syndrome – results of operative treatment in 30 children. Adv Neurosurg 18:164–169

Respiratory Insufficiency Due to Perinatal Lesion of the Spinal Cord: An Inevitable Course of Events?

J. Uekötter[1], K. von Wild[2], Z. Hoovey[1], and D. Palm[3]

Introduction

Delivery techniques such as extraction and complex turnover maneuvers from the breech position are the primary cause of severe intrapartal spinal lesions [1, 3, 6, 7]. Children suffering from cervical spinal cord injury usually reveal the symptoms of spinal shock. They often present with asphyxia, mistakenly interpreted as a newborn's respiratory distress syndrome. Depending on the kind of lesion and its location paralysis, particularly of the limbs, the trunk, or respiratory muscle system, dominate the clinical appearance. Over 5 years three patients have been seen with cervical spinal cord injuries caused by severe birth trauma. Since the course of events of all three cases was similar, one of the cases is outlined here in detail.

Case Report

Following a normal pregnancy without complications, the patient had been delivered on time from a complete breech position by the delivery technique according to Veit and Smellie. The Apgar score was used for the assessment. This is based on a 0–10 scale (from poorest to best): after 1 min, 6 points; after 5 min, 7 points; after 10 min, 8 points (thus a newborn with Apgar score of 2 has asphyxia). Immediately after delivery a suspicious whimpering and a state of general muscle hypotonia were recognized. He was noted to be pale. He cried immediately but very weakly. Hemoglobin 1 h after birth was 12.6%. His general vigor seemed to be poor and activity less than average.

Cranial computed tomography showed intracerebral hemorrhage located temporo-occipitally, right-sided supratentorially, and in the posterior fossa (Fig. 1). The discovery of the bleeding led to immediate consultation with a pediatrician. On the 2nd day clonic seizures and repeated apnea were noted. General muscle tone was very poor. The boy had shallow breathing with reduced respiratory excursions. Electroencephalography revealed abnormalities with irregularity and increase in beta-wave activity. Electromyography and neurography showed no

[1] Department of Pediatrics, Clemenshospital, Duesbergweg 124, 48153 Münster, Germany.
[2] Department of Neurosurgery, Clemenshospital, Duesbergweg 124, 48153 Münster, Germany.
[3] Department of Neuropediatrics, University of Münster, Albert-Schweizer-Str. 33, Münster, Germany.

Advances in Neurosurgery, Vol. 22
B. L. Bauer, M. Brock, M. Klinger (Eds.)

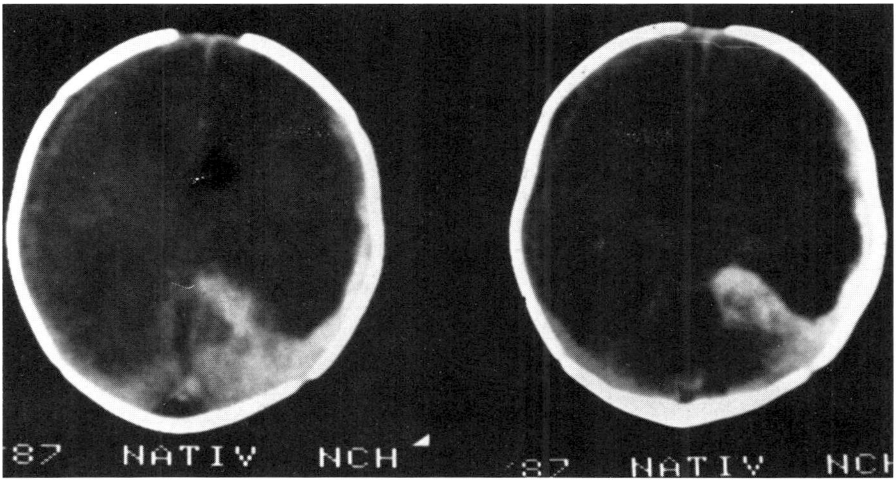

Fig. 1. Computed tomography head scan obtained in 1st day of life showing intracerebral hemorrhage in the right temporo-occipital region

specific signs of neuromuscular disorders. Due to severe chronic respiratory insufficiency and general flaccidity of the muscle the boy was admitted at the age of 13 months to our hospital for further diagnosis and treatment.

Clinical Findings on Admission

The 13-month-old boy was in very poor general condition. His height was 71 cm (28 inches) and weight 2870 g (16.5 lbs), which was far below the 3rd percentile for his group. Hypotonia was present in all extremities. He lay with arms flexed and wrist extended, legs limply assuming a frog position. There was atrophy of the hands and flexor muscle of the forearms. Biceps and triceps reflexes were diminished. Head control was very poor. The chest was underdeveloped and showed no intercostal activity but only diaphragmatic breathing motion. He whimpered and had expiratory and inspiratory grunt. In the legs, although they were limp, the deep tendon reflexes were increased. Anal sphincter tone was poor and urine dribbled. Cranial computed tomography now showed a partially hypodense mass involving the right temporo-occipital region of the brain (Fig. 2).

Clinical Development

The severe endocrine disorder repeatedly led to recurrent pneumonias and the formation of segmental atelectasis (Fig. 3); congenital malformations of the respiratory tract had been excluded by bronchoscopic and bronchographic examination.

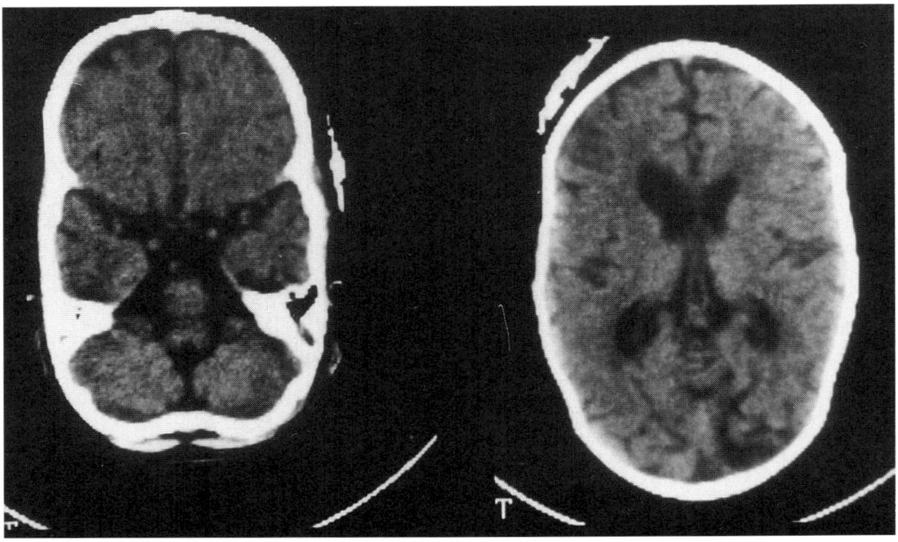

Fig. 2. Cranial computed tomography scan at the age of 13 month revealing hypodense mass involving right temporo-occipital region

The conclusion of the clinical investigation, viewed in combination with the electromyographic and electroneurographic findings, suggested a cervical spinal cord laceration in terms of a cross-section syndrome. After clinical stabilization magnetic resonance imaging was performed of the neck and the thoracic region. This revealed a cystic mass lesion within the spinal cord extending from C6 to T3, while the lower end of the cystic formation suggested an intramedullary origin and the cranial upper border an extramedullary mass of liquid-filled cystic tissue. Except for some coat-shaped, fringe-like band of fibers close to the edge of the

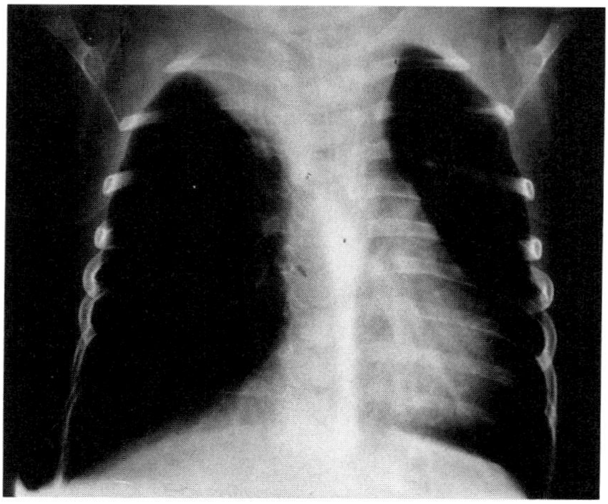

Fig. 3. X-ray study of the chest revealing segmental atelectasis of the right upper lobe; the right lung seemed to be emphysematous

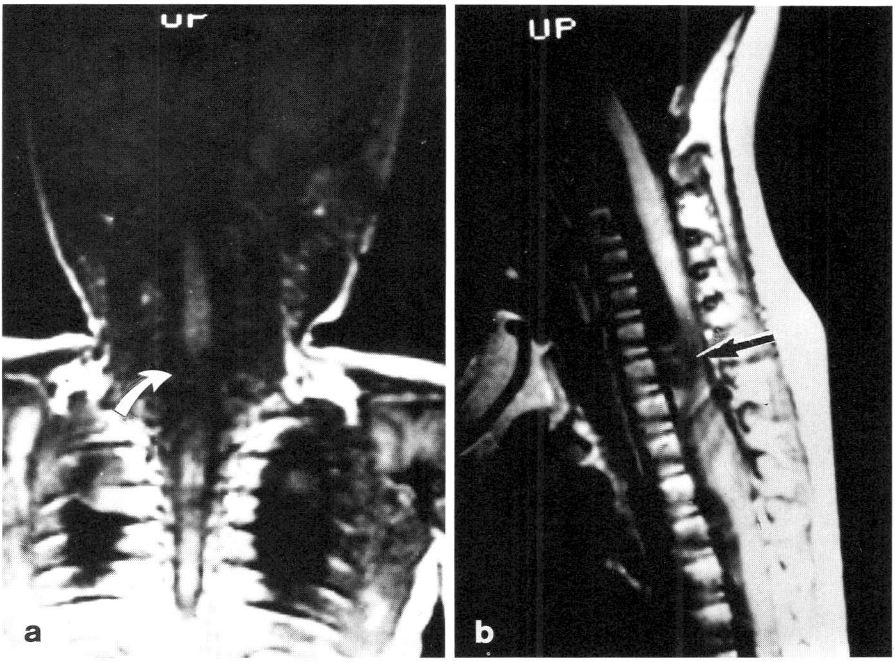

Fig. 4 a, b. Magnetic resonance imaging at the age of 13 months demonstrating severe spinal cord injury at the C6-T3 level. **a** Coronal T1-weighted image *(arrow)*. **b** Sagittal image *(curved arrow)*

medulla it was almost impossible to trace the spinal cord at all. The caudal lower cervical spinal cord and the scans revealed a complete ending of the neural fibers because of a vast depot of granulation tissue (Fig. 4).

We diagnosed a lower cervical spinal cord injury and intramedullary hemorrhage with reactive intraspinal cyst formation due to severe birth trauma. Because of the recurring life-threatening respiration troubles and the persistency of severe general muscular hypotonia it was decided to attempt a decompression of the cervical spinal cord and to reestablish the cervicothoracic passage of the CSF by a microsurgical approach. Preceding the operation intense interdisciplinary consultation was carried out and parental approval was gained. A plastic laminectomy was performed from C5 to T1, followed by the opening of the dura, displaying cystic, altered granulation tissue. At the level of C5 a posttraumatic cyst of the cervical spinal cord with a funnel-shaped expansion toward C6–7 and complete interruption of the medullary fibers on the level of T1 was exposed.

The cyst was removed by microsurgical technique as radical as the circumferential structures would allow, merging into a broad passage for CSF to recirculate between the cranial subarrachnoidal space and lower thoracic region. After stripping the adhering fixations of the granulation tissue, the scar tissue reaching from C5 to C8 was removed. The postoperative course was uneventful. After 12 weeks of inpatient treatment the boy was dismissed in a greatly improved overall condition, importantly, without symptoms of respiratory distress. The impression was emphasized by a further physical examination carried out after a further 15 months.

At the age of 28 months the boy was able to eat. He could turn from the front onto his back and sit up. Fundamentally improved spontaneous motoric and upper limb activity was observed. The respiratory state, pulmonary complications, and endocrine disorder were no longer present. Infections of the respiratory tract showed an uncomplicated, normal healing process. Although general muscular tension still appeared diminished, there was substantial improvement compared to the preoperative state.

The boy is now 6 years old and depends on a wheelchair because of the irreversible paralysis of his legs. There is also incontinence due to the vesical paralysis. He has now entered elementary school and is showing normal intellectual development.

Discussion

This case study presents a boy suffering from a delivery-induced intracranial bleeding and laceration of the cervical spinal cord leading to a transversal section syndrome. The life-threatening pneumonias and endocrine disorder were provoked by insufficient neural supply to the thoracic and respiratory muscles. Koch and Eng [5] have examined 14 children suffering from delivery-induced spinal cord injuries. Eight children died within the first year, and six survived for 2 years with various neurological deficits. Chronically reccurring pneumonias and general muscular hypotonia of tetraspasticity have been seen with rather light and discrete trauma to the spinal cord. After operative decompression a normal function of the upper body, especially the respiratory muscles and the upper limbs, has been observed.

Deliveries from breech positions associated with intracranial hemorrhage of the posterior fossa should suggest the possibility of a cervical spinal cord lesion, especially in case of an initial shock or respiratory distress syndrome. The presumption of a primary asphyxia causing a reactive secondary hypoxic brain defect can delay the correct diagnosis of the spinal cord injury. With the aid of ultrasound [2] and magnetic resonance imaging it is possible to reach the diagnosis of medullary injury in newborns [4, 5]. In the case of delivery-induced cervical cord lesion it is recommended to consider neurosurgical decompression and microneurolysis if the child reveals neurological deficits and respiratory distress 4–6 weeks after birth. This approach lessens the risk of secondary deficits and trauma of the spinal cord caused by external pressure and encourages CNS plasticity in terms of flexibility by regenerating the residual neurological fibers and allowing them to regain their initial function. Finally this concept could spare the child respiratory insufficiency and chronic pneumonias and improves the possibility of early rehabilitation efforts.

References

1. Bucher HU, Bolthauser E, Friedrich J, Isler W (1979) Birth injury to the spinal cord. Helv Paediatr Acta 34:517
2. Bundscherer F, Freudl K, Lindner R, Richter K (1993) Sonographische Diagnostik einer geburtstraumatischen Halsmarkläsion. Monatsschr Kinderheilkd 141:581
3. Crothers B, Putnam MC (1927) Obstetrical injuries on spinal cord. Medicine (Baltimore) 6:41
4. Hoovey Z, Uekötter J, von Wild K (1990) Zur Diagnostik und Therapie chronisch rezidivierender Ateminsuffizienz infolge geburtstraumatischer Halsmarkzerreissung. In: Lütsching (ed) Aktuelle Neuropädiatrie. Springer, Berlin Heidelberg New York, p 418
5. Koch BM, Eng GM (1979) Neonatal spinal cord injury. Arch Phys Ned Rehabil 60:378
6. Stern WE, RAnd RW (1959) Birth injuries to the spinal cord. A report of 2 cases an review of the literature. Am J Obstet Gynecol 78:498
7. Towbin A (1969) Latent spinal cord on brain stem injury in newborn infants. Dev Med Child Neurolog 11:54

Effect of Four Intravenous Anesthetic Agents on Motor Evoked Potentials Elicited by Magnetic Transcranial Stimulation

J. Nadstawek[1], M. Taniguchi[2], U. Langenbach[2], F. Bremer[1], and J. Schramm[2]

Introduction

Transcranial motor cortex stimulation is now being used increasingly to examine patients with motor pathways affection. Two methods of transcranial stimulation are available [5]. Transcranial magnetic stimulation is newer than electric stimulation. For this reason, there is less information available on the intraoperative use and the influence of anesthetics of magnetic stimulation [1, 3, 4, 6, 9, 10]. The aim of this study was to investigate the influence of four different intravenous anesthetics on magnetically evoked compound muscle action potential (magnetic MEP) in humans. Before intraoperative monitoring with magnetic MEP is attempted, compatibility of this modality with anesthetic agents must be established.

Patients and Methods

Sixty-nine patients (ASA I or II; 19–68 years old, mean 43.1 ± 10.6) undergoing lumbar nucleotomy were included in this study after written consent. Pacemaker carriers and patients with seizure history were excluded. The study was approved by the local ethics committee. All patients were premedicated with 0.5 mg atropine, 25 mg promethazine, and 50 mg pethidine. For induction of anesthesia patients received randomized propofol ($n = 22$), etomidate ($n = 13$), methohexital ($n = 19$) or thiopental by a continuous infustion (IVA-Pump, version 3.0, Imperial Chemic Industries PLC, Cheshire, UK) with increasing infusion rates every 15 s up to a minimal anesthesia level in 15 min [7, 8]. The minimal blood concentration required to reach a surgical depth was defined as 1.5 μg/ml for propofol, 0.3 μg/ml for etomidate, 3.0 μg/ml for methohexital, and 10.0 μg/ml for thiopental. Transcranial magnetic stimulation was delivered by a Magstim 200 magnetic stimulator with a 14-cm diameter coil. The maximum intensity of the evoked magnetic field was 2.0 T; this lasted 2 ms. The coil was centered at Cz, and the current flowed in a counterclockwise fashion through the coil. Stimulation intensity was set at 100% of the maximum output of the stimulator as long it was tolerable by the patient. Magnetic MEPs were recorded from the surface of the musculus abductor pollicis brevis. The recording electrodes were placed 4 cm apart in a belly-tendon fashion,

---

[1] Klinik für Anästhesiologie und spezielle Intensivmedizin, Sigmund-Freud-Str. 25, 53105 Bonn, Germany.
[2] Neurochirurgische Klinik, Sigmund-Freud-Str. 25, 53105 Bonn, Germany.

Advances in Neurosurgery, Vol. 22
B. L. Bauer, M. Brock, M. Klinger (Eds.)

and the ground electrode was placed on the ventral side of the forearm, 10 cm proximal to the wrist point. A Nicolet Pathfinder I (Nicolet Biomedical Instruments, Madison, WI) was used for data aquisition and storage. The amplifier was set as follows: bandpasss filter, 30–3000 Hz; sensitivity, 50–100 μV/div; analysis time, 50 ms. MEP examination was performed preoperatively, after premedication and every 2 min during introduction of anesthesia. Between each, the patient's level of consciousness was assessed. Statistical significance calculations were performed by the Wilcoxon/Mann-Whitney test.

Results

No statistical difference in amplitude or latency of MEP between the preoperative values and the values after premedication was found. Regarding the average duration for induction of anesthesia no statistical differences were found among the four groups (propofol, 14.3 ± 2.5 min; etomidate, 12.8 ± 2.9 min; methohexital, 13.6 ± 2.9 min; thiopental, 15.0 ± 2.9 min). During anesthesia induction, the amplitude decreased continuously in all groups. In 47 of the 69 cases the MEP disappeared completely before the patient fell asleep. Figure 1 presents the incidence of perserved MEP response at this moment in each group. The propofol group showed significantly lower incidence of MEP preservation (14%) than methohexital (53%) and etomidate (57%). Thiopental showed similar suppression but not statistically compared to the other groups. Dose-related changes of MEPs during induction with etomidate and thiopental are shown in Fig. 2. The amplitudes were markedly diminished at the end of the induction period. The etomidate group had

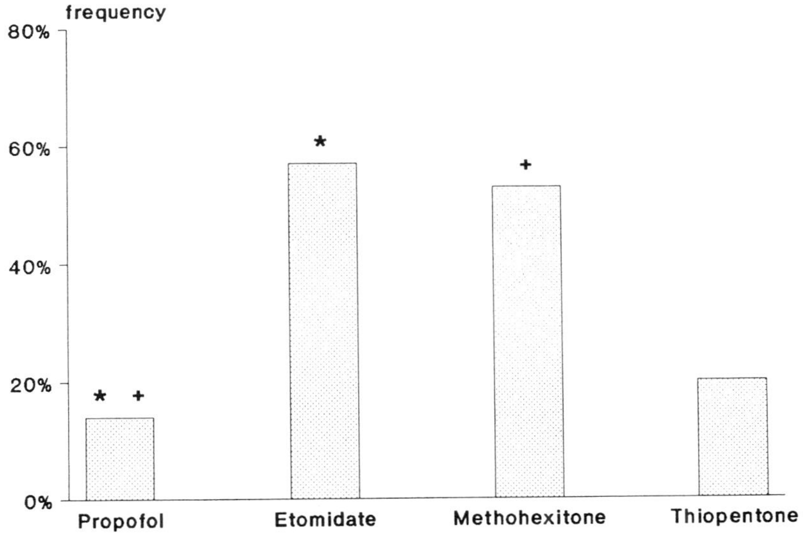

Fig. 1. Preservation of MEP after anesthesia induction with propofol, etomidate, methohexitone, and thiopental, *, +, $p < 0.05$

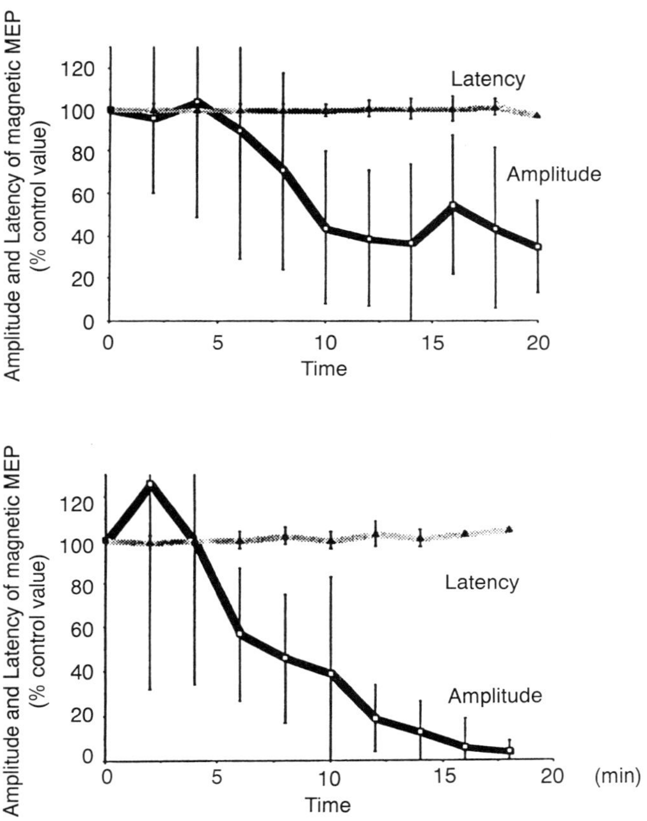

Fig. 2 a, b. Amplitude and latency of MEPs during anesthesia induction. **a** With etomidate. **b** With thiopental

MEPs of the largest amplitude. There were no significant changes in latencies during induction of anesthesia among the groups.

Discussion

Several authors have noted that the magnetic MEP is very susceptible to general anesthesia, making intraoperative monitoring with this technique difficult [2, 6]. MEP tend not to be preserved with volatile anesthetics [6, 10]. Only nitrous oxide has been reported to have little influence on magnetic MEP [6, 9]; anesthesia with nitrous oxide alone, however, is impossible because it does not provide a surgical level of anesthesia. Magnetic MEP has only limited feasibility with the agents described in this study. Dose-dependent suppression of MEP was seen in all drug groups. In 47 of the 69 cases the MEPs were abolished before a surgical level of anesthesia was reached. The etomidate group showed the least suppression of MEP and allowed successful MEP recording after anesthesia induction in 57% of cases. However, because of its negative effects on the cortisol synthesis etomidate is not indicated for total intravenous anesthesia. Propofol and thiopental suppressed MEP and therefore are not suitable for intraoperative magnetic MEP monitoring. After methohexital, which allows MEP monitoring in only 53% of cases, a prolonged recovery period can be expected.

In conclusion, reliable intraoperative monitoring of magnetic MEPs under intravenous anesthesia with a conventional stimulation coil was difficult. The low incidence of successful MEP recording induced with etomidate (57%) and in methohexital (53%) even in the cases without motor pathway involvement indicates insufficient feasibility of the magnetic MEP as a reliable tool for intraoperative monitoring. The use of a more effective stimulation technique, including the use of a more advanced stimulus coil for magnetic stimulation or transcranial electric stimulation, seems necessary for successful monitoring of MEP under general anesthesia.

References

1. Edmonds HL, Paloheimo MPJ, Backman MH, Johnson JR, Holt RT, Shields CB (1989) Transcranial magnetic motor evoked potentials (tcM-MEP) for functional monitoring of motor pathways during scoliosis surgery. Spine 14:683–686
2. Ghaly RF, Stone JL, Levy WJ (1989) Effects of three anesthetic agents on transcranial magnetic motor potentials. J Clin Neurophysiol 4:356–357
3. Jellinek D, Jewkes D, Symon L (1991) Noninvasive intraoperative monitoring of motor evoked potentials under propofol anesthesia: effects of spinal surgery on the amplitude and latency of motor evoked potentials. Neurosurgery 29:551–557
4. Jellinek D, Platt M, Jewkes D, Symon L (1991) Effects of nitrous oxide on motor evoked potentials recorded from skeletal muscle in patients under total intravenous anesthesia with intravenously administered propofol. Neurosurgery 29:558–562
5. Merton PA, Morton HB (1980) Stimulation of the cerebral cortex in the intact human subject. Nature 285:227
6. Schmid UD, Boll J, Liechti S, Schmid J, Hess CW (1992) Influence of some anesthetic agents on muscle responses to transcranial stimulation: a pilot study in humans. Neurosurgery 30:85–92
7. Schüttler J, Schwilden H, Stoeckel H (1983) Pharmacokinetics as applied to total intravenous anaesthesia. Anaesthesia 38 [Suppl]:53–56
8. Schüttler J, Kloos S, Schwilden H, Stoeckel H (1988) Total intravenous anaesthesia with propofol and alfentanil by computer-assisted infusion. Br Anaesth 43:341–345
9. Zentner J, Kiss I, Ebner A (1989) Influence of anesthetics-nitrous oxide in particular on electromyographic response evoked by transcranial electrical stimulation of the cortex. Neurosurgery 24:253–256
10. Zentner J, Albrecht T, Heuser D (1992) Influence of halothane, enflurane and isoflurane on motor evoked potentials. Neurosurgery 31:298–305

Winning Poster Presentations

Episodes of Cerebral Maloxygenation in Comatose Patients

A. von Helden[1], G.-H. Schneider[1], A. Unterberg[1], and W. R. Lanksch[1]

Introduction

Prevention of secondary cerebral ischemia is a main objective in the treatment of comatose patients. In spite of considerable progress made by monitoring of intracranial pressure (ICP), arterial blood pressure, and cerebral perfusion pressure (CPP), episodes of cerebral maloxygenation still occur [3, 8, 11–13]. Measurement of cerebral blood flow would add valuable information, but available methods are not suitable for bedside use and yield only intermittent values. Monitoring of venous oxygen saturation in the jugular bulb allows continuous assessment of cerebral oxygenation [1, 4, 6, 13]. Normal values of jugular venous oxygen saturation ($SJVO_2$) range between 55% and 75%. A $SJVO_2$ of less than 55% is considered critical and one of 50% or below indicates an insufficient cerebral oxygenation. This coincides with an increase in the arteriovenous lactate difference. This study investigated the occurrence and frequency of episodes of desaturation in comatose patients and analyzed possible causes of cerebral maloxygenation. Additionally, pCO_2 and CPP were systematically varied in some patients to study the effects on $SJVO_2$.

Material and Methods

Patient Population. A total of 54 comatose patients were studied. Of these, 28 had suffered a severe head injury (SHI), 14 had an intracerebral hematoma (ICH), and 12 were comatose following subarachnoid hemorrhage (SAH) graded IV or V according to Hunt and Hess [7]. The mean age was between 40 and 62 years (Table 1). The mean Glasgow Coma Score was 5, ranging from 3 to 8. $SJVO_2$, mean arterial blood pressure (MAP), and the resulting CPP were continuously monitored. Additionally, arterial oxygen saturation (SAO_2) and endtidal CO_2 were recorded. All patients were managed by a standardized protocol including early intubation and ventilation, prompt evacuation of space-occupying hematomas and early aneurysm surgery. Intracranial hypertension (> 20 mmHg) was treated aggressively with sedation, relaxation, mannitol, THAM (tris-(hydroxymethyl)-aminomethan), and hyperventilation.

[1] Department of Neurosurgery, Rudolf Virchow Medical Center, Free University of Berlin, Augustenburger Platz 1, 13353 Berlin, Germany.

Advances in Neurosurgery, Vol. 22
B. L. Bauer, M. Brock, M. Klinger (Eds.)

Monitoring of $SJVO_2$. To monitor $SJVO_2$ a fiberoptic catheter (Oximetrics 3, Abbott, Wiesbaden) was inserted percutaneously into the internal jugular vein. The correct position of the catheter tip in the jugular bulb was checked by X-ray. Recalibration of fiberoptic measurements was performed at least every 12 h. Arterial and jugular venous blood samples were taken to determine pO_2, pCO_2, pH, and lactate content.

Desaturation Episodes. Episodes of desaturation were defined as a $SJVO_2$ of 50% or below over a period of at least 15 min [11–13]. Frequency and occurrence were analyzed retrospectively in the different groups of patients, and possible causes of maloxygenation were evaluated.

$SJVO_2$, Hyperventilation, and CPP. The effects of hyperventilation or a lowered CPP on cerebral oxygenation were studied systematically in the different subgroups of patients. PCO_2 was lowered by increasing inspiratory tidal volume and ventilation frequency over a period of 20 min. To investigate the influence of decreased CPP, MAP was lowered by infusion of urapidil over 20 min.

Results and Discussion

Desaturation Episodes. In 28 patients with severe head injury 60 episodes of desaturation were observed over 128 days of monitoring. Over 63 days of monitoring 59 episodes of insufficient cerebral oxygenation were recorded in patients with ICH, and there were 49 of these episodes in patients with SAH (Table 1). An original tracing of a desaturation episode is demonstrated in Fig. 1. Within the first 2 days after the insult 58% of the desaturation episodes occurred. Patients who survived the acute phase had a second peak on the fourth and fifth days. In 86% of the patients with ICH and 74% of those with SAH at least one desaturation episode was observed, while "only" 54% of the SHI patients were afflicted. Other studies reported a similar percentage of desaturation episodes in SHI patients [11, 12]. These findings suggest an even higher risk of cerebral maloxygenation periods in patients comatose due to SAH and ICH. As shown by other groups, the frequency of desaturation episodes is related to neurological outcome [11, 12]. Thus, the main causes of desaturation were analyzed more closely. Possible causes of desatu-

Table 1. Desaturation episodes in comatose patients ($SJVO_2 \leq 50\%$ for more than 15 min)

	ICH ($n = 14$)	SAH ($n = 12$)	SHI ($n = 28$)
Age, mean	62	50	40
Age, range	(36–82)	(27–68)	(4–79)
Frequency of desaturation episodes	59	49	60
Days of monitoring	63	65	128

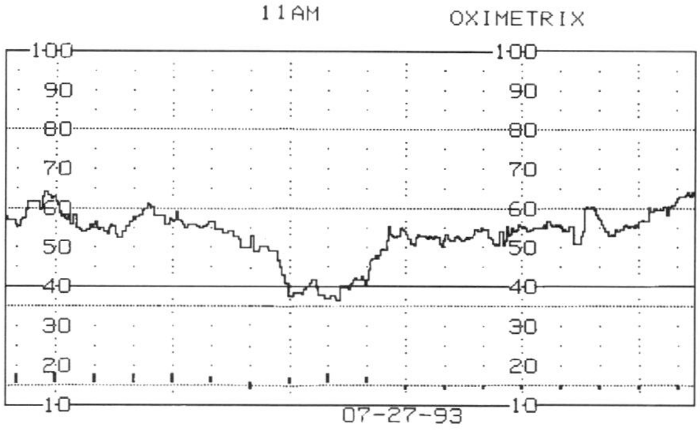

Fig. 1. Desaturation episode ($SJVO_2 < 50\%$ for more than 15 min) in a patient with severe head injury, caused by a fall in blood pressure and respective CPP. This episode of cerebral maloxygenation was treated by raising arterial blood pressure

ration were discovered by retrospective analysis in approximately 65%. The majority of episodes of maloxygenation were associated with hyperventilation (28%) or insufficient CPP (21.5%).

Effects of Hyperventilation and Changes in CPP on $SJVO_2$. Controlled moderate hyperventilation with lowering of the pCO_2 from a mean of 35 to 28 mmHg resulted in a significant decrease in $SJVO_2$ in all patients but two. In five of eight patients with ICH $SJVO_2$ fell below the critical level of 55%, in one case even below 50%. In SHI patients hyperventilation was followed by a decrease in $SJVO_2$ below 55% in 6 of 15 cases; two patients showed signs of cerebral maloxygenation ($SJVO_2 < 50\%$; Fig. 2). Similar results were found in the SAH group. This demonstrates that a hyperventilation maneuver even considered moderate resulted in a critical drop in $SJVO_2$ in 50% of all patients. Again, this finding stresses the critical use of hyperventilation to control intracranial hypertension [9, 10]. According to our results, hyperventilation should be installed with caution only; a pCO_2 below 30 mmHg should only be tolerated with $SJVO_2$ monitoring. Figure 3 demonstrates the effect of a moderate decrease in CPP on $SJVO_2$. MAP was lowered from 103 to 84 mmHg, which decreased CPP from 90 to 72 mmHg [13]. This resulted in a decrease in $SJVO_2$ below 55% in four of eight patients with ICH (Fig. 3). In comparison, six patients of the SHI group showed a reduction in $SJVO_2$ after lowering of MAP, but in no case was a critical level reached. The importance of sufficient CPP is well known, while a safe threshold is still uncertain [2, 8, 12].

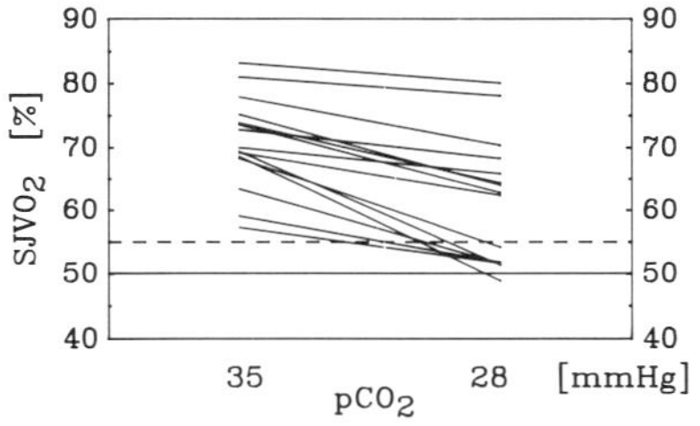

Fig. 2. $SJVO_2$ reaction to moderate hyperventilation in 15 patients with severe head injury. All but two patients showed a decrease in saturation. In six patients a critical $SJVO_2$ (< 55%) was observed; in one patient saturation fell below 50%, indicating insufficient cerebral oxygenation

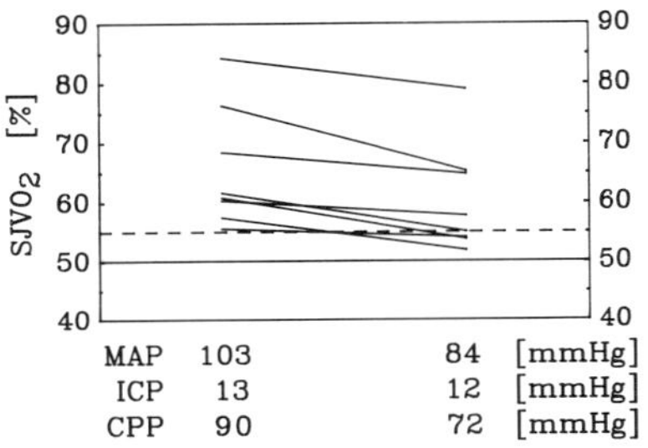

Fig. 3. $SJVO_2$ reaction to moderate reduction of CPP in eight patients with ICH. Lowering of MAP was followed by a $SJVO_2 < 55\%$ in four cases

Our findings indicate an impaired cerebral autoregulation in 57% of all comatose patients and a considerably greater susceptibility of patients with ICH than with SHI. These patients obviously need a higher CPP than the recommended 60–70 mmHg to ensure adequate cerebral perfusion [2, 13].

Conclusions

Continuous monitoring of $SJVO_2$ enables early detection and tailored treatment of insufficient cerebral oxygenation in comatose patients. To prevent secondary ischemia, hyperventilation therapy should be installed cautiously, and a sufficient CPP must be secured.

Acknowledgments. The excellent technical assistance of Mrs. R. Duisberg and Mrs. J. Kopetzki is highly appreciated.

References

1. Andrews PJD, Dearden NM (1990) Validation of Oximetrics 3 for continuous monitoring of jugular bulb oxygen saturation after severe head injury: comparison with IL 282 in vitro cooximeter. Br J Anaesth 64:393P–394P
2. Chan KH, Miller JD, Dearden NM et al. (1992) The effect of changes in cerebral perfusion pressure upon middle cerebral artery blood flow velocity and jugular bulb venous oxygen saturation after severe brain injury. J Neurosurg 77:55–61
3. Cruz J, Allen SJ, Miner ME (1985) Hypoxic insults in acute brain injury. Crit Care Med 4:284
4. Cruz J (1988) Continuous versus serial global cerebral haemometabolic monitoring: application in acute brain trauma. Acta Neurochir Suppl (Wien) 42:35–39
5. Cruz J, Miner ME, Allen SJ et al. (1990) Continuous monitoring of cerebral oxygenation in acute brain injury: injection of mannitol during hyperventilation. J Neurosurg 73:725–730
6. Dearden NM (1991) Jugular bulb venous oxygen saturation in the management of severe head injury. Curr Opin Anaesth 4:279–286
7. Hunt WE, Hess RM (1968) Surgical risk as related to time of intervention in the repair of intracranial aneurysims. J Neurosurg 28:14–20
8. Miller JD, Sweet RC, Narayan R et al. (1978) Early insults to the injured brain. JAMA 240:439–442

9. Muizelaar JP, Marmarou A, Ward JD et al. (1991) Adverse effects of prolonged hyperventilation in patients with severe head injury: a randomized clinical trial. J Neurosurg 75:731–739
10. Patel PM (1993) Hyperventilation as a therapeutic intervention: do the potential benefits outweigh the known risks? J Neurosurg Anaesthesiol 51(1):62–65
11. Prakash S, Robertson CS, Narayan RK et al. (1992) Transient jugular venous oxygen desaturation and neurological outcome in patients with severe head injury. J Neurosurg 76:398A
12. Sheinberg M, Kanter MJ, Robertson CS et al. (1992) Continuous monitoring of jugular venous oxygen saturation in head-injured patients. J Neurosurg 76:212–217
13. Unterberg A, Von Helden A, Schneider G-H, Lanksch WR (1993) Monitoring of jugular venous oxygen saturation in patients with intracerebral hematomas. In: Lorenz R, Klinger M, Brock M (eds) Advances in neurosurgery, vol 21. Springer, Berlin Heidelberg New York, pp 29–33

Depth Electrodes in the Presurgical Evaluation of Epilepsy

D. Van Roost[1], A. Hufnagel[2], and L. Solymosi[3]

Introduction

The use of depth electrodes in the presurgical evaluation of epilepsy remains a matter of debate in view of subdural recordings, which seem to offer equally valuable information without penetrating the brain. We therefore verified our implantation procedure regarding its invasiveness and benefit.

Clinical Material and Methods

From January 1990 to March 1993 and with increasing frequency we have implanted depth electrodes in addition to subdural strip electrodes in 44 patients with medically intractable complex partial seizures who needed intracranial electroencephalographic (EEG) recording for the localization of the epileptogenic focus. The electrode insertion is implemented through a rigid cannula, which is guided stereotactically through the length axis of the hippocampus, the electrode tip thus reaching the amygdaloid nucleus. Computed tomography is the only imaging procedure that we use for stereotactic coordinate determination. The target is chosen medially to the tip of the temporal ventricle horn. The trajectory parallels the floor of the middle cranial fossa, the skull entry point thus being located around the occipitoparietal bone junction about 3 cm from the midline (Fig. 1). The catheterlike, 1-mm-thick silastic electrode (AD-TECH Medical Instrument, Racine, WI, USA) carries ten cylindric contacts of a nickel-chromium alloy, distributed in line over the distal 4 cm. The pair of bilateral depth electrodes remains for about 14 days, part of this time being covered by prophylactic antibiotics. The electrodes serve for EEG recording and for eliciting typical seizures by electric stimulation.

[1] Neurochirurgische Universitätsklinik, Sigmund-Freud-Str. 25, 53127 Bonn-Venusberg, Germany.
[2] Universitätsklinik für Epileptologie, Sigmund-Freud-Str. 25, 53127 Bonn-Venusberg, Germany.
[3] Neuroradiologie, Radiologische Universitätsklinik, Sigmund-Freud-Str. 25, 53127 Bonn-Venusberg, Germany.

Advances in Neurosurgery, Vol. 22
B. L. Bauer, M. Brock, M. Klinger (Eds.)

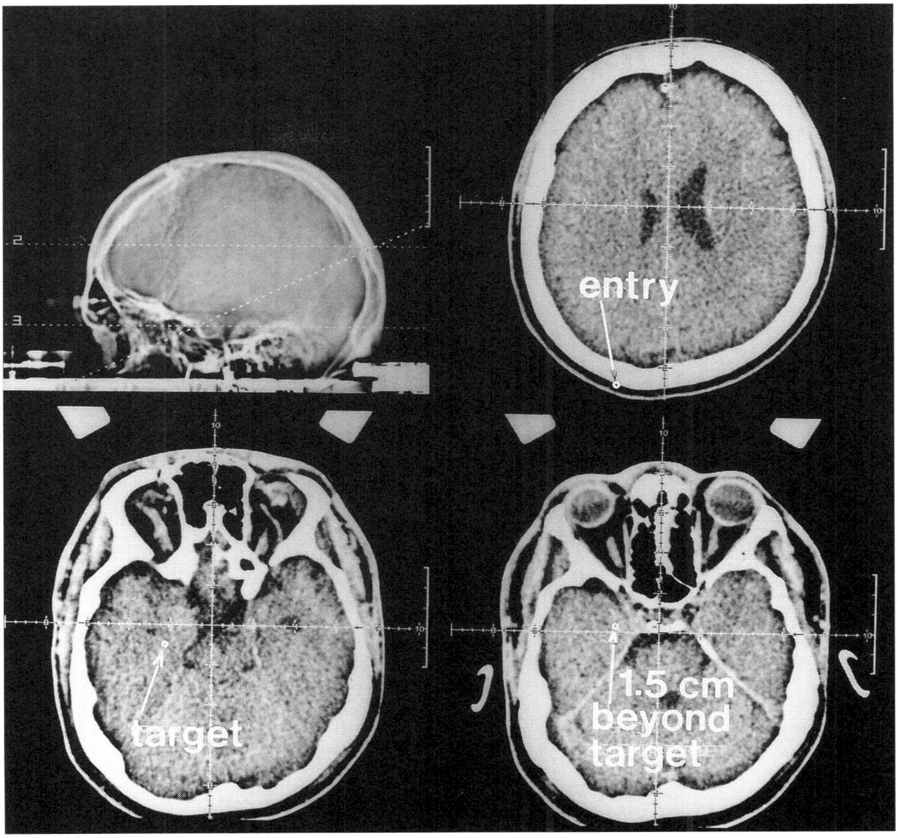

Fig. 1. Planning of the computed tomography based stereotactic insertion of an amygdalohippocampal depth electrode. The scout view shows the trajectory projected on a sagittal plane, running parallel to the floor of the middle cranial fossa, intersected by horizontal lines at the levels of target and skull entry. The target is chosen medially to the tip of the temporal ventricle horn. The electrode tip reaches the amygdaloid nucleus 1.5 cm beyond the target

Results

In about two thirds of the patients who were assessed by magnetic resonance imaging (MRI) perfect depth electrode positions were found (Fig. 2). In the other patients, who invariably had their implantation according to an earlier trajectory planning procedure, the electrodes were found to lie slightly superior to the hippocampus. The positions of the mesiotemporal subdural strip electrodes were also controlled by MRI. The accurate location of both depth electrodes and subdural strip electrodes allowed direct comparison of their diagnostic yield.

Frontal seizures produced no epileptic activity or identical information in both depth and subdural electrodes. In parietal seizures a temporal involvement was

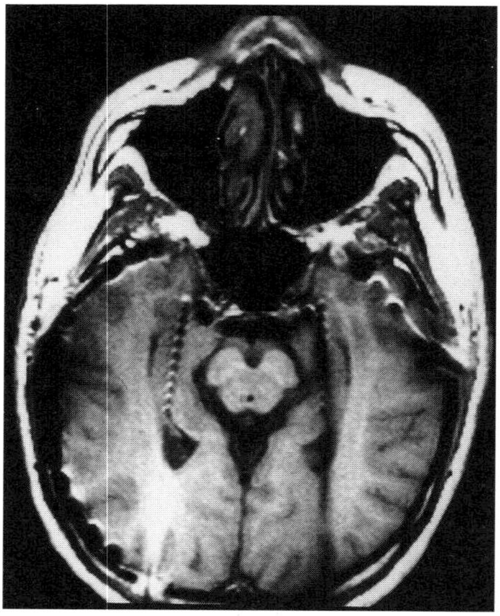

Fig. 2. MRI showing the position of a pair of amygdalohippocampal depth electrodes in an axial (temporal) plane

once observed in the depth electrode only. A laterotemporal seizure onset was unequivocally recognized. Mesiotemporal seizures sometimes showed their onset up to 15 s earlier in the depth electrodes, and some subclinical seizures and auras were recognized in the depth recording only. Finally, an important number of secondary (contralateral) foci were seen only or predominantly in the depth electrodes. Summarizing, the information obtained from subdural recordings and depth electrodes was identical in about two-fifths of the patients, whereas in approximately three-fifths of the patients the depth electrodes brought about additional information.

Regarding complications, we observed one asymptomatic ventricular bleeding and treated one patient with subdural and depth electrodes for an aseptic meningitis. Consequences for the traversed healthy brain tissue may be drawn from resected hippocampus specimens, which at histopathological examination [13] generally showed minute, sharply circumscribed defects and reactive astrogliosis with an overall diameter of 1 mm along the electrode path. One instance of nonbacterial chronic inflammation was observed.

Discussion

As scalp EEG is inaccurate for the localization of seizure foci in about one-third of patients [8], intracranial EEG recording is necessary if resective surgery is being considered. Basically three different approaches to depth electrode placement for chronic recording in the mesial temporal structures are in use. The first, introduced by Bancaud et al. [1], approaches the mesial temporal structures laterally and needs a multitude of parallel probes that puncture the temporal lobe(s) to survey the anteroposterior extension of the hippocampus [1, 6, 10]. The second approach is from a frontocoronal burr hole, which, similar to the former approach, needs several (divergent) probes per side [4] or is combined with subdural electrodes [12]. The approach that we have adopted was proposed by Spencer [7] and traverses the mesial temporal structures lengthwise, so that these can be covered by one multicontact electrode per side. The development of flexible electrodes has rendered this procedure even less invasive. However, for the survey of all brain areas from which complex partial seizures can originate additional depth or subdural electrodes are needed here as well.

Stereotactic angiography [6, 7] or direct cortex inspection, for example, through somewhat larger burr holes [5], have been used to minimize the risk of vascular injury and hemorrhage. MRI is increasingly being used for the determination of the stereotactic coordinates [5, 6].

The overall complication rate of depth electrode implantation, as compiled from 14 smaller series totaling 879 patients, is 4.3%, comprising mainly hemorrhages (with permanent deficit in seven cases) and infections, but no deaths [11]. Other series report a mortality up to 1.5% [2, 3]. The implantation of depth electrodes was not reported to cause any increase of seizure frequency [12].

As to the diagnostic yield of depth electrodes, our results are consistent with those of others, who report that depth electrodes are more sensitive than subdural recordings in detecting auras and subclinical seizures [10], and that depth electrodes show seizures of hippocampal origin earlier than subdural electrodes [9, 10].

Conclusion

Our computed tomography guided stereotactic implantation of amygdalohippocampal depth electrodes can be regarded as a safe procedure which yields EEG information that is never contrary to that drawn from subdural recordings but is often complementary and corroboratory. In some instances, however, the information from the depth electrodes can be complementary and weakening as well. An estimation of the percentage of patients in whom the depth electrodes played the decisive role in view of the surgical treatment cannot as yet be given. More experience is needed in the interpretation of hippocampal depth EEG recordings, which sometimes show unusual features with indistinct value.

References

1. Bancaud J, Talairach J, Bonis A, Schaub C, Szikla G, Morel P, Bordas-Ferer M (1965) La stéréo-électroencéphalographie dans l'épilepsie. Informations neuro-physiologiques apportées par l'investigation fonctionelle stéréotaxique. Masson, Paris
2. Cahan L, Sutherling W, McCullough M, Rausch R, Engel J (1984) Review of the 20-year UCLA experience with surgery for epilepsy. Clev Clin Q 51:313–318

3. Engel J, Crandall P, Rausch R (1983) The partial epilepsies. In: Rosenberg RN et al. (eds) The clinical neurosciences, vol 2. Churchill Livingstone, New York, pp 1349–1380
4. Flanigin HF, Smith JR (1987) Depth electrode implantation at the Medical College of Georgia. In: Engel J Jr (ed) Surgical treatment of the epilepsies. Raven, New York
5. McCarthy G, Spencer DD, Riker RJ (1991) The stereotactic placement of depth electrodes in epilepsy. In: Lüders H (ed) Epilepsy surgery. Raven, New York, pp 385–393
6. Olivier A, Marchand E, Peters T, Tyler J (1987) Depth electrode implantation at the Montreal Neurological Institute and Hospital. In: Engel J Jr (ed) Surgical treatment of the epilepsies. Raven, New York, pp 595–601
7. Spencer DD (1987) Depth electrode implantation at Yale University. In: Engel J Jr (ed) Surgical treatment of the epilepsies. Raven, New York, pp 603–607
8. Spencer SS, Spencer DD, Williamson PD, Mattson RH (1982) The localizing value of depth electroencephalography in 32 patients with refractory epilepsy. Ann Neurol 12:248–253
9. Spencer SS, Spencer DD, Williamson PD, Mattson RH (1990) Combined depth and subdural electrode investigation in uncontrolled epilepsy. Neurology 39:74–79
10. Sperling MR, O'Connor MJ (1989) Comparison of depth and subdural electrodes in recording temporal lobe seizures. Neurology 39:1497–1504
11. Van Buren J (1987) Complications of surgical procedures in the diagnosis and treatment of epilepsy. In: Engel J Jr (ed) Surgical treatment of the epilepsies. Raven, New York, pp 465–475
12. Van Veelen CWM, Debets RMC, Van Huffelen AC, Van Emde Boas W, Binnie CD, Storm Van Leeuwen W, Velis DN, Van Dieren A (1990) Combined use of subdural and intracerebral electrodes in preoperative evaluation of epilepsy. Neurosurgery 26:93–101
13. Wolf HK, Campos MG, Zentner J, Hufnagel A, Schramm J, Elger CE, Wiestler OD Surgical pathology of temporal lobe epilepsy. Surg Pathol (in press)

Microsurgical Anatomy of the Cisterna Quadrigemina and Cisterna Velum Interpositum

S. Hussein[1], D. Woischneck[1], and U. Niemeyer[1]

Introduction

The cisterna quadrigemina is the only cistern with both supra- and infratentorial components. It is used as a route for several neurosurgical operations, especially for surgery in the pineal region [1, 5, 10], splenium [11], and trigonum collaterale [4]. The cisterna velum interpositum as a sail placed in the roof of the third ventricle must be passed to reach the middle and dorsal parts of the midline. This cistern is the ventral border in extirpating trigonal lesions [3, 4]. On the basis of anatomical studies we analyzed the variations of these two cisterns in regard to the surgical procedures mentioned above.

Material and Methods

In 50 brains shortly after removal the vascular system was rinsed with Ringer's solution. In 35 preparations the posterior cerebral artery (PCA) was selectively injected with Epoxide resin. In the other 15 brains the vena cerebri magna was injected with a gelatine ink mixture. We examined the brains under the operation microscope and statistically analyzed the findings.

Results

The cisterna quadrigemina forms the dorsal part of the cisterna ambiens and has an infra- and supratentorial extension. The ventral border is provided by the lamina tecti. Medially one finds the glandula pinealis and rostral pulvinar thalami (Fig. 1). The lateral border is traditionally formed by the pulvinar thalami and crus fornicis. In our material, additionally the caudal parts of the gyrus lingualis were always part of this border (Fig. 2). The cisternal roof consists of the splenium corporis callosi. Here, the arachnoidal separation between the cisterna quadrigemina and the cisterna pericallosa is visible (Fig. 2).

The vascular content of the quadrigeminal cistern is complex. In the middle parts the vena cerebri magna (Galeni) is suspended in a thickened trabecular sys-

---

[1] Neurochirurgische Klinik, Medizinische Hochschule Hannover,
Konstanty-Gutschow-Str. 13, 30623 Hannover, Germany.

Advances in Neurosurgery, Vol. 22
B. L. Bauer, M. Brock, M. Klinger (Eds.)

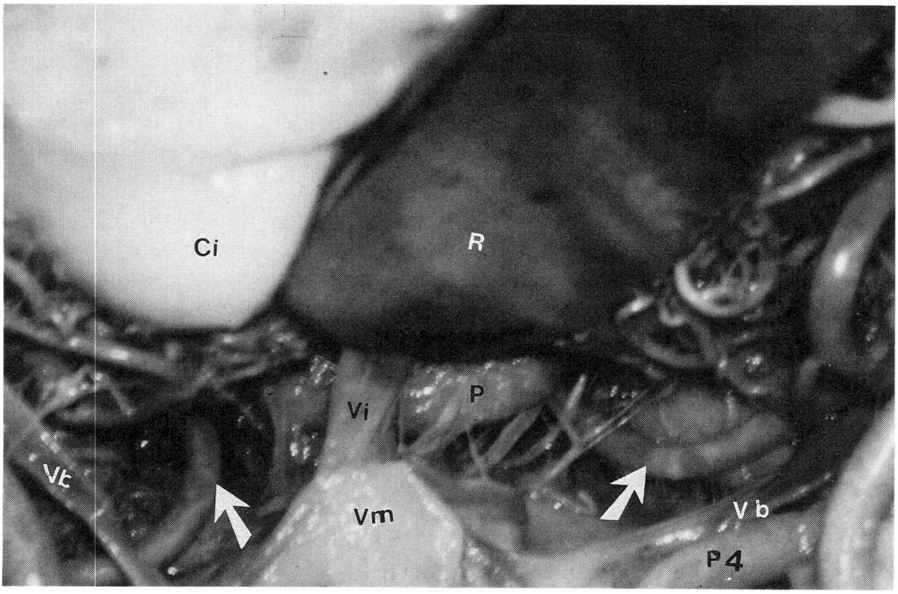

Fig. 1. Dorsal view into the cisterna quadrigeminae (the lamina tecti is oriented upwards by retractor, *R*). *CI*, Colliculus inferior; *P4*, segment of PCA; *P*, pinealis; *VI*, vena cerebri interna; *Vm*, vena cerebri magna; *Vb*, vena basalis (Rosenthali); *arrows*, arteria choroidea posteromedialis

tem. In 17 cases we found the confluence of the internal cerebral veins to vena cerebri magna to be in the cistern. The length of the vena cerebri magna varies due to its variable point of origin; in one case it was only 3 mm.

The P3/P4 segment of PCA in 34 brains on both sides was situated in the lateral portion of the quadrigeminal cistern. In the cisternal floor we found the branches of the ramus superior of the arteria cerebelli superior and vena supraculminalis; here, the cistern continues into the cistern of the vermis cerebelli superior.

The middle parts of the quadrigeminal cistern are filled with the arteriae choroideae posteromediales. These arteries pass the pineal gland and run into the third ventricle. In 58 hemispheres they passed rostrally and in 12 caudally to vena basalis (Rosenthali) (Figs. 1, 2). In one hemisphere we found a doubling of the arteria choroidea posteromedialis. The peripheral branches of this vessel always reached at least the interventricular foramen. The vascular supply of several adjacent structures by this artery was extremely variable: the lamina tecti (in 38%), comissura posterior (30%), habenulae (10%), fornix (45%), and thalamus (70%). The upper floor contained branches of the arteriae laminae quadrigeminae (Fig. 1). In all cases we found the dorasal arachnoidea extremely thick and opaque and made up in different layers.

Rostrally, above the pulvinar thalami, the cisterna quadrigemina continues into the sail-like cisterna velum interpositum (Figs. 2, 3). This cistern, as the roof of the

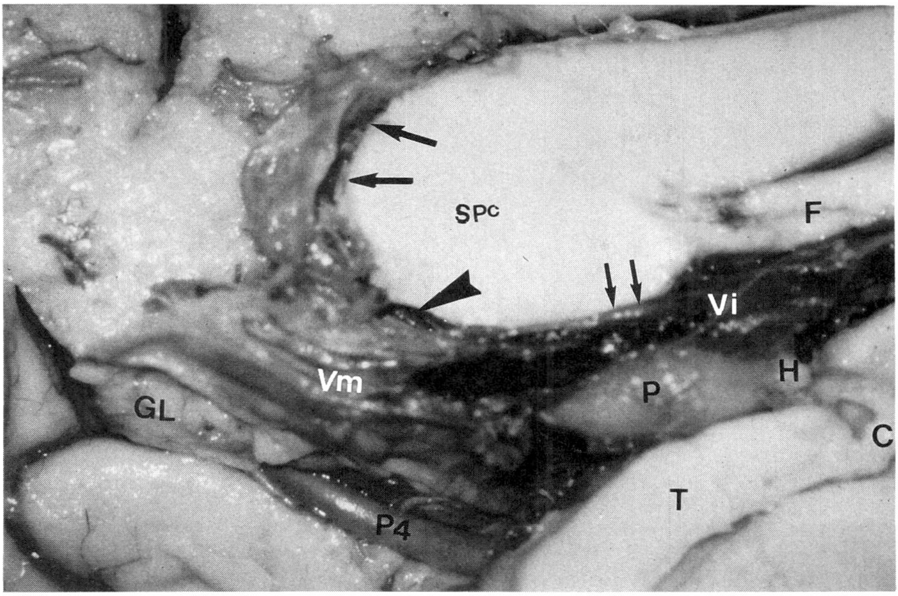

Fig. 2. Lateral view into cisterna quadrigemina (median slice). *V*, Vena cerebri magna; *Vi*, vena cerebri interna; *C*, commissura posterior; *T*, lamina tecti; *F*, corpus fornicis; *P*, pinealis; *P4*, calcarina in cisterna quadrigemina; *GL*, gyrus lingualis; *small arrows*, arteria choroidea posteromedialis; *arrow*, arterial pericallosa posterior

third ventricle, contains the arteriae choroidea posteromediales, which supply the thalamus and plexus choroideus. Especially in this part of the cistern these arteries show many variations (Fig. 3). Additionally, the cisterna velum interpositum contains the vena cerebri interna with its branches from the lateral ventricles (atrial veins), coming through the fissura choroidea. Between the two sheets of the cistern one finds the plexus of the first and second ventricles. The lateral cisternal border is formed by the taenia choroidea between the thalamus and fornix. Here both arachnoidal sheets stick together closely.

Discussion

To summarize our results concerning the cisterna quadrigemina, we divide it into three floors; the upper and middle floor are rostrally adjacent to the cisterna velum interpsoitum, lateral to the fissura choroidea between the crura fornices and pulvinar thalami and tela choroidea. The lower floor lies infratentorially and continues into the cisterna vermis cerebelli.

The upper part contains the venae cerebri internae and vena cerebri magna, which is enfolded into an own arachnoidal cistern [7]. The middle floor contains the venae basales and arteriae choroidea posteromediales. As reported by Fujii [2],

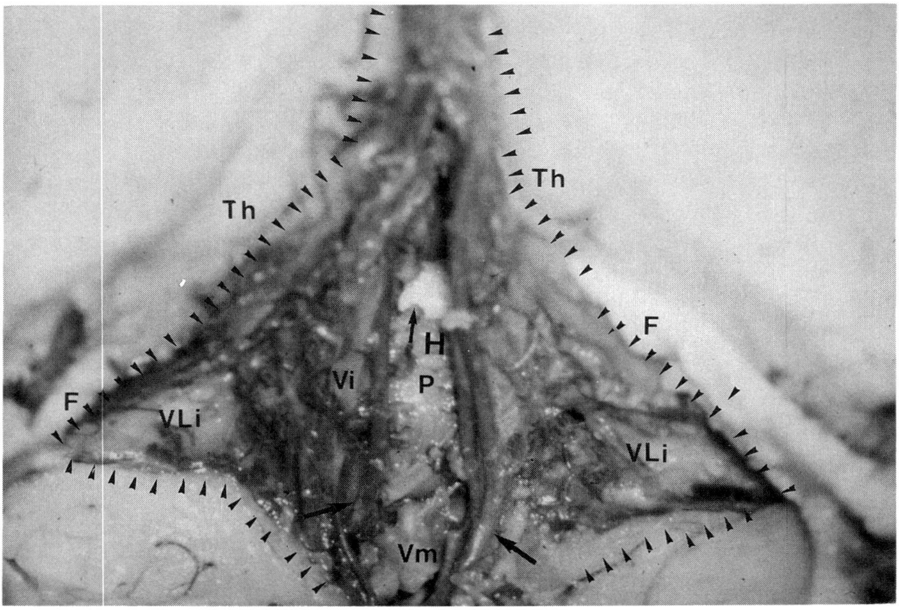

Fig. 3. View on cisterna velum interpositum (*small arrows*). In the arachnoidal cavity we find structures of the tela choroidea in the roof of the third ventricle. *Th*, Thalamus; *P*, pinealis; *H*, commissura habenularum; *VLI*, vessels of the dorsal part of fissura choroidea; *Vi*, vena cerebri interna; *Vm*, vena cerebri magna; *F*, crus fornicis; *large arrows*, arteria choroidea posteromedialis and branches

the vein lies beneath the artery. On this floor the pineal gland forms the ventral border. The lower floor lies intratentorially [8, 9] and contains the vena vermis cerebelli in the midline and additionally the rami superiores of the arteriae cerebelli superiores.

A common operative approach through the cisterna quadrigemina is, according to Krause [10], the supracerebellar-infratentorial route to the pineal region. Approaches along the dorsal interhemispheric route to the lateral mesencephalon or medial parts of the atrium ventriculi also pass the quadrigeminal cistern. After CSF release from the cistern even lesions in the lateral atrium can be reached because of the better retraction of the occipital lobe (transtrigonal operations [3, 4]). Thus by preparation of the quadrigeminal cistern lesions in basal structures can be reached up to 30 mm paramedian, which is not possible by infratentorial approaches.

Alternatively, it is possible to reach lesions of the laterorostral mesencephalon after a subtemporal craniotomy with aperture of the laterosuperior parts of the quadrigeminal cistern (Fig. 4). The cistern forms the dorsal border of such an operation.

The narrow cisterna velum interpositum is the route to the middle and dorsal parts of the third ventricle by a transcallosal operation [1]. This procedure is lim-

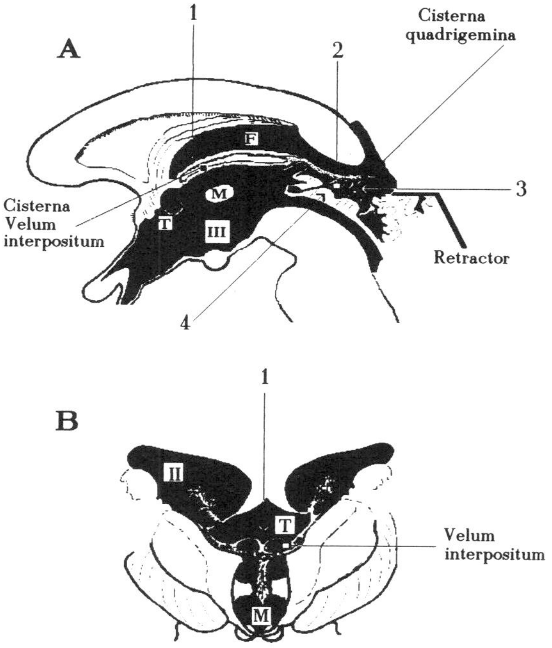

Fig. 4 A, B. Operative approaches to cisterna quadrigemina and cisterna velum interpoditum. *1*, Transcallosal, transventricular approach; *2*, dorsal supratentorial interhemisphery artery; *3* infratentorial supracerebellar artery; *F*, foramen interventriculare; M, massa intermedia; *T*, fissura transversa; *II, III*, second and third ventricle

ited by the thalamus and fornix [6]; it is facilitated hydrocephalus. If there is an intraventricular component, even tumors of the pinealis can be reached in this way [11].

References

1. Dandy WE (1936) Operative experiences in cases of pinealis tumor. Arch Surg 33:19–46
2. Fujii K, Lenkey KL, Rhoton AL (1980) Microsurgical anatomy of the choroideal arteries, of the lateral and third ventricle. J Neurosurg 52:165–188
3. Krause G, Zülch KJ (1951) Pinealistumore. Zentral Neurochir 11:4–5
4. Lavyne MH, Petterson RH (1983) Subarachnoidal trans-velum interpositum approach to mid third ventricular tumors. J Neurosurg 12:86–94
5. Liliequist B (1959) The subarachnoidal cisterns. Anatomical and roentgenologic study. Acta Radiol Suppl 185:1–108
6. Hussein S (1990) Die Trigonale Region. Habilitationsschrift, Medizinische Hochschule Hannover
7. Hussein S, Woischneck D (1990) Topographie des Atrium ventriculi und ihre mikrochirurgische Bedeutung. Neurochirurgia (Stuttg) 33:8–10
8. Matsumo M, Rhoton LA, Peace D (1988) Microsurgical anatomy of the posterior fossa cisterns. Neurosurgery 23:58–80

9. Omo M, Rhoton LA, Burry M (1984) Microsurgical anatomy of the tentoriell incisura. J Neurosurg 60:365–399
10. Pendel G (1986) Pineal and midbrain lesions. Springer, Vienna New York
11. Yasargil MG, Jenin KK, Anlic J (1976) Arteriovenous malformations of the splenium of corpus callosum: microsurgical treatment. Surg Neurol 5:5.14

Diagnostic Value of Somatostatin Receptor Scintigraphy in the Pre- and Postoperative Management of Glioma Patients

C. Luyken[1], G. Hildebrandt[1], B. Krisch[2], K. Scheidhauer[3], and N. Klug[1]

Introduction

Somatostatin receptors (SR) have been identified in vitro in normal brain tissue, neuroendocrine tumors, and cerebral gliomas of WHO grades 1 and 2 by autoradiography and with somatostatin-gold conjugates [1, 2, 4]. In vivo SR detection has become possible by scintigraphy with the somatostatin analogue octreotide radiolabeled with ^{111}In [2, 4, 5]. It was thought that the expression of SR in cerebral gliomas correlates with low malignancy and in vivo somatostatin receptor scintigraphy (SRS) might offer an alternative grading system for cerebral gliomas [3]. The aim of this study was to evaluate whether SRS can improve the preoperative determination of tumor nature or the postoperative management of patients with cerebral gliomas.

Patients and Methods

A total of 86 patients were examined with 94 cerebral lesions (Table 1). Nineteen had cranial gliomas (WHO grade 2, $n = 8$; grade 3, $n = 3$; grade 4, $n = 8$; Table 1), five cerebral metastases (one carcinoma of the breast, one adenocarcinoma of the lung, one bronchial carcinoma, two of unknown origin), and one a brain abscess. After written consent was obtained, the ^{111}In-radiolabeled somatostatin analogue DTPA-octreotide was injected intravenously as 10- or 20-μg bolus, corresponding to 110 or 220 MBq ^{111}In. Gamma-camera images of the head were obtained using digital planar (128 x 128 matrix, four views) and single photon emission computed tomography (SPECT; 64 x 64 matrix) using a large field of view gamma-camera (Philips) and a double-head gamma-camera (Picker) fitted with medium-energy parallel-hole collimators. Peaks were set to 173 and 247 keV with 20% windows. Acquisition parameters for planar images were 5 min per view and 64 projections of 20 s each for the SPECT studies. Images were obtained 4–6 and 24 h postinjection. Scintigrams were assessed independently by two observers without

[1] Department of Neurosurgery, University of Cologne, Joseph-Stelzmann-Str. 9, 50931 Köln, Germany.
[2] Department of Nuclear Medicine, University of Cologne, Joseph-Stelzmann-Str. 9, 50931 Köln, Germany.
[3] Department of Anatomy, University of Kiel, Neue Universität, Olshausenstr. 40, 24098 Kiel, Germany.

Advances in Neurosurgery, Vol. 22
B. L. Bauer, M. Brock, M. Klinger (Eds.)

Table 1. Results of somatostatin receptor analysis in patients with different cerebral lesions

Histology	In vivo: ^{111}In-labeled DTPA-octreotide (*n*/positive signal)	In vitro: gold-ligand technique (*n*/binding sites)
Meningioma grades 1–3	39/39	2/2
Pituitary adenoma	8/18	1/1
Glioma grades 3, 4	11/11	5/6
Glioma grade 2	0/8	5/5
Neurinoma	0/5	
Cerebral metastases	5/5	3/4
Tumors of the orbit	2/4	
Neurofibroma	2/2	
Brain abscess	1/1	0/1
Cystic brain lesion	0/1	
Total	68/94	16/19

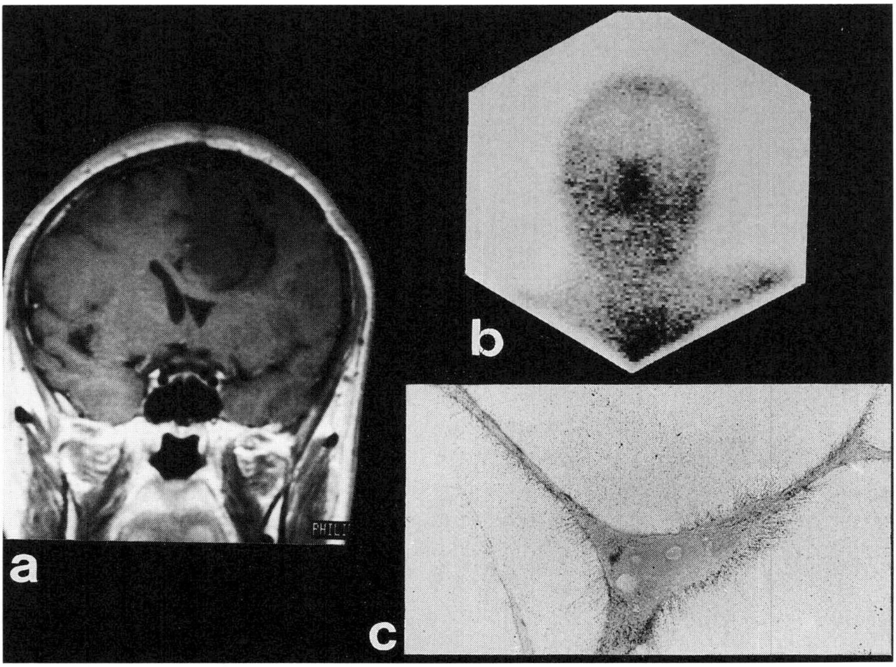

Fig. 1 a–c. Oligodendroglioma grade 2, located in left frontal lobe. **a** Coronal Gd-enhanced MRI showing the mass effect of the hypointense lesion. **b** Anterior planar view of the head, performed with a gamma-camera 24 h after intravenous injection of 110 MBq ^{111}In-labeled octreotide showing no focal increased uptake of the radiopharmaceutical within the tumor area. **c** Electron microscopy of a cultured glia cell from intraoperatively removed tumor tissue after incubation with 1 n*M* somatostatin-inhibitory factor–gold conjugate outlines fine, black silver deposits on the cell surface, indicating bound somatostatin-gold knowledge of the results of other imaging modalities – computed tomography or magnetic resonance imaging (MRI). Three of the patients with gliomas grade 4 were additionally examined with ^{99m}Tc-DTPA scintigraphy.

Tumor specimens were classified according to the WHO grading system. Part of our findings were compared to results from the same tumor kept in culture and submitted to in vitro assays for study of somatostatin binding sites by means of somatostatin-gold as ligand. Immunohistochemistry was performed using an antibody against glial filament acid protein (GFAP) to confirm the glial nature of the cultivated cells [2].

Results

None of the patients with glioma grade 2 and intact blood-brain barrier (no Gd enhancement in MRI; Fig. 1 a) showed local enhanced tracer uptake in SRS (Fig. 1 b), whereas in vitro somatostatin binding sites were observed (Fig. 1 c) (Table 1). Every patient with glioma grade 3 or 4 and disturbed blood-brain barrier (Gd enhancement in MRI; Fig. 2 a) demonstrated a positive signal in SRS (Fig. 2 b). The

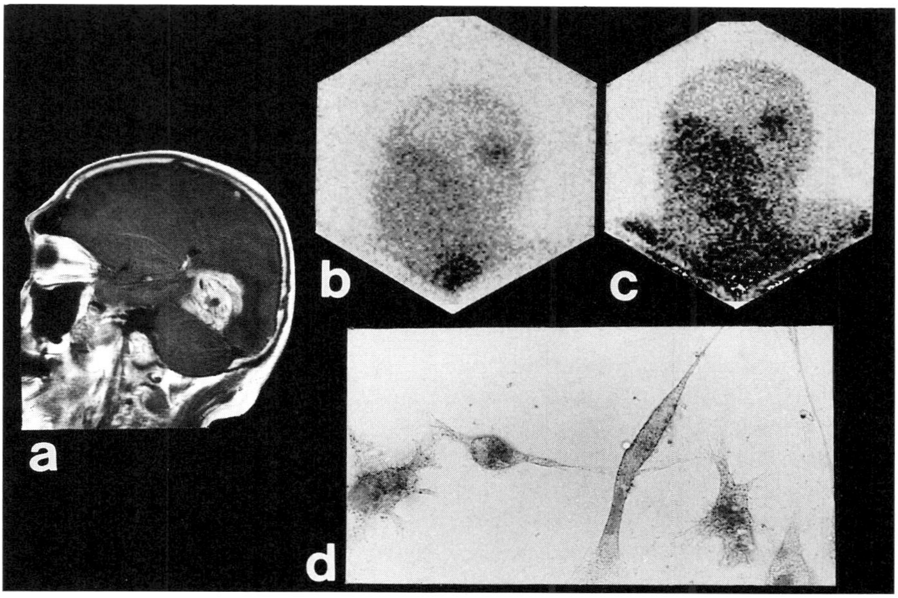

Fig. 2 a–d. Glioma grade 4 located in the right temporo-occipital region. **a** Sagittal (paramedian right projection) contrast-enhanced MRI demonstrates the hyperintense lesion in the right temporal and occipital lobe. **b** Lateral planar view of the head after intravenous injection of indium-labeled octreotide shows increased focal uptake in the tumor area. **c** Lateral planar view of the head after intravenous injection of ^{99m}Tc-DTPA displays enhanced focal tracer in projection of the tumor. **d** Light microscopic visualization of somatostatin binding sites on the surface of cultured tumor cells after incubation with 1 n*M* somatostatin-inhibitory factor–gold conjugate and silver intensification

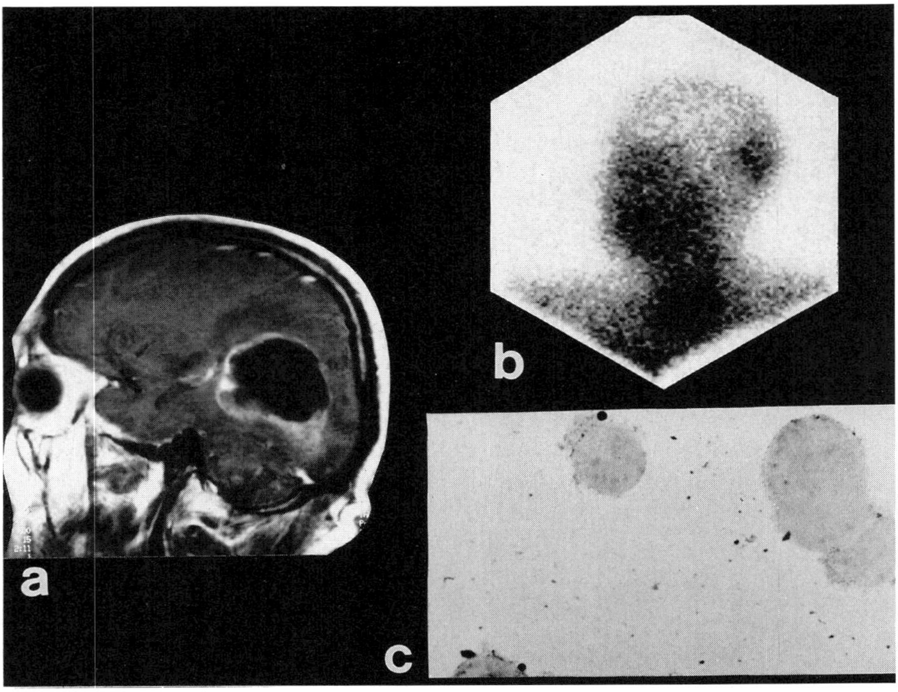

Fig. 3 a–c. Metastasis of a bronchial carcinoma located in the right occipital lobe. **a** Sagittal contrast-enhanced MRI outlines a circular hyperintense lesion with central hypodense area. **b** Lateral planar view after intravenous injection of indium-labeled octreotide demonstrates enhanced focal tracer uptake within the tumor area. **c** Light microscopy of the cultured metastatic tissue incubated with somatostatin-gold conjugate without somatostatin binding sites on the cell surface

three patients additionally examined with ^{99m}Tc-DTPA (Fig. 2 c) showed an enhanced focal tracer uptake with analogue intensity. Five of six tumor samples showed somatostatin binding sites in vitro (Fig. 2 d, Table 1). All patients with metastases and disturbed blood-brain barrier (Gd-labeled MRI) (Fig. 3 a) demonstrated enhanced focal tracer uptake in SRS (Fig. 3 b). In vitro four of five showed SR binding sites on the cell surface. The metastases of the bronchial carcinoma did not show somatostatin binding sites (Fig. 3 c). The brain abscess with Gd enhancement in MRI (Fig. 4 a) showed a positive signal in SRS (Fig. 4 b) but in vitro no SR on the cell surface (Fig. 4 c).

Discussion

In contrast to Lamberts [3, 4] and Reubi [5, 6] no patient in our study with glioma of grade 2 showed enhanced tracer uptake in SRS, although in vitro in all cultured

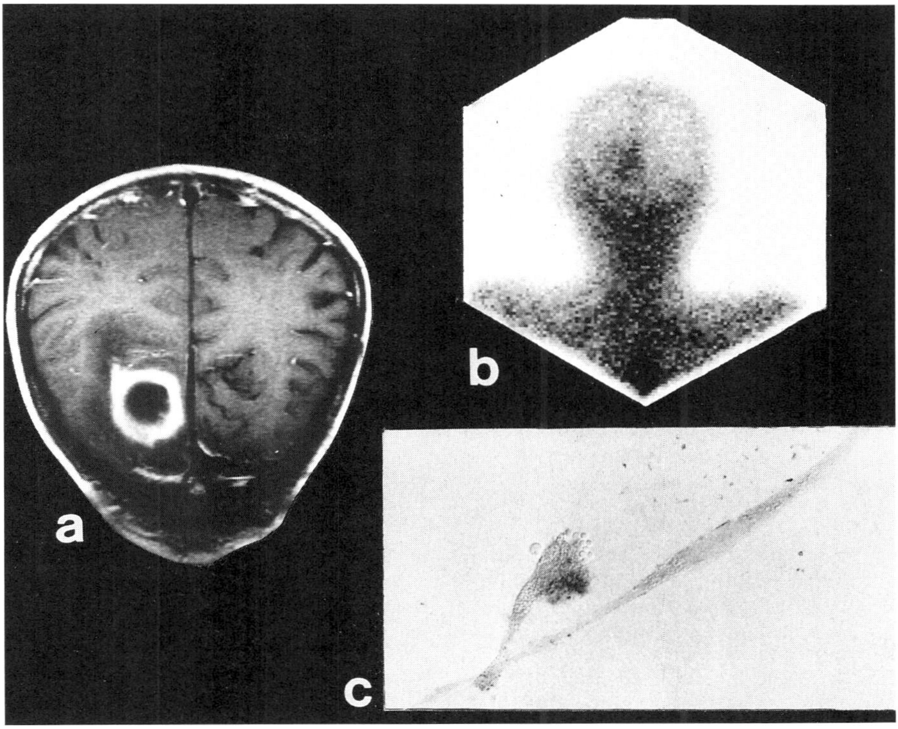

Fig. 4 a–c. Streptococcal brain abscess located in the left occipital lobe. **a** Coronal Gd-enhanced MRI outlines a circular hyperintense lesion with central hypodense area. **b** Anterior planar view after intravenous injection of indium-labeled octreotide reveals enhanced focal tracer uptake within the abscess area. **c** Light microscopy of the abscess tissue from which fibroblasts were cultivated does not show somatostatin binding sites on the cell surface after incubation with somatostatin-gold ligand

tumor samples of glioma grade 2 somatostatin binding sites were detected. These findings can be explained by the fact that the intact blood-brain barrier is not penetrated by somatostatin and its analogue octreotide. In gliomas of grade 3 or 4 the results of the SRS seem to correlate with the in vitro findings. However, the SR-unspecific scintigraphy with ^{99m}Tc-DTPA showed a positive signal with analogue tracer uptake within the tumor area. Even inflammatory altered tissue (brain abscess) and cerebral metastases with contrast-labeled MRI showed a positive signal in SRS with no difference to the malignant gliomas in tracer uptake intensity. In all probability the results of the SRS are caused by the peritumoral edematous lesion, where lymphocytes and macrophages were found. The tracer uptake might be caused by phagocytosed indium into macrophages or by known somatostatin binding sites on lymphocytes. A reliable confirmation of SR is only possible in vitro using the gold-ligand technique in which the SR on every single cell is evident. In conclusion, in vivo SRS does not improve tumor classification nor does it provide any additional information for the pre- or postoperative management of patients with gliomas.

References

1. Bakker WH, Albert R, Bruns C, Breemann WAP, Hofland LJ, Marbach P, Pless J, Pralet D, Stolz B, Koper JW, Lamberts SWJ, Visser TJ, Krenning EP (1991) [^{111}In-DTPA-D-Phe^{1}]-Octreotide, a potential radiopharmaceutical for imaging of somatostatin receptor-positive tumours: synthesis, radio-labeling and in vitro validation. Life Sci 49:1583–1591
2. Krisch B, Buchholz C, Mentlein R (1991) Somatostatin binding sites on rat diencephalic astrocytes. Light microscopic study in vitro and in vivo. Cell Tissue Res 263:253–263
3. Lamberts SWJ, Krenning EP, Reubi JC (1991) The role of somatostatin and its analogs in the diagnosis and treatment of tumors. Endocr Rev 12:450–482
4. Lamberts SWJ, Koper J, Reubi JC, Krenning EP (1992) Endocrine aspects of diagnosis and treatment of primary brain tumors. Clin Endocrinol 37:1–10
5. Reubi JC, Kvols L, Krenning EP, Lamberts SWJ (1990) Distribution of somatostatin receptors in normal and tumor tissues. Metabolism 39:78–81
6. Reubi JC, Laissue J, Krenning EP, Lamberts SWJ (1992) Somatostatin receptors in human cancer: incidence, characteristics, functional correlates and clinical implications. J Steroid Biochem Mol Biol 43:27–35
7. Scheidhauer K, Hildebrandt G, Luyken C, Schomäcker K, Klug N, Schicha H (1993) Somatostatin receptor scintigraphy in brain tumors. Horm Metab Res Suppl Ser 27:59–62

Secondary Growth of a Primary Brain Tissue Necrosis from a Focal Lesion

J. Eriskat[1], L. Schürer[2], O, Kempski[3], and A. Baethmann[1]

Introduction

Traumatic brain injury is associated with the development of secondary brain damage, such as brain edema, intracranial hypertension, and cerebral ischemia [1]. A novel aspect is that a primary necrosis of brain parenchyma evolving from a focal cerebral insult may be subjected to secondary growth. Experiments utilizing different methods of brain injury have consistently confirmed an increase in size of the resulting tissue necrosis within 24 h, amounting to 50% in rats [3, 7, 10] and even 300% in rabbits [11]. It is not clear yet, however, whether the phenomenon reflects a delayed but irreversible primary process which is resistant to treatment or a manifestation of secondary brain damage, thus serving as a potential target of therapeutic inhibition. Confirmation of the latter would require more detailed information on the time course as well as extent of lesion growth on a quantitative basis – the point of the present experimental investigations.

Materials and Methods

In male Sprague-Dawley rats (278 ± 39 g b.w., $n = 59$) ether anesthesia was introduced after premedication with 0.25 mg atropin subcutaneously to reduce salivation. Anesthesia was maintained then by intraperitoneal chloral hydrate (360 mg/kg b.w.). The animals breathed room air enriched with oxygen. The skull was positioned in a stereotactic frame. For exposure of the left parietal cerebral cortex a craniotomy of 3-mm diameter was made with a dental drill under continuous cooling and using an operating microscope. The dura remained intact and was frequently moistened with isotonic saline. The freezing insult was induced by a metal probe (diameter of 1 mm) attached to a cylinder cooled to – 68 °C by a dry ice/acetone mixture. The cooling probe was fixed to a stereotactic device powered by a computer-controlled stepper motor for maximum precision of

[1] Institut für Chirurgische Forschung, Klinikum Großhadern, Marchioninistr. 15, 81366 München, Germany.
[2] Neurochirurgische Klinik, Klinikum Großhadern, Marchioninistr. 15, 81366 München, Germany.
[3] Institut für Neurochirurgische Pathophysiologie, Klinikum der Johannes-Gutenberg-Universität, Langenbeckstr. 1, 55101 Mainz, Germany.

Advances in Neurosurgery, Vol. 22
B. L. Bauer, M. Brock, M. Klinger (Eds.)

placement and duration of the freezing insult. The focal cold injury was induced according to Klatzo et al. [6] through the cranial burr hole over a freezing period of 10 s. Morphological analysis of the resulting lesion demonstrated confinement of the insult to the cerebral cortex. Body temperature was monitored and maintained during anesthesia between 37.5 °C and 38.0 °C by a servocontrolled heating pad.

The animals were assigned to one of six experimental groups with different survival periods after trauma (5 min, 3, 6, 12, 18, and 24 h) for examination of progression of the lesion during the posttraumatic course. Animals sacrified immediately after trauma were rapidly thoracotomized for perfusion fixation of the brain through the left cardiac ventricle, starting with isotonic saline for 30 s followed by 2% buffered paraformaldehyde (pH 7.4) for 20 min. Animals of other experimental groups surviving longer periods were allowed to recover from anesthesia after surgical closure of the scalp. Anesthesia was induced again after respective survival periods for perfusion fixation of the brain as described above. Following in situ fixation of the brain, the animals were decapitated, and the head was placed in 10% formalin over night at 4 °C. The brain was subsequently removed carefully and stored again in 10% formalin prior to preparation for histology following dehydration and embedding in paraffin. Coronal serial sections of the brain of 3–5 mm thickness were made at 100-mm intervals throughout the lesion area. The sections were stained with cresyl violet according to Nissl. The area of necrosis was measured planimetrically in all sections containing lesion. The maximal lesion area was determined from these data, and the areas of necrosis of the total brain were utilized for calculation of the necrosis volume by the basic volume estimator [9]. Data are given as mean ± standard error of the mean. Differences between groups were tested by the Kruskall-Wallis test with Conover's multiple comparison [8].

Results

Kinetics of the spread of necrosis and the calculated necrosis volume is summarized in Table 1. The maximum area of necrosis increased within 3 h by approximately 20%, from 0.75 ± 0.06 to 0.90 ± 0.05 mm^2, while growth of necrosis was not observed between 3 and 12 h after trauma. Thereafter, the area of necrosis increased further between 12 and 24 h, from 0.85 ± 0.05 to 1.09 ± 0.08 mm^2 ($p < 0.05$). The maximal area of necrosis altogether increased within 24 h after trauma by 45% ($p < 0.001$). The volume of necrosis calculated on the basis of the serial brain sections increased from 0.78 ± 0.09 mm^3 5 min after trauma to 1.09 ± 0.08 mm^3 24 h after trauma. Hence, the increase in necrosis volume was also 45% within the posttraumatic observation period. Due to the greater statistical scatter of individual data, the differences between results obtained at 5 min and at 24 h after trauma are not statistically significant.

Table 1. Maximal area and volume of necrosis of brain parenchyma in rats with focal cold injury

Survival	n	Maximal lesion area (mm^2)	Lesion volume (mm^3)
5 min	9	$0.75 \pm 0.06^{***}$	0.78 ± 0.09
3 h	8	0.90 ± 0.05	1.02 ± 0.09
6 h	10	$0.85 \pm 0.05^{**}$	0.97 ± 0.11
12 h	7	$0.85 \pm 0.05^{**}$	1.04 ± 0.10
18 h	10	$0.94 \pm 0.06^{**}$	1.07 ± 0.07
24 h	15	1.09 ± 0.08	1.13 ± 0.09

* $p < 0.05$ versus 5 min; ** $p < 0.01$ versus 24 h; *** $p < 0.001$ versus 24 h

Discussion

The focal cold lesion utilized in this study approximates cerebral contusion, a frequent and relevant manifestation of primary brain damage in severe head injury. It produces a well-standardized and sharply demarcated necrosis of cerebral cortex, which may become hemorrhagic within 24 h after injury. The freezing lesion also causes disruption of the blood-brain barrier and vasogenic brain edema [6], important aspects of traumatic brain injury.

The primary lesion induced by freezing of the cerebral cortex for 10 s was limited to the gray matter of cerebral cortex, making possible an accurate distinction between irreversibly damaged and surviving perifocal brain parenchyma in histological preparations. In addition, growth of the area of necrosis in the histological sections was tested by assessment of the density of viable nerve cells in perifocal brain tissue areas (data not shown). The findings confirm that lesion growth following the primary insult must be attributed to progressive extinction of brain parenchyma and not to mere expansion of the necrotic area by swelling.

As to the mechanisms mediating growth of the primary lesion, microcirculatory as well as cytotoxic processes seem to be involved. One may relate it to impairment of the arterial blood supply of the initially intact, deeper cortical layers resulting from damage to the supplying blood vessels by cold injury. Another hypothesis concerns activation and release of cytotoxic mediator compounds, such as excitatory amino acids, free fatty acids, or platelet-activating factor [1, 2, 4, 5] from the area of necrosis which flood perifocal tissue, causing its secondary destruction.

Conclusion

The present findings confirm that a primary brain tissue necrosis increased in rats within 24 h by 45%. Spread of necrosis is not limited to the first few posttraumatic hours postinsult but progresses over a delayed period between 12 and 24 h. Although underlying mechanisms are presently unknown, it is surmised that vascular and cytotoxic processes are involved. Identification of the growth of a primary brain tissue lesion from trauma as manifestation of secondary brain damage requires that it can be inhibited by therapeutic methods. Respective findings would have clinical relevance.

Acknowledgments. This research was supported by Deutsche Forschungsgemeinschaft (Ba 452/6–7). The technical and secretarial assistance of Evi Duncan, Ann Hedblom, Helga Kleylein, and Monika Stucky is gratefully acknowledged.

References

1. Baethmann A, Maier-Hauff K, Kempski O, Unterberg A, Wahl M, Schürer L (1988) Mediators of brain edema and secondary brain damage. Crit Care Med 16:972–978
2. Baethmann A, Maier-Hauff K, Schürer L, Lange M, Guggenbichler C, Vogt W, Jacob K, Kempski O (1989) Release of glutamate and of free fatty acids in vasogenic brain edema. J Neurosurg 70:578–591
3. Eggert HR, Kiessling M, Kleihues P (1985) Time course and spatial distribution of neodymium:yttrium-aluminium-garnet (Nd:YAG) laser-induced lesions in the rat brain. Neurosurgery 16:443–448
4. Frerichs KU, Lindsberg PJ, Hallenbeck JM, Feuerstein GZ (1990) Platelet-activating factor and progressive brain damage following focal brain injury. J Neurosurg 73:223–233
5. Hayes RL, Jenkins LW, Lyeth BG (1992) Neurotransmitter-mediated mechanism of traumatic brain injury: acetylcholine and excitatory amino acids. J Neurotrauma 9[Suppl 1]:S173–S187
6. Klatzo I, Piraux A, Laskowski EJ (1958) The relationship between edema, blood-brain barrier and tissue elements in a local brain injury. J Neuropathol Exp Neurol 17:548–564
7. Lindsberg PJ, Frerichs KU, Burris JA, Hallenbeck JM, Feuerstein G (1991) Cortical microcirculation in a new model of focal laser-induced secondary brain damage. J Cereb Blood Flow Metab 11:88–98
8. Theodorsson-Norheim E (1986) Kruskall-Wallis test: BASIC computer program to perform nonparametric one-way analysis of variance and multiple comparisons on ranks of several independent samples. Comput Methods Programs Biomed 23:57–62
9. Uylings HBM, Van Eden CG, Hofman MA (1986) Morphometry of size/volume variables and comparison of their bivariate relations in the nervous system under different conditions. J Neurosci Methods 18:19–37
10. Vonhof S. Autoradiographische Untersuchungen des Gehirns über das sekundäre Nekrosewachstum nach primären Trauma. Thesis, Ludwig-Maximilians-Universität, Munich (in preparation)
11. Wyrwich W. Die Entwicklung einer sekundären Hirngewebsnekrose nach primären Trauma. Thesis, Ludwig-Maximilians-Universität, Munich (in preparation)

Allogeneic Neurografting in the Rat Model of Parkinson's Disease: Effect of the Grafting Technique on the Functional and Morphological Integration of the Transplant

U. J. Knappe[1], A. Brandis[2], A. Jödicke[3], G. F. Walter[2], M. Samii[4], R. Schönmayr[5], and G. Nikkah[6]

Introduction

The experimental model of Parkinson's disease in the rat is based upon the unilateral injection of 6-hydroxydopamine (6-OHDA) into the substantia nigra, resulting in a selective degeneration of dopaminergic neurons. Lesioned rats show an abnormal D-amphetamine induced rotation response ipsilateral to the lesion site [6]. Transplantation of fetal dopaminergic neurons into the denervated caudate putamen (CPU) may restore dopamine levels and normalize the behavioral deficits. However, questions remain open regarding the influence of surgical parameters on the functional and morphological integration of the grafts. Furthermore, while most studies have been performed in a syngeneic graft setting [1], the clinical application would require allogeneic material [7]. To evaluate the influence of the transplantation technique on the functional and morphological integration of grafted dopaminergic cells the conventional stereotactic procedure was compared to a new microimplantation approach in an allogeneic transplantation protocol.

Materials and Methods

Animals. Rats of the DA strain served as donors and rats of the Lewis 1W strain as recipients. These strains differ in both class I and II MHC antigens and non-MHC antigens. No immunosuppression was used.

Lesion. Thirty-one adult female Lewis 1W rats received a stereotactic injection of 6-OHDA into the right substantia nigra and median forebrain bundle at the fol-

[1] Neurochirurgische Klinik, Universitätskrankenhaus Eppendorf, Martinistr. 52, 20251 Hamburg, Germany.
[2] Institut für Neuropathologie, Medizinische Hochschule Hannover, Konstanty-Gutschow-Str. 8, 30625 Hannover, Germany.
[3] HNO-Klinik, St. Gertraudenkrankenhaus, Paretzer Str. 12, 10713 Berlin, Germany.
[4] Medizinische Hochschule Hannover, Neurochirurgische Klinik, Krankenhaus Nordstadt, Haltenhoffstr. 41, 30167 Hannover, Germany.
[5] Neurochirurgische Klinik, Horst-Schmidt-Kliniken, Ludwig Erhard Str. 100, 65199 Wiesbaden, Germany.
[6] Neurochirurgische Klinik, Krankenhaus Nordstadt, Haltenhoffstr. 41, 30167 Hannover, Germany.

Advances in Neurosurgery, Vol. 22
B. L. Bauer, M. Brock, M. Klinger (Eds.)

lowing coordinates (in millimeters, with reference to bregma and dura): (a) 2.5 μl 6-OHDA (3.6 μg/μl in 0.2 mg/ml L-ascorbate saline) at anterior-posterior (AP) 4.4, lateral (L) 1.2, vertical (V) 7.8 [tooth bar (TB) – 2.4]; (b) 3 μl 6-OHDA at AP – 4.0, L 0.8, V 8.0 (TB +3.4).

Functional Test. Rotational response was determined after intraperitoneal injection of D-amphetamine (2.5 mg/kg b.w.) and monitored over a period of 90 min. Rotation tests were performed 2–4 weeks after 6-OHDA lesion and 3, 6, and 12 weeks after transplantation.

Transplantation. Fetal ventral mesencephalon (VM) was obtained from DA rats on embryonic day 14. After removal of the leptomeninges, mechanical dissection, and incubation with trypsin (0.1%) and DNase (0.05%) a single cell suspension with 10^5 cells/μl resulted [5]. In the conventional method (macrografts) the grafts were injected as a single deposit of 1 μl through a steel cannula of 500 μm in outer diameter. The stereotactic coordinates were AP +1.0, L +3.0, and V 4.5 (TB 0). The target area was the right dorsolateral CPU. The micrografts were implanted through a glass cannula with an outer diameter of 50–70 μm as four deposits of 250 nl each along two punctuations into the dorsolateral and dorsomedial CPU. The coordinates were AP +1.0, L +2.5 and +3.5, and V 5.0 and 4.1 (TB 0).

Histology. Specimens were examined 1 and 3 weeks ($n = 4$/group), 6 weeks ($n_{micro} = 4$, $n_{macro} = 5$), and 12 weeks ($n_{micro} = 4$), $n_{macro} = 2$) after transplantation. Serial cryostat sections of the grafts were immunohistochemically stained for tyroxine hydroxylase (TH) to visualize surviving dopaminergic neurons and for glial fibrillary acidic protein to determine the astroglial reaction of the host (streptavidine-biotin method with DAB as chromogene).

Results

D-amphetamine Test. A diminution of pathological right turns was more pronounced in the macrografts than in the micrografts. However, the graft-induced amelioration varied considerably among animals within the same group (Fig. 1). Net left rotations were only observed in the two rats with macrografts 12 weeks posttransplantation.

Histology. Both macrografts and micrografts survived well without signs of rejection. TH staining showed maturation of dopaminergic neurons with axonal outgrowth and innervation of the surrounding CPU at 12 weeks after transplantation (Fig. 2). While macrografts tended to increase in volume by time (Fig. 2 a), this phenomenon was not observed in the micrografts, which remained slender and well integrated into the host tissue (Fig. 2 b). Macrografting resulted in considerable tissue damage with hemorrhage, necrosis, and cellular reaction along the needle track and to a lesser extent at the graft-host interface in the CPU. In contrast

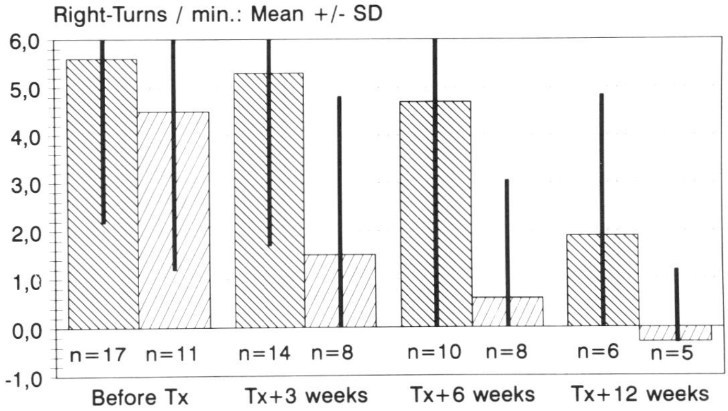

Fig. 1. Functional integration of the grafts. Amelioration of pathological right turns is more evident in the macrografts (▨) than in the micrografts (▧). *Tx*, Transplantation

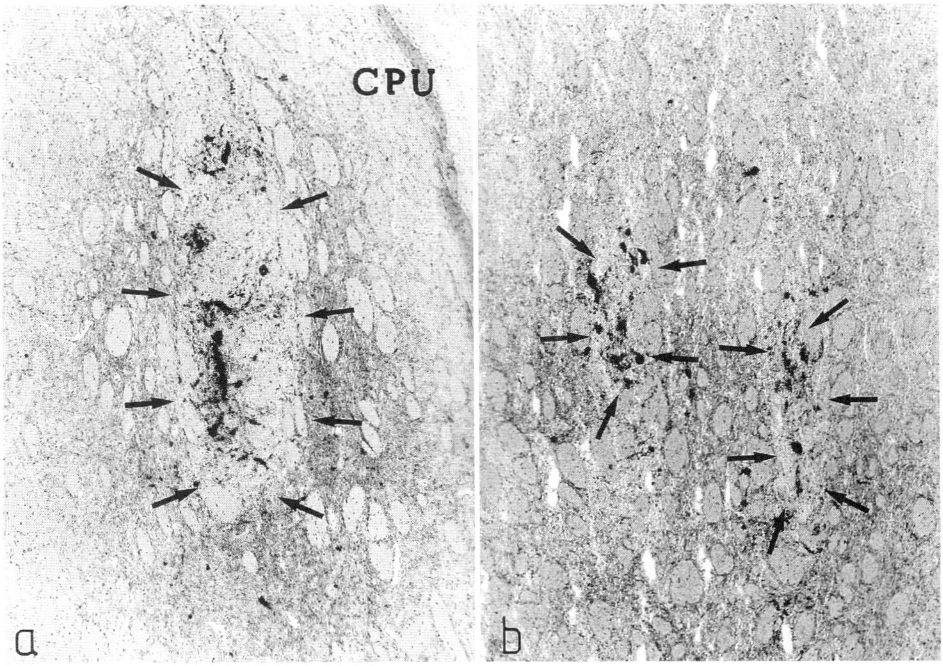

Fig. 2 a, b. TH expression. **a** Macrograft 12 weeks after transplantation: mature dopaminergic neurons within the graft which forms a distinct mass in the CPU (*arrows*). x 100. **b** Two micrografts 12 weeks after transplantation: dopaminergic neurons within well-integrated transplants (*arrows*). x 100

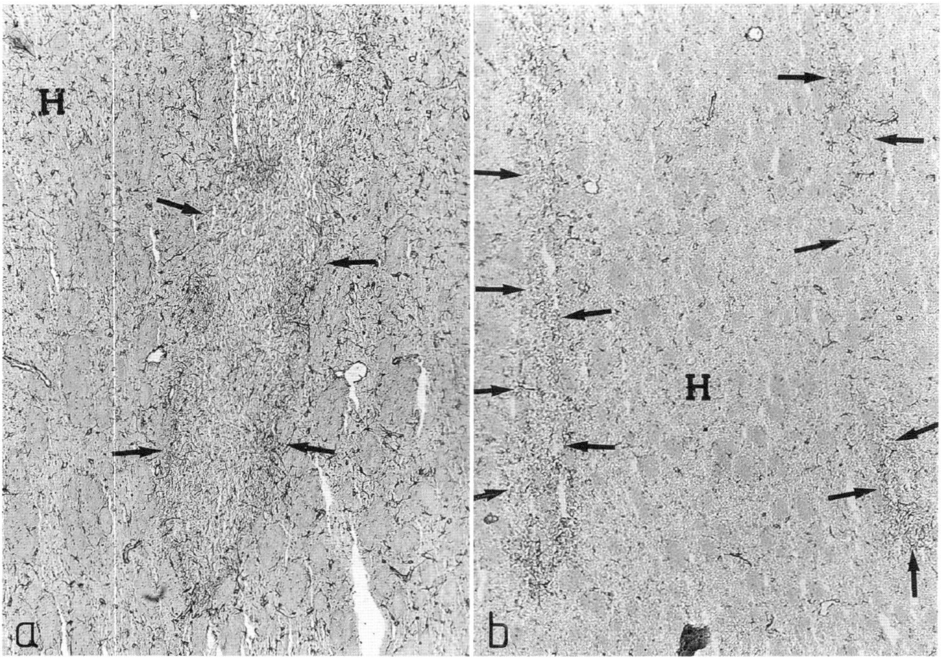

Fig. 3 a, b. Glial fibrillary acid protein expression. **a** Macrograft 3 weeks after transplantation: glial fibrillary acidic protein reactivity is pronounced at the graft-host (*H*) interface and forms a distinct border (*arrows*). **b** Two micrografts 6 weeks after transplantation: glial reaction is less obvious than in **a** and is restricted to loosely arranged astrocytes surrounding the grafts (*arrows*)

the micrografting technique produced no major tissue trauma, the injection sites being identified only by the presence of some siderophages. Accordingly, the astroglial reaction tended to be more pronounced in the macrografts and reached its maximum 3 weeks after transplantation. Reactive gliosis was observed along the needle tracks and as a broad rim around the grafts (Fig. 3 a). Astroglial reaction in the micrografts was delayed and reached its maximum 6 weeks after transplantation. Compared with the macrografts the rim of the reactive astrocytes around the transplants was thinner and of loose texture.

Discussion

The main finding of the present study was that the response of glial fibrillary acidic protein within and around the micrografts was less intense and delayed compared to the macrografts. However, without any immunosuppression there were no obvious signs of allograft rejection in either group. It has been shown previously that the micrograft technique promotes the survival of dopaminergic neurons threefold

[4, 5]. It is suggested that cellular and humoral events induced by the implantation trauma may have an adverse effect on the survival and functional integration of grafted dopaminergic neurons.

The lack of a glial barrier and of a well-defined demarcation of the micrografts may have a positive effect on the migration of afferent and efferent axons. This is critical in larger CNS lesions [3].

To obtain effects on the D-amphetamine induced rotations a local level of dopamine must be attained in the dorsolateral CPU [2]. Compared to other studies (e.g., [1, 4]) our macrografts with a volume of 1 μl are small; however, they caused a considerable decrease in pathological right turns. The micrografts with a volume of 250 nl each were distributed in the dorsolateral and dorsomedial CPU and therefore apparently did not attain the required threshold value for dopamine. However, the distribution of small graft volumes in the target area is important for complex sensorimotor performances [4].

Conclusions

The new micrograft technique can reduce the implantation trauma within the host tissue and enhances the survival of grafted dopaminergic neurons in the rat Parkinson's disease model. These findings may also contribute to the further development of transplantation strategies for patients with Parkinson's disease.

References

1. Björklund A, Stenevi U, Schmidt RH, Dunnett SB, Gage FH (1983) Intracerebral grafting of neuronal cell suspensions. I. Introduction and general methods of preparation. Acta Physiol Scand 522:1–7
2. Björklund A (1992) Dopaminergic transplants in experimental parkinsonism: cellular mechanisms for graft-induced functional recovery. Curr Opin Neurobiol 2:683–689
3. Das GD (1986) Neural transplantation in spinal cord under different conditions of lesions and their functional significance. In: Das GD, Wallace RB (eds) Neural transplantation and regeneration. Springer, Vienna New York, pp 1–62
4. Nikkhah G, Duan W-M, Knappe UJ, Jödicke A, Björklund A (1994) Restoration of complex sensorimotor behavior and skilled forelimb use by a modified nigra cell suspension transplantation approach in the rat parkinson model. Neuroscience (in press)
5. Nikkhah G, Cunningham MG, Jödicke A, Knappe UJ, Björklund A (1994) Improved graft survival and striatal reinnervation by microtransplantation of fetal nigral cell suspensions in the rat Parkinson model. Brain Res (submitted)
6. Ungerstedt U (1971) Postsynaptic supersensitivity after 6-hydroxydopamine induced degeneration of the nigro-striatal dopamine system. Acta Physiol Scand [Suppl] 367:69–93
7. Widner H, Tetrud J, Rehncrona S, Snow B, Brundin P, Gustavii B, Björklund A, Lindvall O, Langston JW (1992) Bilateral fetal mesencephalic grafting in two patients with Parkinsonism induced by 1-methyl-4-phenyl-1,2,3,6-tetrahydropyridine (MTPT). N Engl J Med 327:1556–1563

Subject Index

Springer-Verlag and the Environment

We at Springer-Verlag firmly believe that an international science publisher has a special obligation to the environment, and our corporate policies consistently reflect this conviction.

We also expect our business partners – paper mills, printers, packaging manufacturers, etc. – to commit themselves to using environmentally friendly materials and production processes.

The paper in this book is made from low- or no-chlorine pulp and is acid free, in conformance with international standards for paper permanency.

Printing: Druckerei Zechner, Speyer
Binding: Buchbinderei Schäffer, Grünstadt